SYSTEMIC PATHOLOGY / THIRD EDITION

Volume 10   The Cardiovascular System
Part A: General Considerations and Congenital Malformations

SYSTEMIC PATHOLOGY / THIRD EDITION

General Editor W. St C. Symmers

Volume Editors

M. C. Anderson **Female Reproductive System**

I. D. Ansell **Male Reproductive System**

M. E. Catto and A. J. Malcolm **Bone, Joints and Soft Tissues**

B. Corrin **The Lungs**

M. J. Davies and J. Mann **The Cardiovascular System: Part B**

C. W. Elston and I. O. Ellis **Breasts**

I. Friedmann **Nose, Throat and Ears**

K. Henry and W. St C. Symmers **Thymus, Lymph Nodes, Spleen and Lymphatics**

P. D. Lewis **Endocrine System**

B. C. Morson **Alimentary Tract**

K. A. Porter, R. C. B. Pugh and I. D. Ansell **The Kidneys/The Urinary Tract**

W. B. Robertson **The Cardiovascular System: Part A**

D. Weedon **The Skin**

R. O. Weller **Nervous System, Muscle and Eyes**

S. N. Wickramasinghe **Blood and Bone Marrow**

D. G. D. Wight **Liver, Biliary Tract and Exocrine Pancreas**

For Churchill Livingstone

Publisher: Timothy Horne
Copy Editor: Ruth Swan
Indexer: J. Sampson
Sales Promotion Executive: Douglas McNaughton

SYSTEMIC PATHOLOGY / THIRD EDITION

General Editor W. St C. Symmers

Volume 10

The Cardiovascular System

Part A: General Considerations and Congenital Malformations

EDITOR

W. B. Robertson BSc MD FRCPath

Director of Studies, Royal College of Pathologists; Professor Emeritus in Histopathology, University of London at St George's Hospital Medical School, and Honorary Consultant in Pathology, St George's Hospital, London, UK

AUTHORS

R. H. Anderson BSc MD FRCPath

Joseph Levy Professor of Paediatric Cardiac Morphology, National Heart and Lung Institute, Royal Brompton National Heart and Lung Hospital, London, UK

A. E. Becker MD

Professor of Pathology, Department of Cardiovascular Pathology, Academic Medical Center, Amsterdam, The Netherlands

W. B. Robertson BSc MD FRCPath

CHURCHILL LIVINGSTONE
EDINBURGH LONDON MADRID MELBOURNE NEW YORK AND TOKYO 1993

CHURCHILL LIVINGSTONE
Medical Division of Longman Group UK Limited

Distributed in the United States of America by Churchill
Livingstone Inc., 650 Avenue of the Americas, New York,
N.Y. 10011, and by associated companies, branches and
representatives throughout the world.

First published 1993

ISBN 0-443-03096-0

British Library of Cataloguing in Publication Data
A catalogue record for this book is available from the British
Library.

Library of Congress Cataloging in Publication Data
A catalog record for this book is available from the Library of
Congress.

The
publisher's
policy is to use
**paper manufactured
from sustainable forests**

Printed and bound in Great Britain by
Butler & Tanner Ltd, Frome and London

Preface

The decision by Churchill Livingstone to publish the third edition of Systemic Pathology in an expanded format, devoting a volume to each organ-system, has enabled authors to deal with their subjects more comprehensively and in greater depth than was possible in previous editions. This, however, raised a problem with the volume on the cardiovascular system as preliminary planning of the volume revealed that the final estimated number of pages of text would exceed by far that of other volumes in the series. The publishers therefore agreed that it should be published in two parts, A and B, but thereby raised the further question of the content of each part. All the contributors to both parts are new to Systemic Pathology and a corporate decision was taken to adopt a radical approach to the presentation of disorders of the cardiovascular system. In most textbooks of pathology congenital cardiac lesions, in defiance of temporal events, are dealt with after acquired lesions of the cardiovascular system and it was decided to reverse this order. This decision was taken, not just to give greater prominence in Part A to congenital lesions, but to allow consideration of normal anatomy and physiology of the system at a logical early stage rather than as adjuncts to morphological descriptions of disease processes and entities as is usual in other texts. Similarly, Part A includes also the general principles of the pathophysiology of the cardiovascular system, together with the subjects of systemic hypertension and pulmonary hypertension, all of which provide an essential background for acquired lesions of the heart and blood vessels which are dealt with in Part B.

Despite the generally acknowledged fact that diseases of the cardiovascular system, as a group, are the major cause of death in Westernized societies, there has been a remarkable decline of interest by pathologists in cardiovascular pathology. In the middle decades of the current century, it would have been unusual to visit a pathology department and not find at least one member of staff, probably more, engaged in research on atherosclerosis, human or experimental, or in the equally contentious subject of coronary (ischaemic) heart disease or in other cardiovascular diseases. Cardiologists and cardiovascular surgeons now bemoan the lack of support given to their subject by pathologists. There would appear to be little response, as yet, to this *cri de coeur*; the pun aside, trainee pathologists should take note. It may be that the lessening of interest in autopsy pathology allied to the burgeoning sciences of cell and molecular biology are attracting trainee and practising pathologists into the fields of neoplasia, immunologically determined disorders and other aspects of pathology where modern technology would seem more easily applied. Does this imply that cardiovascular pathology is considered to be stranded in traditional morbid anatomy and histopathology? If that be the reason, then it reflects badly on the leaders of our branch of the medical profession.

Professor Symmers, in his preface to Volume 1 of the second edition of Systemic Pathology, raised the pertinent question of the future of such texts because of the cost of their production. Certainly, with the resources of modern libraries, word-processing, photocopying, computerized search facilities and the like, allied to the profusion of specialized medical journals, the research worker, other than the beginner, has little need for textbooks. Nonetheless, there is still a demand from practising and trainee pathologists for texts such as Systemic Pathology as a convenient source of comprehensive and up-to-date information at the bench and from those preparing for postgraduate examinations. To this end, the referencing of chapters has been aimed at providing other sources of detailed information rather than long lists of individual scientific publications which the average reader has little time or inclination to consult.

The three authors of part A of the volume owe much to many people, too numerous to mention by name, but they are particularly indebted to the series editor, Professor W. St C. Symmers, who read and commented upon draft manuscripts of each chapter in his usual perceptive and helpful manner. The editor of Part A (WBR) would like to thank Professor M. J. Davies and Professor N. Woolf for their generosity in allowing access to their departments and facilities to enable him to prepare illustrations for his contributions. The contributions of RHA would not have been possible without the co-operation of Siew Yen Ho and the technical support and assistance of Christine Anderson, Felicity Gil, Aldrin Sweeney and Lucienne Kilpatrick. Those of AEB depended on the electronmicrographs provided by Koert P. Dingemans DSc and the secretarial work of Marsha I. Schenker. Lastly, but by no means leastly, acknowledgement must be made to Mr Timothy Horne and his staff at Churchill Livingstone for their help, patience and forbearance when, due to a variety of reasons, delays occurred in the submission of material for publication.

Wimbledon, London   W.B.R.

Contents

SECTION THREE   The Vascular System: Basic Principles

The Heart: Basic Principles

Normal cardiac anatomy

INTRODUCTION

The heart is the major structure in the middle component of the inferior mediastinum. Although more or less a median structure, it lies in the mediastinum in such a way that two-thirds of its bulk are to the left of the midline behind the second to the sixth costal cartilages, with the left-sided portion extending to the mid-clavicular line in the fifth interspace (Fig. 1.1). On each side the heart abuts on the lungs, and the pleural cavities overlie the right side of the heart as far as the midline. On the left side, in contrast, the lung and pleura are drawn away from the middle so that, in the area of the cardiac notch, the surface of the heart comes to lie directly against the rib cage, separated from it only by the pericardial coverings.

The heart is enclosed by the pericardium, which is a tough fibrous sac with a serosal lining (Fig. 1.2). The inner serous layer is firmly adherent to the heart, forming the epicardium; the outer layer is fused to the fibrous sac. The pericardial cavity, therefore, is between the fibrous pericardium and the surface of the heart. The vagus and phrenic nerves are intimately related to the pericardium, running posteriorly and anteriorly respectively to the pulmonary hilum on each side (Fig. 1.3). The recurrent laryngeal branch of the vagus turns back around the arterial ligament on the left side but around the subclavian artery on the right.

On removing the heart from the pericardial cavity, but retaining it in the anatomical position, it will be seen that the right border is occupied by the right atrium while the inferior surface is

3

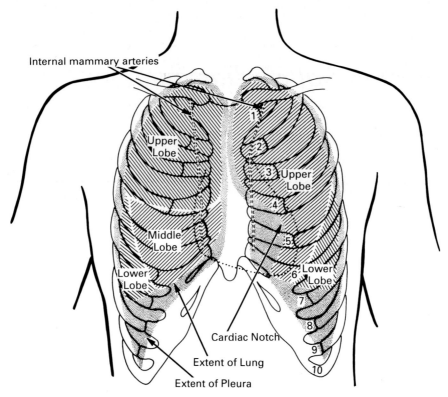

Fig. 1.1 The surface markings of the normal heart relative to the lungs and ribs.

formed by the right ventricle (Fig. 1.4). The left ventricle comes to the anterior surface only as a thin strip between the anterior interventricular groove and the obtuse margin, while only the appendage of the left atrium can be seen from the front. The aorta springs from the middle of the cardiac base, being to the left of the pulmonary trunk. The left atrium is a posterior structure and is anchored by the four pulmonary veins. Further description of the heart is best approached by taking each of the cardiac chambers and describing its individual features, taking note also of the septal structures and the sub-systems of the heart.

THE MORPHOLOGICALLY RIGHT ATRIUM

Throughout the text, we will use the term 'morphologically' to describe the cardiac chamber with the recognized features of the given chamber in the normal heart. As will be seen, this is frequently necessary in the setting of congenitally malformed hearts since the chambers are often not to be found in their anticipated location. The normal right atrium possesses a smooth-walled component (the venous sinus) which receives the superior and inferior caval veins along with the coronary sinus, a vestibule which surrounds the right atrioventricular junction, a septal surface, and a prominent broad-based triangular appendage. The septal surface is characteristic, having the prominent rim of the oval depression (fossa ovalis) opposite the mouth of the inferior caval vein (Fig. 1.5). This arrangement promotes the flow of the richly oxygenated placental blood into the left atrium during fetal life. Surprisingly little of the supposed 'septum' separates the right and left atrial chambers. The true septal area is confined to the floor of the oval fossa and its immediate environs. The significance of this

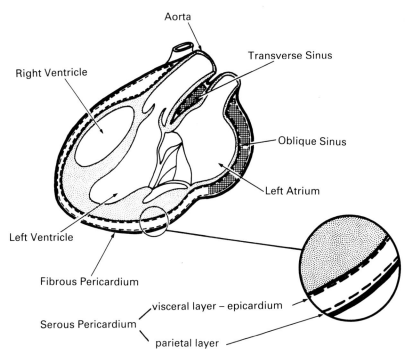

Fig. 1.2 The arrangement of the normal pericardial cavity and the location of its transverse and oblique sinuses.

feature will become clear when we describe the anatomy of interatrial communications (see Ch. 6). Although the septal surface is a typical feature of the right atrium, it cannot be used in final adjudication of atrial morphology since the septum itself can be absent. Similarly, the obvious connexions of the great veins together with the arrangement of their venous valves are ruled out as characteristics for definition since these connexions can themselves be anomalous. The most constant feature of the morphologically right atrium, and hence the best marker of its morphological rightness, is the shape of the appendage together with the anatomy of its junction with the smooth-walled atrium. The appendage has the shape of a broad-based triangle (Fig. 1.6). Its junction with the venous component is marked internally by the prominent terminal crest (crista terminalis) from which arise the pectinate muscles (Fig. 1.7). The pectinate muscles in the right atrium extend all round the atrioventricular junction and reach the sinus beneath the orifice of the inferior caval vein (the sub-Eustachian sinus).

The site of the terminal crest is marked externally by the terminal groove (sulcus terminalis). This is significant since it houses the sinus node (see below).

THE MORPHOLOGICALLY LEFT ATRIUM

Like the right atrium, the left atrium possesses a venous component, a vestibule leading to the atrioventricular junction, a septal surface, and an appendage (Fig. 1.8). Again, it is the appendage which is the most constant feature and which is best used for identification of morphological leftness. The left appendage is a tubular structure with several bends along its length (Fig. 1.9). It has a narrow junction with the smooth-walled atrium. This junction is not marked by a terminal crest or groove. The pectinate muscles in the left atrium are confined within the appendage, extending to only a limited extent round the atrioventricular junction. The larger part of the left atrium is formed by the extensive venous

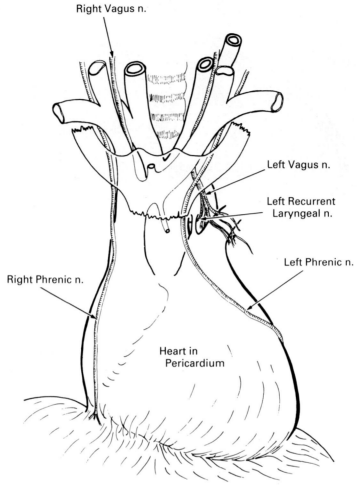

Right Vagus n.

Left Vagus n.

Left Recurrent
Laryngeal n.

Left Phrenic n.

Right Phrenic n.

Heart in
Pericardium

Fig. 1.3 The relationship of the vagus and phrenic nerves to the pericardial sac.

component, anchored at its corners by the connexions of the four pulmonary veins. The septal surface comprises the flap valve of the oval depression. Typically, there are several rough ridges along the atrial roof at the point where the flap valve overlaps the left atrial aspect of the infolded interatrial roof (the rim of the oval fossa).

THE MORPHOLOGICALLY RIGHT VENTRICLE

The ventricles are traditionally described as having sinus and conus portions. We find this approach to be wanting in several respects. First, it is difficult to find clear anatomical boundaries between these two supposed ventricular components. Second, and more important, it is not possible to account for all types of ventricle found in malformed hearts on the basis of a normal ventricle possessing only two components. Our preference is to describe the normal ventricles as having three parts. These three portions are the inlet component, the apical trabecular component, and the outlet component. They are particularly well seen in the morphologically right ventricle (Fig. 1.10). The inlet component extends from the atrioventricular junction to the

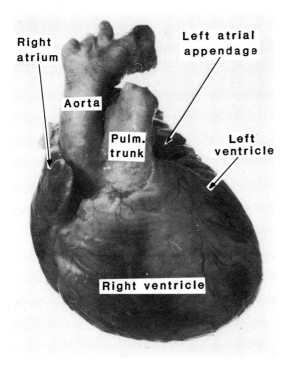

Fig. 1.4 This heart has been photographed in the usual anatomical position, showing the relationship of the cardiac chambers to the frontal silhouette.

distal attachments of the tendinous cords (chordae tendineae) of the tricuspid valve. The outlet component is the smooth-walled tube of muscle which supports the three semilunar leaflets of the pulmonary valve. The apical trabecular component extends out from the two parts surrounding the valves and reaches to the apex. This part is coarsely trabeculated and exhibits, on its septal surface, the particularly prominent and characteristic muscular structure which we term the septomarginal trabeculation. Others describe this structure as the 'septal band'. It is the apical trabecular component which is the most constant and characteristic part of the morphologically right ventricle. In addition to its own coarse trabeculations, the ventricle also possesses a series of septoparietal trabeculations which extend from the anterior surface of the septomarginal trabeculation on to the parietal wall of the ventricle (Fig. 1.11). Another muscle bundle, the moderator band, is prominent and crosses from the septomarginal trabeculation to the anterior papillary muscle and thence to the parietal wall. The other ventricular components have specific features in the normal heart which aid in the recognition of the morphologically right

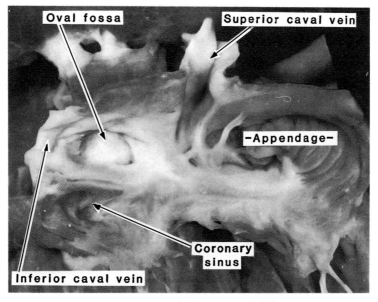

Fig. 1.5 The features of the internal aspect of the morphologically right atrium.

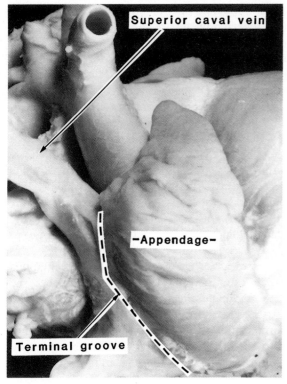

Fig. 1.6 The most characteristic feature of the external appearance of the morphologically right atrium is the shape of its appendage and the broadness of its junction with the venous atrial component.

ventricle. The morphologically tricuspid valve, as its name indicates, has three leaflets. These are found in septal, inferior and anterosuperior position and are separated one from another by the anteroseptal, supero-inferior and inferoseptal commissures, respectively (Fig. 1.7). The inferior leaflet takes its origin exclusively from the diaphragmatic parietal wall of the ventricle and is often called the mural leaflet. Each commissure has, by convention, been defined previously in terms of its support by a prominent papillary muscle topped by a fan-shaped commissural cord. This approach is less than perfect, since it transgresses the morphological method of defining structures in terms of their own intrinsic morphology. The commissures, therefore, are best considered as the breaches in the leaflet skirt extending from the central point of closure of the valve to its circumferential margin. Only the circumferential extent of these junctional commissures is seen by the pathologist when the atrioventricular junction is laid open, but their full extent can readily be reconstituted. The commissures are located anteroseptally, anterosuperiorly and inferiorly. In the tricuspid valve, they are not always supported by the corresponding papillary muscle. In terms of the muscular support, the

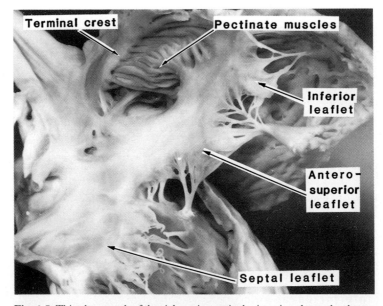

Fig. 1.7 This photograph of the right atrioventricular junction shows the three-leaflet arrangement of the tricuspid valve. It also demonstrates well the terminal crest and pectinate muscles of the right appendage.

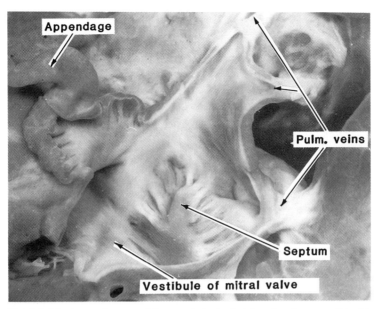

Fig. 1.8 The internal aspect of the morphologically left atrium is seen well in this dissection.

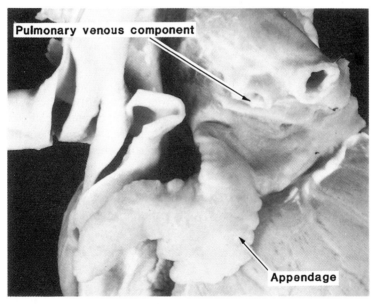

Fig. 1.9 The morphologically left atrium has a characteristically narrow appendage (compare with Fig. 1.6).

anterior muscle is the largest and usually springs directly from the body of the septomarginal trabeculation. The complex of cords supporting the anteroseptal commissure is dominated by the medial papillary muscle (of Lancisi), a relatively small muscle which springs either as a single band or as a small sprig of cords from the posterior limb of the septomarginal trabeculation. The support given to the commissure is reinforced by further sprigs which arise from the septum. The inferior

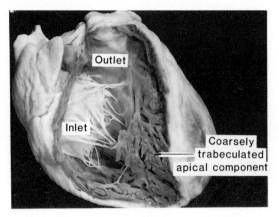

Fig. 1.10 The morphologically right ventricle is best described in terms of inlet, outlet and apical trabecular components. The coarse nature of the apical part is the most constant feature in normal and abnormal ventricles.

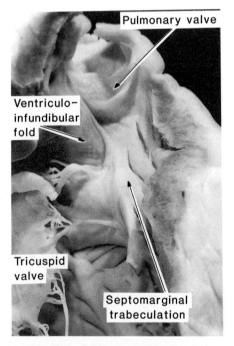

Fig. 1.11 This view of the outlet component of the morphologically right ventricle shows the ventriculo-infundibular fold between tricuspid and pulmonary valves along the septomarginal and septoparietal trabeculations.

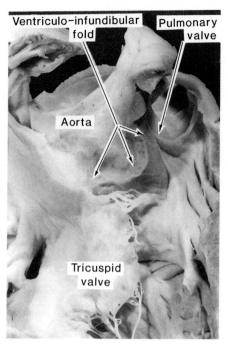

Fig. 1.12 This dissection of the heart shown in Fig. 1.11 reveals that the supraventricular crest is almost exclusively composed of the ventriculo-infundibular fold (the inner heart curvature).

muscle, the most insignificant, is usually single. It, too, may be represented by several small muscles. The most characteristic and distinguishing feature of the tricuspid valve is the direct attachment of cords from the septal leaflet into the septum.

Cordal attachments to the septal surface are never seen in the morphologically left ventricle except when the tricuspid valve straddles and inserts on to the left ventricular septal aspect. The major feature of the outlet of the morphologically right ventricle is that it is a complete muscular structure. The muscular shelf which separates the tricuspid and pulmonary valves in the roof of the ventricle is called the supraventricular crest (crista supraventricularis). It is made up of the inner curvature of the heart wall. We call this structure the ventriculo-infundibular fold (Fig. 1.12).

THE MORPHOLOGICALLY LEFT VENTRICLE

As with the right ventricle, we describe the left ventricle in terms of inlet, apical trabecular and outlet components (Fig. 1.13). The inlet component contains the mitral valve and extends from the atrioventricular junction to the attachments

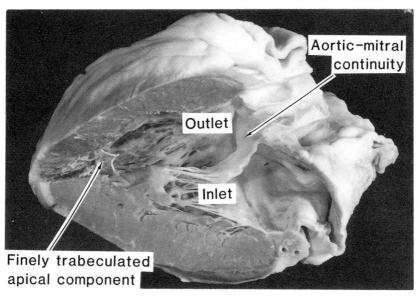

Fig. 1.13 This dissection shows the features of the morphologically left ventricle, notably its fine apical trabeculations (compare with Fig. 1.10).

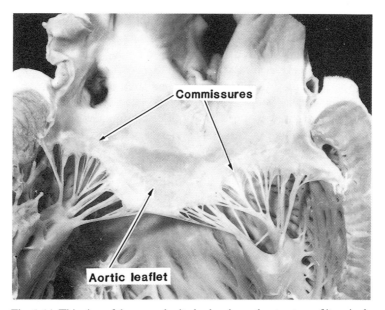

Fig. 1.14 This view of the opened mitral valve shows the structure of its paired papillary muscles. The 'spread' of the muscles, however, is artefactual (see Fig. 1.15). Note also the dissimilar morphology of the aortic and mural leaflets (the valve has been opened through the middle of the mural leaflet).

of the prominent papillary muscles. The valve has two leaflets of markedly dissimilar shape and circumferential length. The more anteriorly located leaflet is square in shape and takes up only one-third of the annular circumference (Fig. 1.14). Because of the obliquity of location of

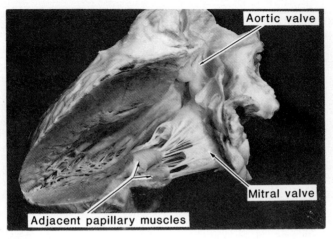

Fig. 1.15 This dissection of the 'in situ' arrangement of the mitral valve shows how the papillary muscles are adjacent when the ventricle is in its natural position.

the valve, the leaflet is not strictly anterior. Its most characteristic feature is its fibrous continuity with the leaflets of the aortic valve. For this reason we prefer to call it the aortic leaflet. The other leaflet is long and thin, taking up two-thirds of the annular circumference. It is attached throughout its length to the diaphragmatic wall of the ventricle and we describe it as the mural leaflet. Others call it the posterior leaflet. The commissure between the leaflets is oriented in postero-medial and anterolateral position. Its two ends are traditionally described as separate commissures, although they are the extremities of one continuous junction (a 'commissure', defined literally, is a junction). The two ends of the commissure are supported by prominent papillary muscles. Although often illustrated in texts of cardiac pathology as widely spread, the two papillary muscles have their origins very close together. This is readily demonstrated when the heart is dissected without spreading the atrioventricular junction (Fig. 1.15). A characteristic feature of the left ventricle is that the mitral valve never possesses cordal attachments to the septum. The most characteristic feature, and the one that decides the morphological leftness of the ventricle, is the fine trabecular nature of the apical component. The smooth septal surface also helps in identification, since the morphologically left ventricle never possesses a septomarginal trabecu-

lation or a moderator band. Prominent trabeculations sometimes cross the ventricular cavity as strands. We have never seen these structures arranged in the fashion of the septomarginal trabeculation of the morphologically right ventricle (see above). The major feature of the outlet of the morphologically left ventricle is its abbreviated nature. Part of two leaflets of the aortic valve have muscular attachments to the outlet component. The remainder of the leaflets take origin from the fibrous tissue of the aortic root, part of this being the extensive area of fibrous continuity with the aortic leaflet of the mitral valve (Fig. 1.16). It is the posterior aspect of the roof of the outlet, therefore, which is particularly short. There is no muscular segment of the ventriculo-infundibular fold in the left ventricle such as separates the arterial and atrioventricular valves of the right ventricle (compare Figs 1.12 & 1.16).

THE AORTA

The aorta, the major systemic arterial trunk of the normal heart, has an intrinsic structure not markedly different from that of the pulmonary trunk. It is distinguished from the pulmonary trunk by its branching pattern. The origin at the ventriculo–arterial junction is characterized by the

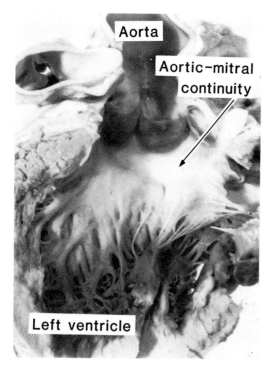

Fig. 1.16 This view of the outlet aspect of the left ventricle shows the fibrous continuity between the leaflets of the mitral and aortic valves.

three sinuses which support the semilunar attachments of the aortic valve. Two of these sinuses usually give rise to the coronary arteries. Always, in our experience, these sinuses have been the ones opposite the pulmonary trunk, irrespective of the origin and relationship of the aorta to the pulmonary trunk. These two sinuses can be termed the adjacent or facing sinuses. The other sinus, which we have never seen giving rise to a coronary artery, is then called the non-facing or non-adjacent sinus (Fig. 1.17). In the normal heart, the sinus giving rise to the right coronary artery can simply be called the right-facing (or right coronary) sinus. Similarly, that giving rise to the left coronary artery is the left-facing (or left coronary) sinus. It helps, however, to use a convention for naming the coronary sinuses which works irrespective of which coronary artery they give origin to and irrespective of the relation of the aorta to the pulmonary trunk. Such a convention is provided by the suggestion of Gittenberger-de-Groot and her colleagues[1] that the observer should consider himself as standing in the non-facing sinus and looking into the two coronary sinuses. The sinus to the right hand is then

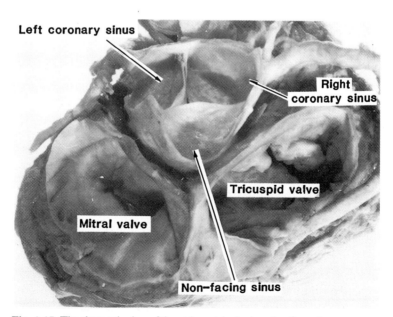

Fig. 1.17 The short axis view of the atrioventricular junction from above shows the relationship of the aortic to the atrioventricular valves and illustrates how the coronary arteries emerge from the aortic sinuses closest to ('facing') the pulmonary trunk.

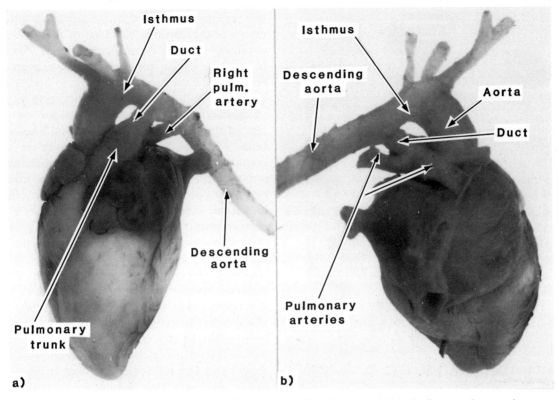

Fig. 1.18 a,b The major flow pathway from the right ventricle to the pulmonary trunk in the fetus continues as the arterial duct. This fetal heart is shown (**a**) from the front and (**b**) from behind. The right and left pulmonary arteries are side branches at this stage of development.

conventionally described as 'Sinus No. 1' while the other is 'Sinus No. 2'. Since it is still possible to forget the definitions of No. 1 and No. 2, we prefer to describe the sinuses in terms of their left-hand and right-hand position. This convention is of most value in assessing hearts with abnormal ventriculo–arterial connexions such as complete transposition (Ch. 20) or double outlet right ventricle (Ch. 21). It will be re-emphasized at those points.

The ascending portion of the aorta in the normal heart gives rise to the brachiocephalic (innominate) artery followed by the left common carotid and left subclavian arteries. The aortic arch then continues at the isthmus, which extends to the junction of the aortic arch with the arterial duct (ductus arteriosus). The duct is a wide channel in the heart of the fetus and the newborn but closes rapidly shortly after birth. It is repre-

sented subsequently by the attachment of the arterial ligament to the underside of the arch (see below). The aortic arch itself then continues as the descending thoracic aorta, which gives rise to the bronchial and intercostal arteries before piercing the diaphragm to become the abdominal aorta.

THE PULMONARY TRUNK

The pulmonary trunk has a very simple branching pattern, dividing into the right and left pulmonary arteries. The trunk in the fetus continues as the arterial duct into the descending aorta, the right and left pulmonary arteries being side branches from the flow pathway from the duct to the aorta (Fig. 1.18). After birth, with closure of the arterial duct, this arrangement rapidly becomes

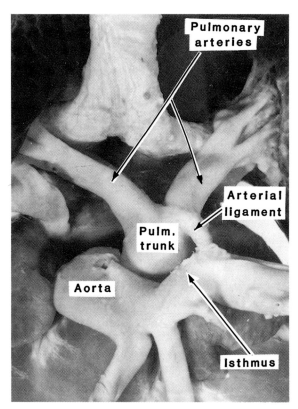

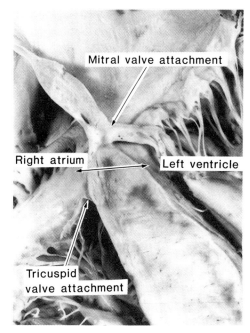

Fig. 1.20 This 'four chamber' section close to the crux of the heart shows how the off-setting of the attachments of the tricuspid and mitral valves results in the formation of a muscular atrioventricular septum (two-headed arrow).

Fig. 1.19 Remodelling of the pulmonary trunk after birth, concomitant with closure of the arterial duct, leads to formation of the pulmonary bifurcation.

moulded into the smooth bifurcation seen in the normal child and adult (Fig. 1.19). The site of the arterial duct is marked by the arterial ligament with the recurrent laryngeal nerve passing around it.

THE NORMAL SEPTAL STRUCTURES

The descriptions of the chambers given above set the scene both for the understanding of normal cardiac anatomy and also for sequential segmental analysis (see Ch. 4). Further details of normal anatomy must be discussed, however, so as to facilitate the interpretation of congenital malformations. The first of these topics is the extent of the normal septal structures. We have already hinted at the relatively small extent of the atrial walls which constitute the interatrial septum. If one simply opens the parietal wall of the right atrium and inspects the opposite surface, the impression is gained of an extensive 'septum'. Dissection shows that most of this area is either composed of infoldings of the atrial wall or else is made up of the atrioventricular septum (see below). The sweep of atrial wall seen anteriorly overlies the aortic root. The so-called 'septum secundum', better considered as the rim of the oval depression, is a characteristic feature of the right atrial septal surface. It is made up predominantly of the infolded atrial roof. The posterior aspect of the oval depression is, usually, the wall of the inferior caval vein. The larger part of the inferior border is the atrioventricular septum. Only a small area is truly a septal structure separating the cavity of the right atrium from that of the left.

The atrioventricular septum has received scant attention in textbooks either of anatomy or of pathology. In the normal heart, it separates the cavity of the right atrium from that of the left ventricle. It has two components, muscular and membranous. The former exists because the proximal attachment of the septal leaflet of the tricuspid valve is considerably further towards the ventricular apex than is the (very limited) attachment of the leaflets of the mitral valve (Fig. 1.20). The atrial and ventricular septal structures overlap in the small area towards the crux of the heart where the two valves are attached opposite to each other. This area of overlap constitutes the muscular atrioventricular septum. Immediately anterior to the muscular area, the subaortic outflow tract is wedged between the mitral valve and the septum. This wedged location lifts the aortic leaflet of the mitral valve away from the septum and explains why the valve has such a limited septal attachment (Fig. 1.21). The medial wall of the aortic outflow tract in this area is a fibrous structure crossed on its right side by the attachment of the septal leaflet of the tricuspid valve. This divides it into supra- and infra-tricuspid components. The whole partition is called the membranous septum. The supra-tricuspid component separates the left ventricle from the right atrium and is, therefore,

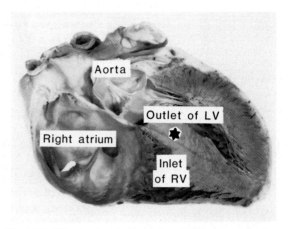

Fig. 1.22 This simulated subcostal section in paracoronal plane shows how the muscular ventricular septum (starred) separates the inlet of the right ventricle from the outlet of the left.

the atrioventricular membranous septum. The infra-tricuspid component of the membranous septum makes up the central point of the ventricular septum. It is small when compared to the vast bulk of the muscular septum, which has a most complex geometric arrangement. The part bordering the inlet of the right ventricle is more or less in the sagittal plane of the body while that separating the outlets is almost in the coronal plane. The septum, therefore, almost bends through a right angle. In addition, it has a considerable inclination as it extends out to separate the two apical trabecular components. This extensive muscular septum is conventionally divided into segments. Some authors divide it simply into inlet and outlet portions.[2] Others use a more complex division based upon arbitrary construction of imaginary lines.[3] Our preference is to follow the tripartite concept of ventricular division and to consider the septum as having three components. This approach must be used with caution because of the wedge position of the normal subaortic outflow tract. The greater part of the septal component beneath the septal leaflet of the tricuspid valve separates the inlet of the right ventricle from the outlet of the left (Fig. 1.22). The largest part of the muscular septum extends out towards the ventricular apices and separates their characteristically trabeculated surfaces. This component is aptly described as the apical trabec-

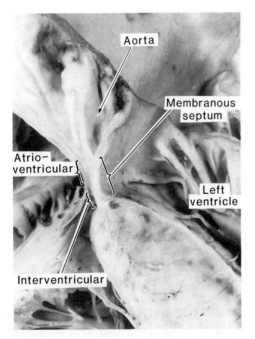

Fig. 1.21 This 'four chamber' section taken anteriorly to the one seen in Fig. 1.20 shows the membranous septum divided into atrioventricular and interventricular components by the attachment of the septal leaflet of the tricuspid valve.

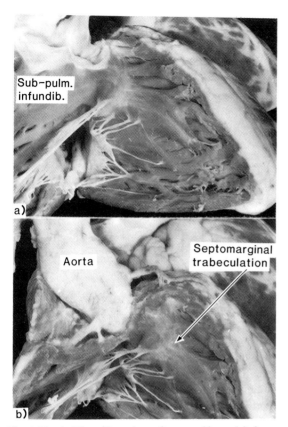

a)

Sub–pulm. infundib.

b)

Aorta

Septomarginal trabeculation

Fig. 1.23 a,b These dissections of a normal heart (**a**) show how the subpulmonary infundibulum can be removed (**b**) without entering the cavity of the left ventricle. This is because it is a discrete structure made up predominantly of the ventriculo-infundibular fold.

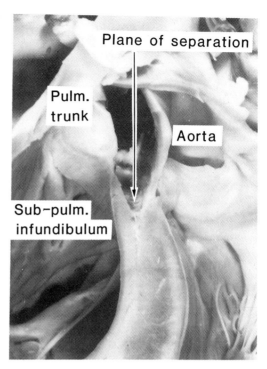

Plane of separation

Pulm. trunk

Aorta

Sub–pulm. infundibulum

Fig. 1.24 This long axis section of the outflow tracts confirms that the subpulmonary infundibulum is a discrete sleeve of outlet musculature (see Fig. 1.23). The normal outlet septum is very small.

ular septum, although we do not mean to imply from this usage that the inlet septum is devoid of trabeculations. The third part of the septum gives most problems in description. Dissection shows that the entirety of the subpulmonary infundibulum can be removed from the heart without entering the cavity of the left ventricle (Fig. 1.23). It is self-evident that no part of the subpulmonary infundibulum thus removed can be part of the outlet septum. Indeed, transections of the ventricular outlets show that only a very small part of the normal septum separates the outlets (Fig. 1.24). This is not to say that the outlet septum does not exist as a major muscular structure in malformed hearts, but rather that it is not represented to so marked an extent in the normal heart.

THE VENO–ATRIAL CONNEXIONS

In the account of the atria, we described the normal arrangement of their venous connexions. At that time, we considered only the nature of the veins connected to each chamber. There is, in addition, a normal and abnormal morphology for these venous connexions. This aspect will be of particular significance when we consider the veno–atrial connexions in patients with atrial isomerism (see Ch. 16). It is important, therefore, to describe with precision their normal arrangement.

There are three venous channels connected to the morphologically right atrium. These are the superior and inferior caval veins and the coronary sinus. They all join the atrium within the confines of the venous sinus (sinus venosus), this part of the chamber being bounded medially by the atrial septum and laterally by the terminal crest. The relationship to the terminal crest is important, as

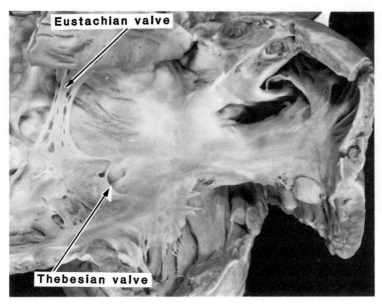

Fig. 1.25 This view of the opened right atrioventricular junction shows the typical arrangement of the Eustachian and Thebesian valves.

this area is indicated externally by the terminal groove. The position of the septum is also visible externally as a deeper groove between the connexions of the caval veins to the right atrium and the right pulmonary veins to the left atrium. This groove, which represents the infolding of the atrial roof at the superior rim of the oval fossa, is often termed Waterston's groove (or Sondergaard's groove) in textbooks of surgical anatomy. When viewed internally, the opening of the superior caval vein is seen to be bounded medially by the superior rim of the fossa (the inner aspect of Waterston's groove) and by the terminal crest laterally. The wall of the inferior caval vein often runs directly into the oval fossa but, sometimes, there is a rim between the two. Laterally it is bounded by the terminal crest. In many hearts, a fold of tissue (the Eustachian valve) springs from the crest in this area and functions as a valvar mechanism (Fig. 1.25). This is a remnant of the more extensive valve which, in fetal life, serves to direct the richly oxygenated placental blood entering through the inferior caval vein into the left atrium through the oval foramen. The opening of the coronary sinus occupies the most postero-inferior corner of the right atrium and is separated by the sinus septum from the oval fossa.

It, also, is guarded in fetal life by a valve (the Thebesian valve). When persisting in postnatal life, this valve extends on to the sinus septum and, in this position, forms a commissure with the Eustachian valve. The commissure itself is then continued as a fibrous strand which buries itself in the sinus septum and runs forward to insert into the central fibrous body. This structure, known as the tendon of Todaro, forms the atrial border of the triangle of Koch. The triangle is important because it contains the atrial component of the specialized atrioventricular conduction axis (see below). More extensive remnants of the valves of the venous sinus often extend in filigree fashion across the cavity of the right atrium to attach to the superior portion of the terminal crest. Called Chiari networks, these remnants are of no functional significance unless present as a solid sheet (see Ch. 6). Although usually small in comparison to the orifices of the caval veins, the mouth of the coronary sinus can be large when it drains a persistent left superior caval vein. Such a venous channel is present during early fetal life but usually becomes absorbed and attenuated during development. Its site is marked by the oblique ligament of the left atrium.

The four pulmonary veins normally connect to

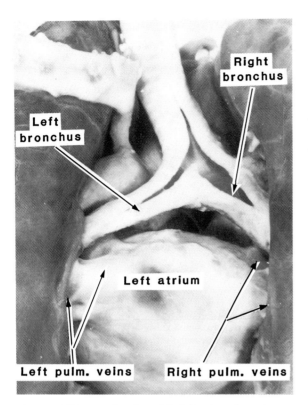

Left bronchus

Right bronchus

Left atrium

Left pulm. veins

Right pulm. veins

Fig. 1.26 This posterior view of the left atrium shows the four pulmonary veins (arrowed) entering the corners of the chamber, anchoring the heart to the mediastinum. Note also the arrangement of the bronchi.

the morphologically left atrium in a constant fashion, each entering a different corner of the posterior atrial wall so that together they enclose a substantial area (Fig. 1.26). The oblique ligament (or a persistent left superior caval vein if present) always runs between the left pulmonary veins and the left atrial appendage. Normally, the right pulmonary veins are separated from the caval veins by Waterston's groove.

THE FIBROUS SKELETON OF THE HEART

Accounts of cardiac anatomy often describe an extensive fibrous skeleton at the atrioventricular junction enclosing the attachments of all four cardiac valves. Careful examination of the normal heart, particularly in infants and children, shows

scant evidence of the existence of such an extensive structure. The best-formed component of the skeleton is the so-called central fibrous body. This is the junction of the fibrous parts of the aortic, mitral and tricuspid valves. It incorporates within its structure the membranous septum together with the strengthened medial end of the area of fibrous continuity between the mitral and aortic valves (Fig. 1.27). This thickened area is called the right fibrous trigone and it forms the roof of the posterior extension of the subaortic outflow tract. The fibrous skeleton continues as a firm structure along the length of the aortic–mitral fibrous continuity, the lateral end also being thickened as the left fibrous trigone. The skeleton continues in most hearts as a firm cord around the entirety of the left atrioventricular junction where it forms the annulus of the mitral valve. Its skeleton is also continued as thinner fibrous plates in the interleaflet triangles between the left and non-coronary leaflets and the non-coronary and right coronary leaflets of the aortic valve (see below). In the heart of the infant and child, there are no crown-like extensions of the skeleton which support the semilunar attachments of the three aortic leaflets. If these exist in the aged heart, they do so as the consequence of accretion of fibrous tissue. Similarly, it is not possible to trace a complete cord-like annulus around the origin of the leaflets of the tricuspid valve. These leaflets are mostly attached to the surface of the ventricular myocardium and are continuous with the fibrofatty tissue of the atrioventricular groove. The leaflets of the pulmonary valve are entirely without skeletal support, arising predominantly from the musculature of the right ventricular infundibulum, although the commissural apices are attached to the fibrous wall of the pulmonary trunk. The fibrous skeleton of the heart, therefore, is confined to the central fibrous body and the area of aortic–mitral fibrous continuity, together with extensions around the mitral orifice and into two of the three interleaflet triangles of the aortic root (Fig. 1.27).

THE CONDUCTION TISSUES

The arrangement of the conduction tissues, being

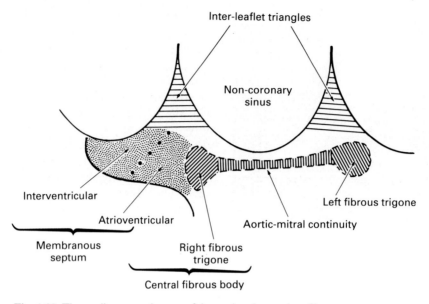

Fig. 1.27 The semilunar attachments of the aortic valve produce fibrous interleaflet triangles. This diagram shows the relationship of those adjoining the non-coronary sinus to the membranous septum and the fibrous continuity with the mitral valve.

an integral part of the anatomy, varies according to the particular morphology of the normal or abnormal heart. The sinus node (or pacemaker) is a cigar-shaped structure lying immediately subepicardially within the terminal groove (Fig. 1.28). Usually it is found lateral to the crest of the atrial appendage and has tailed out towards the orifice of the inferior caval vein. In a minority of cases, it extends in horseshoe fashion across the crest and into the interatrial groove. The artery of supply to the sinus node is a branch of the initial course of the right coronary artery in just over half of all people and of the start of the left circumflex coronary artery in most of the remainder. The artery ascends through the interatrial groove and can enter the node either in precaval or retrocaval fashion (Fig. 1.29). Sometimes it divides to enter from both ends, the two arteries then forming a circle around the superior cavo–atrial junction. Rarely, but of major surgical significance when present,[4–6] the artery can arise more distally from either the right or circumflex arteries and then runs across the right appendage or the roof of the left atrium to reach the node.

The specialized tissues which connect the atrial and ventricular muscle masses are arranged as a continuous axis which extends from the atrioventricular muscular septum, penetrates the atrioventricular membranous septum and branches on the crest of the muscular interventricular septum (Fig. 1.30). The atrial component of the atrioventricular axis is contained exclusively within the triangle of Koch. This landmark is delineated by the tendon of Todaro, the septal attachment of the tricuspid valve and the mouth of the coronary sinus (Fig. 1.31). The atrial specialized tissues within the triangle are composed of a component transitional between atrial and nodal cells together with the compact atrioventricular node. The axis passes through the atrioventricular membranous septum at the apex of the triangle of Koch as the penetrating atrioventricular bundle (of His). It then immediately emerges in the sub-aortic outflow tract beneath the commissure between the non-facing and right coronary leaflets of the aortic valve. The axis then branches almost immediately in the normal heart, usually on the crest of the muscular septum but sometimes to its left side. The left bundle branch then fans out on the smooth aspect of the septum in a continuous

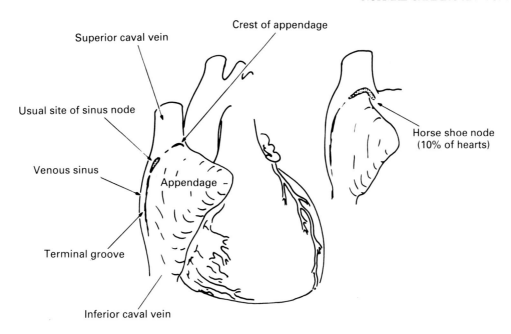

Fig. 1.28 This diagram depicts the site of the sinus node in the normal heart. The inset shows the 'horseshoe' variation found in about one-tenth of individuals.

cascade, splitting into three divisions (anterior, septal and posterior) towards the ventricular apex. The right bundle branch turns back through the septum as a cord-like structure and continues through the substance of the septomarginal trabeculation before crossing in the moderator band and ramifying into the right ventricular myocardium. Sometimes, the axis itself continues as a dead-end tract on the septal crest and ascends towards the facing commissure of the aortic valve. The function of this part of the axis is unknown.

Although the presence of specialized pathways between the sinus and atrioventricular nodes has been postulated,[7] no one yet has provided convincing morphological evidence of their existence. Careful studies of the entirety of the atrial tissues show that the histologically specialized tissues are confined to the sinus and atrioventricular nodes and the rests of nodal tissue that are found around the atrioventricular junctions in the distal insertions of the atrial myocardium into the valve leaflets.[8,9] These rests around the atrioventricular junction are of interest as they are found in most normal hearts. They are, however, sequestrated in the atrial tissues. In normal circumstances, they do not make contact with the ventricular myocardial tissues. Presumably, these were the structures observed by Kent when he suggested that the possibility for atrioventricular conduction in normal hearts existed at several points around the atrioventricular junction.[10] In terms of interatrial conduction, it is now established beyond reasonable doubt[11] that it is the structure of the bundles of working myocardium which determine the preferential spread of activity.

THE CORONARY CIRCULATION

The myocardium is supplied with its own system of arteries, capillaries, veins and lymphatics, all of which must be in working order if the heart is to function normally. The coronary arteries are the first branches of the aorta (Fig. 1.32). There are two major coronary arterial branches from the aorta which arise from two of the three sinuses of Valsalva, permitting the sinuses to be named as right coronary and left coronary, respectively. The

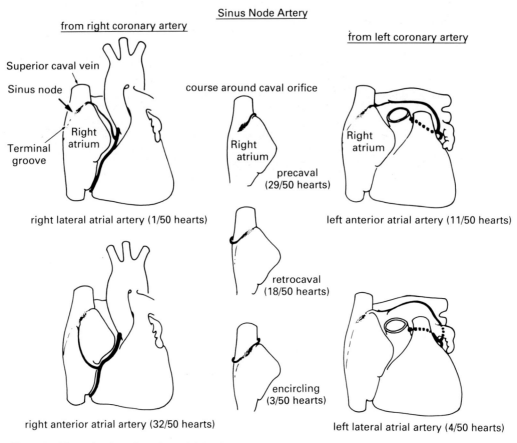

Fig. 1.29 These drawings show the variability in course and origin of the artery to the sinus node in a series of 50 hearts from normal infants. (Note: 2/50 had origins from both left and right coronary arteries.)

coronary arteries usually arise within the expanded portion of the appropriate sinus. Origin of an artery above the commissural ring of the aorta (in other words from the tubular ascending aorta) is considered to be a congenital malformation (see Ch. 23). The two coronary arteries have major differences in their branching pattern once they have emerged from their sinuses and this establishes their distinction as morphologically right or morphologically left. The right coronary artery runs an extensive course around the orifice of the tricuspid valve. It emerges from the right sinus to achieve a position in the transverse sinus above the supraventricular crest of the right ventricle. In this initial part of its course, it usually gives off the sinus nodal artery into the atrial musculature and the infundibular (or conal)

artery into the ventricular muscle mass. The artery then runs to the acute margin of the heart where it gives rise to the acute marginal artery of the right ventricle and, usually, a lateral atrial artery. Continuing around the tricuspid orifice, it gives off a varied number of smaller ventricular branches before, in the majority of hearts, it ends in the posterior interventricular groove. The area of junction of the posterior interventricular and the atrioventricular grooves is generally called the crux of the heart. The posterior inter-ventricular artery is given off at this point in most hearts. When supplying the posterior artery, the right coronary artery itself makes a U-turn into the area of the atrioventricular muscular septum and gives off the artery to the atrioventricular node from the apex of the U. It then continues

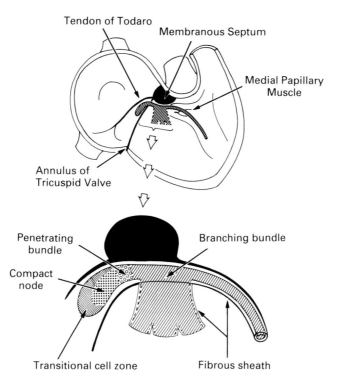

Fig. 1.30 This diagram shows the landmarks of the triangle of Koch (upper) and the components of the atrioventricular conduction axis (lower).

on to the diaphragmatic surface of the left ventricle where it supplies ventricular branches (Fig. 1.33).

The left coronary artery has a shorter course. It emerges into the left margin of the transverse sinus beneath the left atrial appendage and extends for only one or two centimetres before branching into the circumflex and anterior interventricular branches. In a proportion of hearts, the main stem divides into three branches (Fig. 1.34). The third artery was previously described as the intermediate artery. It is now more customary (following the proposals of the National Heart, Lung and Blood Institute, USA)[12] to describe it as the first diagonal branch of the anterior interventricular artery. The anterior artery itself runs down the anterior interventricular groove, often buried, in part, within the musculature. Intramyocardial course of a coronary artery is termed myocardial bridging. The anterior interventricular artery gives off an important series of branches which pass perpendicularly into the anterior septum, the septal perforating arteries. The interventricular artery supplies infundibular branches to the outflow component of the right ventricle, these often anastomosing with the branches from the right coronary artery. It also gives rise to a varied number of diagonal arteries which supply the anterior free wall of the left ventricle. The circumflex artery gives rise to the sinus nodal artery from its initial course in almost half of all hearts. The rest of its course is variable. In some hearts it terminates almost immediately. In these circumstances it often gives off the atrial circumflex artery which runs in the atrial myocardium around the mitral orifice. More usually the circumflex artery continues to the obtuse margin of the left ventricle and breaks up into the obtuse marginal arteries. These are often embedded within the muscle of the left ventricle. In a small proportion of hearts, the circumflex

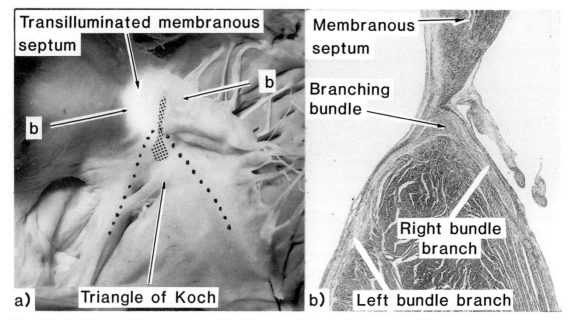

Fig. 1.31 a,b This view of the septal aspect of the right atrium (**a**) shows the landmarks which produce the triangle of Koch. The right-hand panel (**b**) shows a section through the plane b–b, illustrating the location of the atrioventricular conduction axis.

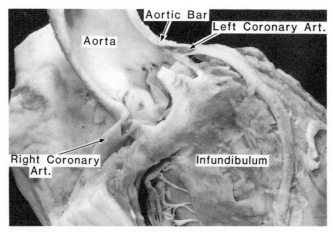

Fig. 1.32 This dissection of the normal heart shows how the coronary arteries are the first branches of the ascending aorta.

artery continues all the way round the mitral orifice and hugs closely the annulus of the valve. It then gives rise to both the posterior interventricular artery and the artery to the atrioventricular node. This arrangement is called left dominance, in contrast to the much more common pattern of right dominance. In still other hearts, both the

right and circumflex arteries may supply the diaphragmatic surface without there being a prominent posterior interventricular artery. The latter arrangement is termed a balanced circulation.

The coronary veins return the blood to the coronary sinus, forming major channels in both

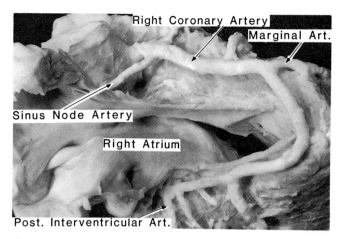

Fig. 1.33 This dissection shows the course of the right coronary artery around the tricuspid orifice.

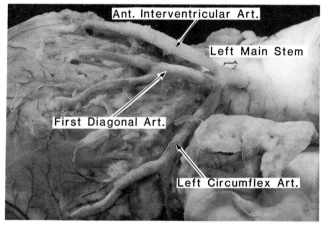

Fig. 1.34 The left coronary artery is a very short structure. In this heart it gives rise to anterior interventricular, circumflex and first diagonal branches.

the interventricular and the atrioventricular grooves. A large tributary is formed in the anterior interventricular groove and is termed the great cardiac vein. It runs round the mitral orifice and expands to form the body of the coronary sinus in the left posterior atrioventricular groove. At the crux, the coronary sinus also receives both the blood returned through the middle cardiac vein, which runs up the posterior interventricular groove, and that from the small cardiac vein. The latter vessel initially accompanies the acute marginal artery and then turns round the orifice of the tricuspid valve in the right atrioventricular groove before terminating in the coronary sinus at the crux (Fig. 1.35).

The heart is supplied by a rich plexus of lymphatics. Very little had been written about these channels until the recent publication of the major volume by Miller.[13] The lymphatic channels run along with the veins but drain the lymph to the pulmonary hilar lymph nodes and also directly into the thoracic duct and the left lymphatic channel.

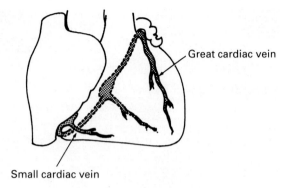

Great cardiac vein

Small cardiac vein

Anterior aspect

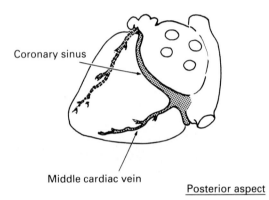

Coronary sinus

Middle cardiac vein

Posterior aspect

Fig. 1.35 The arrangement of the coronary veins is shown diagrammatically from the front (upper) and behind (lower).

REFERENCES

1. Gittenberger-de-Groot AC, Sauer U, Oppenheimer-Dekker A, Quaegebeur J. Coronary arterial anatomy in transposition of the great arteries. A morphologic study. Ped Cardiol 1983; 4: I:15 – 24.
2. Van Praagh R, David I, Van Praagh S. What is a ventricle? The single ventricle trap. Ped Cardiol 1982; 2: 79 – 84.
3. Brandt PWT. Axial angled angiocardiography. Cardiovasc Intervent Radiol 1984; 7: 166 –169.
4. Busquet J, Fontan F, Anderson RH, Ho SY, Davies MJ. The surgical significance of the atrial branches of the coronary arteries. Int J Cardiol 1984; 6: 223 – 234.
5. Nerantzis S, Argoustakis D. An S-shaped atrial artery supplying the sinus node area. Chest 1980; 78· 274 – 278.
6. Kennel AJ, Titus JL. The vasculature of the human sinus node. Mayo Clin Proc 1972; 47: 556 – 561.
7. James TN. The connecting pathways between the sinus node and the A-V node and between the right and the left atrium in the human heart. Am Heart J 1963: 66: 498 – 508.
8. Janse MJ, Anderson RH. Internodal atrial specialised pathways—fact or fiction? Eur J Cardiol 1974; 2: 117 –137.
9. Anderson RH, Davies MJ, Becker AE. Atrioventricular ring specialized tissue in the normal heart. Eur J Cardiol 1974; 2: 219–230.
10. Kent AFS. Researches on the structure and function of the mammalian heart. J Physiol 1983; 14: 233–254.
11. Spach MS, Miller WT III, Barr RC, Gesolowitz DB. Electrophysiology of the internodal pathways: determining the difference between anisotropic cardiac muscle and a specialized tract system. In: Little RC, ed. Physiology of atrial pacemakers and connective tissues. Mount Kisco, New York: Futura 1980: 367–380.
12. The principal investigators of CASS and their associates. The National Heart, Lung, and Blood Institute Coronary Artery Surgery Study (CASS). Circulation 1981; 63: 11–81.
13. Miller AJ. Lymphatics of the heart. New York: Raven Press, 1982.

Pathophysiology of the heart in relation to morphology

INTRODUCTION

The heart functions as a mechanical pump, composed of muscle and driven by electricity. Maintenance of adequate function of this pump depends on a delicate balance between electrical and mechanical factors such as formation and conduction of the cardiac impulse, cellular excitation, contraction and relaxation, and valvar competence.

MORPHOLOGY RELATED TO PHYSIOLOGY

The totality of muscle cells within the heart forms a functional unit to the extent that the organ contracts in synchronous fashion. At the light microscopical level, the cardiac muscle shows a texture of cells without distinct boundaries (Fig. 2.1). For that reason, cardiac muscle has long been considered a syncytium. Ultrastructural studies, however, have shown that an indented line, the intercalated disc, forms the boundary between bundles of cells oriented in parallel and their neighbours (Fig. 2.2). Intercellular junctions are formed at various sites.[1] There are three basic types of these junctions, two of which are important for intercellular adhesion, namely the fascia adherens and desmosomes. The third junctional type is the gap junction or nexus (Fig. 2.3). These nexuses are considered areas of lower electrical impedence and, on that basis, are capable of transmitting an electrical impulse rapidly from one cell to the other. Such transmission is essential for synchronous contraction.

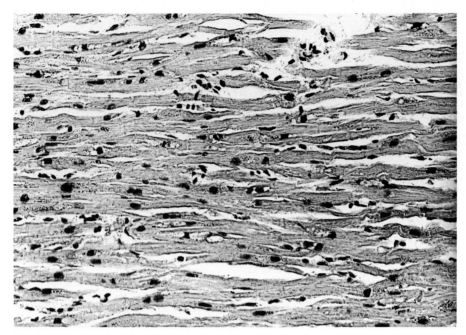

Fig. 2.1 Histological section of normal ventricular myocardium (autopsy case) showing a syncytium-like arrangement of myocardial cells.
Haematoxylin–eosin × 230

Within a cardiac muscle cell, or myocyte, myofibrils are found which are oriented in parallel fashion and more or less in the direction of the cellular long axis.[2] Each cell contains between 300 and 700 myofibrils. Each myofibril is itself composed of two types of myofilaments, actin and myosin. A myosin filament is surrounded by six actin filaments. In one myofibril there are from 200–1000 filaments. Actin and myosin are the contractile proteins; the two together are considered the contractile apparatus within the myocyte.

The sarcomere is the functional unit within the myofibril (Fig. 2.4). It is composed of actin and myosin proteins and is delineated at both sides by a so-called Z line. The actin proteins of adjoining sarcomeres insert into the Z line. The Z lines then form the point of fixation for the actin proteins during muscular contraction, when the myosin filaments slide in between the actin filaments, leading to sarcomeric shortening.

The structure of the cardiac muscle cells is tailored towards the transformation of chemical energy into mechanical processes. To this end, a number of structural components play an impor-
tant role (Fig. 2.5). First is the cell membrane, or sarcolemma, which envelops the myocyte. The outer glycocalyx of this sarcolemma has an affinity for calcium ions, which are crucial for the process of contraction. Moreover, the cell membrane acts as a selective barrier for various ions. Invaginations of the sarcolemma into the cell form the so-called transverse tubular system (T-system). This architectural arrangement ensures an enormous increase in surface area where intracellular organelles and extracellular substances can come into contact.[3] A third structure of significance is the sarcoplasmic reticulum. This forms a longitudinally branching tubular system which is more or less parallel to, and in close contact with, the contractile proteins. The sarcoplasmic reticulum has several sites of contact with the sarcolemma and the T-system. Dilatations of the sarcoplasmic reticulum occur at sites known as sub-sarcolemmal cisterns. The fourth important structural component is the contractile apparatus, already discussed. Finally, abundant mitochondria provide the energy necessary for contraction of the myocyte.

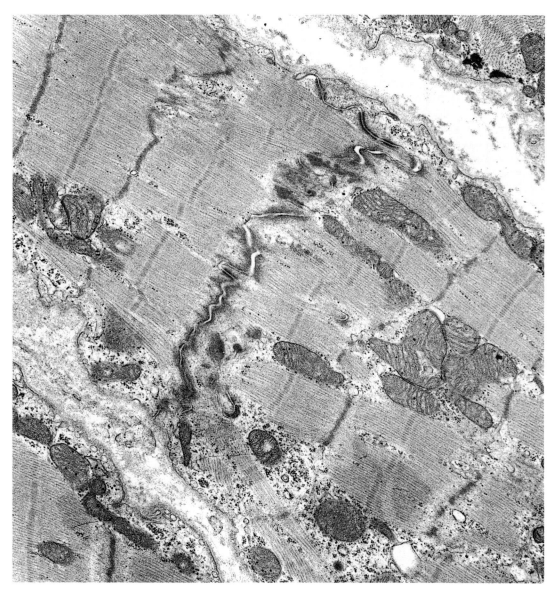

Fig. 2.2 Ultrastructure of ventricular muscle showing the intercalated disc separating two myocytes. Electronmicrograph × 19 000

During contraction and relaxation, coupling occurs between excitation of the cell, which consists of a reversal of the membrane potential, and mechanisms which bring about the contraction.[4] This so-called excitation-contraction coupling is initiated at the moment that an action potential causes depolarization of the sarcolemma. This process is accompanied by complex phenomena of ion exchanges across the membrane (Fig. 2.6). During the initial rapid phase of depolarization, influx of sodium ions occurs. This influx soon stops because of a loss in membrane permeability to these ions. Slow influx of calcium ions then ensues, concomitant with the plateau phase of the action potential. Towards the end of this phase, the permeability for calcium

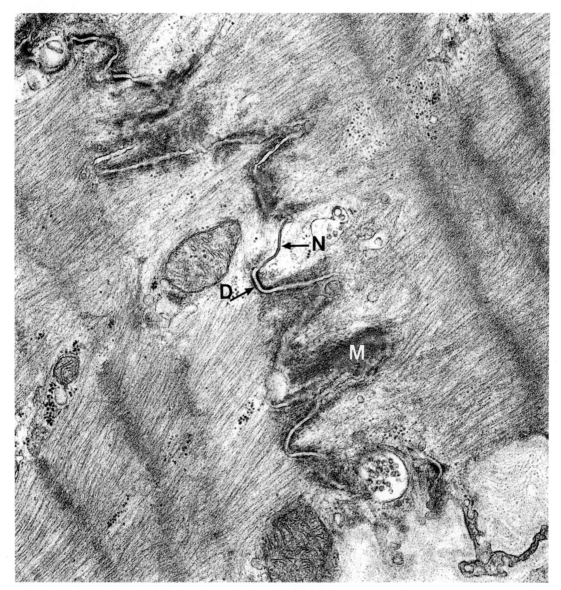

Fig. 2.3 Part of an intercalated disc showing a nexus (N), a desmosome (D) and sites of myofibrillar insertion (M). Electronmicrograph × 33 000

ions also disappears and the membrane becomes increasingly permeable to potassium ions.

The initial trans-sarcolemmal influx of calcium ions takes place by way of voltage-dependent calcium channels. These calcium ions are not immediately available for contraction. They function as a 'trigger' to release activator calcium ions from the sub-sarcolemmal cisterns. These, in turn, mobilize calcium stored in the sarcoplasmic reticulum. Changes in the electrical potential of the sarcolemma of the T-system may also play a role in the release of calcium from the cisterns.

The free calcium ions in the cytosol will bind with a regulatory protein, the troponin/tropomyosin complex, which is bound to actin.[5] By binding to a specific polypeptide of the

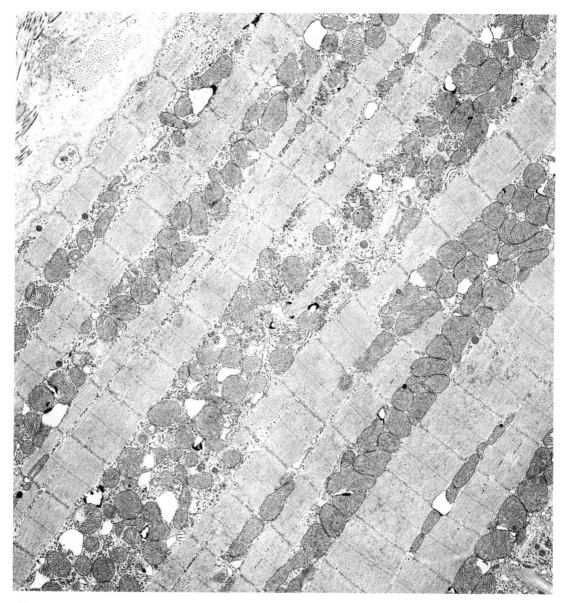

Fig. 2.4 Ultrastructure of ventricular muscle cell, showing the arrangement of myofilaments into sarcomeres, delineated by Z lines.
Electronmicrograph × 9000

tropomyosin protein, a change is induced in the binding sites between troponin and tropomyosin. New bridges are formed between actin and myosin and the result is a shift of actin filaments in between the thicker myosin filaments. This shift towards the centre of the sarcomere results in shortening and, hence, in contraction.

Relaxation occurs when calcium ions dissociate from the contractile apparatus to become, in part, stored once more in the longitudinal tubular system of the sarcoplasmic reticulum. Some calcium ions will also be removed by way of the cell membrane into the extracellular space. The changes in the troponin/tropomyosin complex, associated with the removal of calcium, will prevent the occurrence of new cross bridges

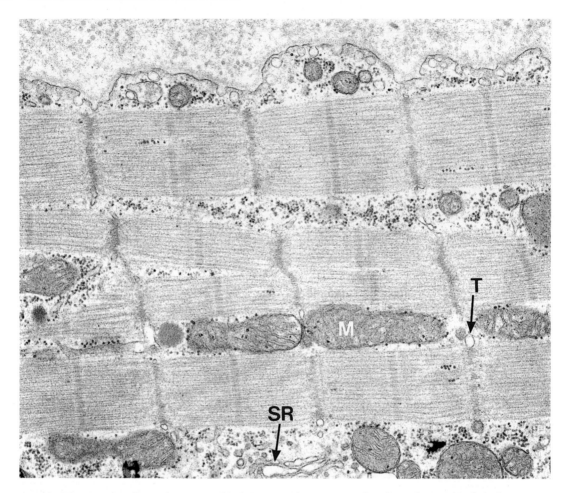

Fig. 2.5 Ultrastructure of part of a myocyte showing structural components that play an important role in the process of contraction/relaxation, such as mitochondria (M), T tubules (T), the sarcoplasmic reticulum (SR), and the contractile proteins organized in sarcomeres. The sarcolemma shows numerous small circular invaginations, known as caveolae or sarcolemmal vesicles.
Electronmicrograph × 27 000

between the actin and myosin filaments. The myocyte relaxes and the heart will enter its diastolic phase.

This classic concept of the excitation-contraction coupling is complicated by the presence within the membrane of calcium channels which are receptor-dependent. In cardiac muscle adrenergic (catecholamine-dependent) receptors are important, with β-receptors, and β_1-receptors in particular, being the most significant. Stimulation, for instance by way of adrenaline, will lead to an activation of adenyl cyclase, which increases the production of cyclic adenosine monophosphate (cAMP). Along this pathway, protein kinases dependent on cyclic adenosine monophosphate are activated: they modulate the intracellular effects of calcium ions. The activated enzymes enhance activator calcium ions and, by so doing, increase contractility of cardiac muscle. The speed with which calcium ions are taken up by the sarcoplasmic reticulum, and the speed of dissociation of the binding sites on troponin, are also modulated. The density of the α-adrenergic receptors in cardiac muscle is less than that in the vessel wall (see Ch. 24).

In this context, cholinergic receptors should

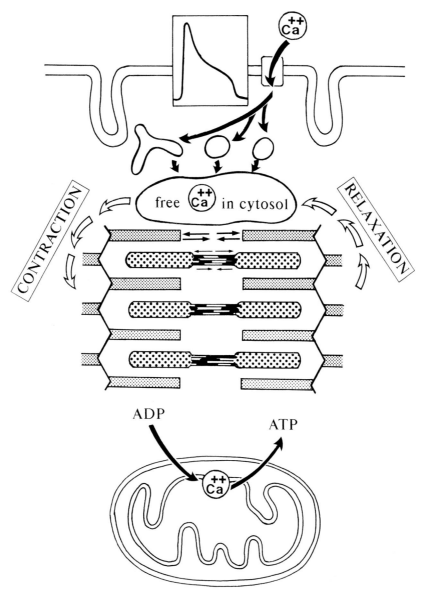

Fig. 2.6 This diagram shows the major influences of calcium during activation of the cardiac myocyte. The upper part of the diagram represents the influx of calcium ions (Ca^{2+}) through the sarcoplasmic reticulum, whence free calcium ions are released into the cytosol. They are then utilized during the processes of contraction and relaxation of the myofibrils, while calcium is also involved at mitochondrial level (bottom) in the conversion of adenosine diphosphate (ADP) into adenosine triphosphate (ATP).
Adapted from Becker A E. Circulatiestoornissen. In: Hoedemaeker Ph J, Bosman F T, Meijer C J L M, Becker A E, eds. Pathologie, 2nd ed. Utrecht: Wetenschappelijke Uitgeverij Bunge, 1991; Ch 2, Fig 2.2.

also be mentioned briefly. The muscarinic receptors, which have an affinity for acetylcholine, may, once activated, increase the permeability of the membrane to potassium ions. This process delays the diastolic repolarization and has a particular effect on the cells of the sinus and atrioventricular nodes leading to a decrease in frequency of the heart beat.

The energy necessary for the interaction between actin and myosin is provided by adenosine triphosphate (ATP). The latter is regenerated from adenosine diphosphate (ADP) in the mitochondria by a process of oxidative phosphorylation. Creatine phosphate is the most important store of energy-rich phosphate, and the enzyme creatine phosphokinase therefore plays an important role in the process of energy-producing metabolism.

Under physiological circumstances, the mitochondria play no part in the movement of calcium ions during excitation-contraction coupling. Under abnormal circumstances, as for instance when there is a high concentration of calcium in the cytosol, this may change. Mitochondrial transport of calcium may then take place, a process which will consume ATP. Hence, oxidative phosphorylation may be inadequate and cellular metabolism will become dependent on anaerobic metabolic processes. Long-lasting ischaemia of the myocytes may be associated with this process of uptake of calcium in the mitochondria.[6]

Apart from the consumption of energy because of the process of contraction, energy will also be consumed to restore the ionic changes that occur during this process. The sodium/potassium pump restores the membrane potential and takes place by way of an energy-consuming enzyme, so-called Na^+K^+-ATPase. The efflux of calcium ions occurs against both an electrical and a concentration gradient. The sarcolemma contains a calcium-dependent ATPase which contributes to an active removal of calcium from the cytosol. Parallel to this, a bidirectional system is operative for exchange of sodium and calcium and is dependent to a large extent on the relative concentrations of the ions inside and outside the myocytes. Mechanisms that inhibit the Na^+K^+ pump will produce, as a side-effect, an increase in concentration of sodium within the cell which will lead to a decrease in the efflux of calcium across the membrane because of competition with the Na^+-Ca^{2+} exchange. Digitalis has such an effect. A regulatory protein, the so-called G-protein, appears also to play an important role in modulating many of these processes.

THE PATHOPHYSIOLOGY OF THE FAILING HEART

Heart failure may occur as soon as parts of the pump are damaged, or once the balance between the various functional processes is disturbed. It is obvious, taking into account the intricacies of the mechanisms that underlie pump function, that many diseases may lead to failing of the heart. These include diseases of the cardiac muscle itself, such as myocardial infarction and myocarditis, abnormal impulse formation and conduction, such as ventricular extrasystoles and tachycardias, and abnormalities of heart valves, such as valvar stenosis or insufficiency.

Basic mechanisms

Taking into account the intricacies of the physiological processes associated with the excitation-contraction coupling, it is clear that dysfunctioning within this chain of events may lead to inadequate pump function.

Abnormal handling of intracellular calcium ions has serious consequences for the myocardium. Evidence in this respect has been obtained from the study of the so-called 'stunned myocardium'.[7] This condition is defined as an acute depression of the contractile function of the cardiac muscle, lasting at least for a few hours to days, which follows temporary occlusion of a coronary artery. Animal experiments have shown that a reduction in the quantity of calcium ions available for activation of the contractile elements plays an important role in this process. The concept is that either a diminished trans-sarcolemmal influx of calcium ions plays a role, or else a reduction in the amount of calcium stored in the sarcoplasmic reticulum (see also Fig. 2.6).

In patients who suffer from chronic heart failure a deficiency in the production of cyclic AMP has been demonstrated, which could have been the result of a change in the activity of the regulatory protein.

It has also been shown that, in heart failure, the β_1-adrenergic receptors are 'down-regulated', leaving a relative surplus of β_2-receptors.[8] In the healthy ventricular muscle, the density of β_1-receptors is highly dominant, while in the failing heart the β_1 fraction makes up less than 50% of the total. The α-adrenergic receptor density does not change significantly, leading to the assumption that an alpha-mediated positive inotropic response plays an important role in maintaining contractility of the failing heart. Experimental therapeutic work is devoted particularly to the upregulation of β-receptor functions.

Furthermore, in patients with chronic heart failure a diminished mitochondrial ATPase activity has been demonstrated, but the question remains whether this reduction is a secondary effect rather than the cause of muscular dysfunction.

Apart from changes in the amount of calcium available for the process of contraction, there could be a role also for changes in the sensitivity of the myofilaments to calcium ions. Such a

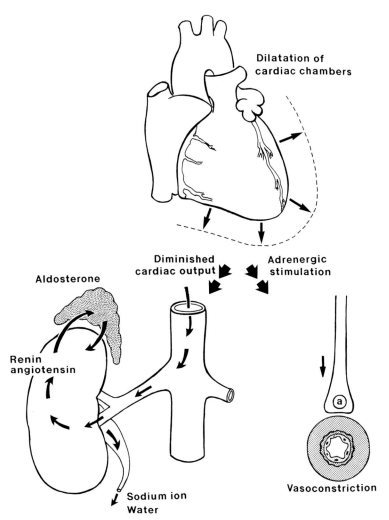

Fig. 2.7 This diagram shows the interaction between heart, kidneys and arterial system in the setting of heart failure. Dilatation of the cardiac chambers leads to stimulation of adrenergic (α) nerves, producing arterial constriction, while diminished cardiac output induces responses in the adrenal glands and kidneys resulting in excretion of sodium ions and water.
Adapted from Becker A E. Circulatiestoornissen. In: Hoedemaeker Ph J, Bosman F T, Meijer C J L M, Becker A E, eds. Pathologie, 2nd ed. Utrecht: Wetenschappelijke Uitgeverij Bunge, 1991; Ch 2, Fig 2.7.

change could be due to a change in the troponin C, but thus far no definitive proof has been obtained.

Finally, it is important to note that the activity of ATPase in cardiac muscle is also dependent on the iso-enzymatic type of myosin present. These myosin iso-enzymes may vary as a consequence of a change in working conditions. Inadequate contraction could be related, therefore, to inadequate energy metabolism associated with a change in the contractile proteins.[9]

It is evident, therefore, that heart failure at the cellular level is a complex biochemical process and that several mechanisms may be active in the disruption of these delicate pathways.

Adaptation to heart failure

Heart failure is defined, from a clinical point of view, as an inability of the cardiac muscle to maintain adequate circulation. The heart muscle, when failing, initiates a chain of events which should be considered as adaptive or compensatory mechanisms of the circulatory system. These mechanisms will dominate the clinical picture of heart failure, particularly since, in the long run, they lose their beneficial effect and turn into harmful processes.

The failing heart will be unable to maintain an adequate circulation and, therefore, to meet the energy demand of tissues and organs. In latent heart failure the circulation becomes insufficient only when the consumption of energy is increased, for instance during stress. In all other forms of heart failure the functional parameters will be abnormal under all circumstances. Inadequacies in circulation will lead to processes which may become evident clinically as congestion of the venous system (backward failure), or insufficient filling of the arterial system (forward failure). Both will lead to adaptation, which will mask the effect of the underlying heart failure on vital organs for as long as possible.

The adaptive mechanisms involved are diverse (Fig. 2.7).[10] Within the heart itself, the chambers may dilate and account for an increased volume, which, in turn, will increase the stroke volume of the heart. At rest, therefore, cardiac output will not necessarily be diminished. The cardiopulmonary baroreceptors will be stimulated, which leads to a modulation, by way of the central nervous system, of the activity of the sympathetic and parasympathetic nervous system. It is important, in this setting, to distinguish between acute and chronic changes. In the latter situation, chronic change, the level of response of the baroreceptors and the autonomic nerve activity with respect to pressure and volume changes will be upregulated, thus diminishing for a time at least, the ill-effects. Long-lasting dilatation of cardiac chambers will be accompanied by hypertrophy of cardiac muscle cells, which leads to an increase in total consumption of oxygen (see Ch. 3).

It is outside the heart, nonetheless, that the most important changes take place. Basically these are all part of the essential homeostatic mechanisms that regulate perfusion of the vital organs. At an early stage of heart failure, the kidneys will diminish their excretion of sodium and water, most likely as a reaction to diminished cardiac output. The adrenergic system is activated, which causes vasoconstriction at several peripheral sites such as the kidneys and the intestines. The renin-angiotensin system is activated, at least at the stage when the compensatory volume increase has not yet taken place. The regulatory mechanism in this instance is, most likely, arterial hypotension. This mechanism may also be responsible for the release of arginine and vasopressin. Baroreceptors play an important role, through activation of the regulatory system located within the central nervous system (see Ch. 24).

Longlasting adaptation in this setting will eventually lead to the situation where the heart will no longer be able to cope with the 'compensatory' expansion of volume. Progressive irreversible heart failure will then occur.

REFERENCES

1. Page E, McCallister LP. Studies on the intercalated disk of rat ventricular myocardial cells. J Ultrastruct Res 1973; 43: 388–411.
2. Fawcett DW, McNutt NS. The ultrastructure of the cat myocardium. I. Ventricular papillary muscle. J Cell Biol 1969; 42: 1–45.
3. Sommer JR, Waugh RA. The ultrastructure of the mammalian cardiac muscle cell—with special emphasis on the tubular membrane systems. A review. Am J Pathol 1976; 82: 192–232.
4. Sommer JR, Johnson EA. Ultrastructure of cardiac muscle. In: Berne RM, Sperelakis N (eds). Handbook of physiology, Section 2, Vol 1. The heart. Bethesda: The American Physiological Society, 1979; 113.
5. Goldstein MA, Schroeter JR, Sass RL. The Z lattice in canine cardiac muscle. J Cell Biol 1979; 83: 187–204.
6. Buja LM, Hagler HK, Willerson JT. Altered calcium homeostasis in the pathogenesis of myocardial ischemia and hypoxic injury. Cell Calcium 1988; 9: 205–217.
7. Weisfeldt ML. Reperfusion and reperfusion injury. Clin Res 1987; 35: 13–20.
8. Bristow MR. Myocardial β-adrenergic receptor downregulation in heart failure. Int J Cardiol 1984; 5: 648–652.
9. Entman ML, Micae L H. Molecular and cellular basis for myocardial failure. In: Parmley WW, Chatterjee K (eds). Cardiology, Vol 2. Philadelphia: Lippincott, 1988; Ch 4.
10. McCall D, O'Rourke R. Congestive heart failure. Mod Concepts Cardiovasc Dis 1985; 52: 55–60.

Pathophysiology of cardiac adaptation

INTRODUCTION

As discussed in the previous chapter, in maintaining circulation of the blood the heart functions basically as a mechanical pump which is driven by electricity.[1] Since part of its propelling force is derived from the positive effects of venous return,[2] the heart also functions as a suction pump. Changes in the conditions under which the heart is called upon to work will always evoke a response, known as adaptation.[3] These adaptive phenomena may be of a purely physiological nature, such as an increase in heart rate, or they may become manifest by alterations of morphology. In this context, an accurate interpretation of morphological features can be achieved only when the pathologist has a full understanding of pathophysiological mechanisms. For instance, a decrease in effective cardiac output may increase the heart rate so as to maintain effective perfusion of the vital organs. At the same time, the increase in the heart rate may cause potential impairment of effective myocardial perfusion because of shortening of the time available for diastolic perfusion. As a consequence, there may be evidence of circumferential subendocardial myocardial infarction although the degree and extent of obstructive coronary arterial disease is minimal. Similarly, adaptive phenomena, evoked as a response to a change in working load, may induce secondary abnormalities which may then, eventually, themselves dominate the clinical presentation. For instance, an increase in left ventricular afterload, as occurs with aortic valvar disease, will cause myocardial hypertrophy. At the same time, it will invoke an overall increase in myocardial consumption of oxygen which must be provided by increased flow within the coronary arteries. Under such circumstances the flow may be insufficient to supply the needs so that myocardial ischaemia may ensue, particularly when the volume load of the left ventricle is increased, leading to left ventricular dilatation. In this way, a vicious circle can be induced, which started as simple adaptation to a change in the working conditions of the heart, but which leads eventually to overt pathological changes, and even to unexpected sudden cardiac death. The pathologist, therefore, when evaluating an abnormal heart, whether the abnormal state is congenital or acquired, has to place the observed changes within their appropriate perspective. For that, the pathologist must be acquainted with both the physiology and the pathophysiology of the heart.

The morphology of cardiac adaptation is limited. The cardiac chambers may dilate, consequent upon an increased volume load, or the wall may thicken as an expression of an increased work load. Clinicians often refer to these changes as remodelling of the heart. Such adaptation (or remodelling) depends on several factors. Time plays an important role. For example, adaptation in response to a sudden rise in volume load on the left ventricle, as in a patient with ruptured cords of the mitral valve, differs from adaptation in a patient who develops a gradually progressive mitral insufficiency on the basis of rheumatic heart disease. Transitions in the isotypes of cardiac myosin may occur in response to a variety of stimuli, although the significance of these changes in the human heart remains unclear.[4] The speed of myocardial contraction[5] and oxygen consumption[6] are directly related to such transitions, thus suggesting that they play a role in the process of remodelling.

Little is known, at present, about the role in adaptation of the fine fibrillar meshwork of connective tissue that wraps around individual cells of the myocardium. This extracellular matrix constitutes a tensile element that resists stretch and provides a restoring force that may cause individual myocardial cells to return to their original length after contraction.[7] In this respect, distinctions must be made between the endomy-sium, the perimysium and the epimysium (Fig. 3.1). The *endomysium*, surrounding individual cells, is composed of a meshwork of collagen fibres, the so-called weave. This meshwork is connected by way of struts to the basal lamina of the myocytes. Neighbouring weaves are interconnected through single strands of collagen. Weaves and struts play an important role in safeguarding the integrity of the myocardium during myocardial diastole. The weaves are anchored in the *perimysium*, which connects groups of myocytes and is composed of coiled collagen fibres.[7] These coils are arranged along the length of small groups of myocytes and are interconnected so as to inhibit myocardial overstretching during the phase of end-diastole. The coils also function so as to store energy during systole, providing, in this way, the basis for considering the heart as a suction pump.[2] The *epimysium* then enwraps several of the bundles of myocardial cells grouped by the perimysium and is oriented parallel to the long axis of the muscle fibres. The overall extracellular matrix provides considerable strength to resist over-distension of the myocardium when the pressure within the chamber rises. The amount of fibrous tissue increases concomitant with adaptive changes;[8] it is not yet known whether such fibrosis is a permanent feature.

Myocardial remodelling, therefore, is a process that involves all the cellular tissues of the heart, affecting them at subcellular as well as cellular levels. Although probably reversible, at least in part, these adaptive changes may introduce secondary alterations, such as increase in total consumption of oxygen, that render the heart prone to ischaemic injury.

MYOCARDIAL GROWTH

From the earliest stages of intra-uterine life the heart must support the fetal circulation, thus requiring functional organization of the myocytes very early in gestation. Initially cellular multiplication occurs, but soon cellular enlargement becomes the most important contribution to the augmentation of the myocardial mass. Myocytic

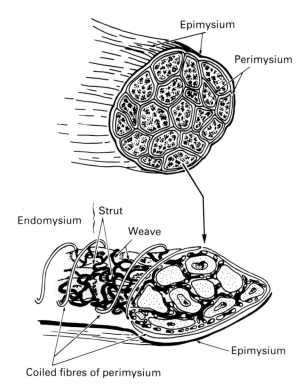

Fig. 3.1 Drawing illustrating the relationship between myocytes and the connective tissue components (epi-, peri- and endomysium).

guarantee optimum functional capacity. Secondly, fetal myocytes have the capacity to adapt to abnormal circumstances by hypertrophy. The myocytes increase their bulk by expanding and enlarging those cellular organelles which are responsible for consumption of oxygen and for synthesis and utilization of adenosine triphosphate. Sub-systems around the myocytes, such as the vascular network and the fine fibrillar matrix of connective tissue, also adapt to supplement these changes.

At present, little is known of intra-uterine remodelling and its functional implications, although the myocardium in a congenitally malformed heart may function differently from that in the normal heart. This may be important when considering myocardial vulnerability in the postnatal state, such as the susceptibility to hypoxia.

The transition from the fetal to the adult circulatory pathways is accompanied by a progressive increase in the volume loads affecting both sides of the heart. There is a particularly marked increase in the pressure load on the left ventricle. These functional changes cause further enlargement of myocytes so that the left ventricle rapidly outgrows the right (Fig. 3.2). At the cellular level, the composition of myocytic organelles changes rapidly after birth. There is a significant increase in the fractional volumes of mitochondria and myofibrils and these achieve their adult levels shortly after birth. This change is accompanied by a proportional increase in the capacity of the coronary vascular bed.

enlargement, moreover, is accompanied by growth of accompanying capillaries.

In this context, two important aspects merit further consideration. First, during intra-uterine development the growing myocardium adapts to the presence of cardiac malformations so as to

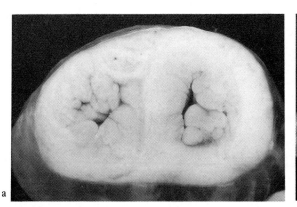
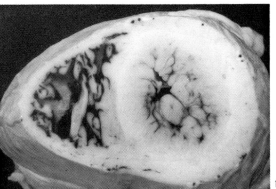

Fig. 3.2 a,b Cross-sections through the heart at the level of the ventricular papillary muscles enabling contrast of the left and right ventricular wall thicknesses in a newborn infant (**a**) and a one-year old infant (**b**).

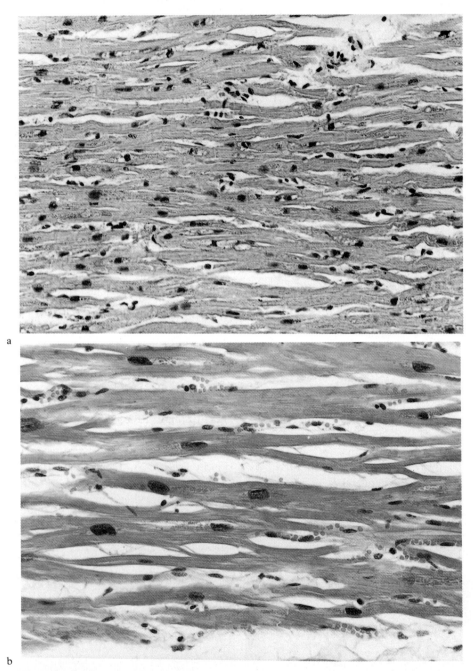

Fig. 3.3 a,b Microscopical view of myocytes in normal (**a**) and hypertrophied (**b**) left ventricle. Haematoxylin–eosin × 230

The normal maturation of the myocardium is a well-balanced adaptive event in which the myocytes, including their cellular organelles, and the capillary microvasculature grow in proportion to the load of work. Abnormalities, if present, will cause an exaggeration of this adaptive response. In consequence the myocardium may then be rendered vulnerable to ischaemic damage.

Indeed, congenitally malformed hearts may already exhibit myocardial damage at birth.[9]

HYPERTROPHY

Hypertrophy of the heart is defined as an increase in the myocardial mass due to enlargement of the myocytes (Fig. 3.3). Ultrastructurally, the hypertrophied myocyte can be seen to contain an increased volume of mitochondria (Fig. 3.4), these organelles being responsible for consumption of oxygen and synthesis of adenosine triphosphate. There is also an increase in the amount of contractile proteins in the myofibrils; it is these contractile proteins that utilize the adenosine

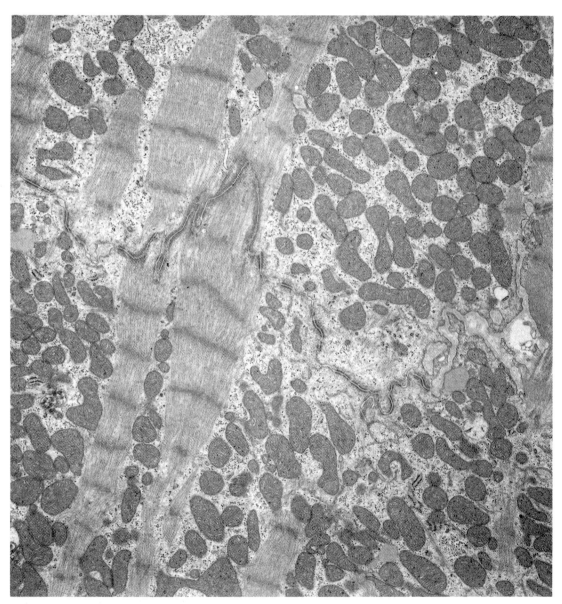

Fig. 3.4 Electron microscopical aspect of hypertrophied myocardium showing an increase in volume of mitochondria. × 12 000

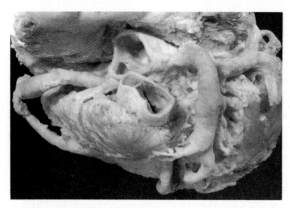

Fig. 3.5 Gross aspect of heart with hypertrophy of the ventricular muscle mass, revealing adaptive dilatation of the main coronary arteries.

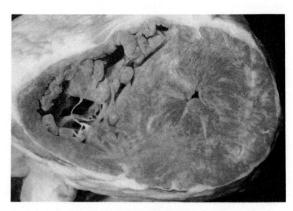

Fig. 3.6 Pressure load hypertrophy. Cross-section of the heart showing marked left ventricular hypertrophy *without* dilatation of the left ventricular cavity.

triphosphate.[10] Myocardial hypertrophy itself is accompanied by dilatation of the main coronary arteries (Fig. 3.5) and expansion of the capillary network, ensuring in this way the maintenance of an adequate supply of oxygen. As a consequence of hypertrophy, there is a rise in the total demand for oxygen by the myocardium which, clinically, may become of the utmost significance.

In descriptive terms, adaptive myocardial hypertrophy has been categorized as concentric or eccentric. The adaptive response described as 'eccentric' is not to be confused with the asymmetrical variant of hypertrophy observed in hypertrophic cardiomyopathy. The latter is an abnormal condition in its own right, and not a phenomenon of remodelling. In this respect, therefore, the term 'eccentric' as applied to the adaptive phenomenon is less than perfect, since the hypertrophy induced is symmetrical and in that respect is also 'concentric'. The difference conveyed by the terms as presently used is that the 'eccentric' form of hypertrophy is also accompanied by chamber dilatation, whereas the 'concentric' form is not. It may be preferable to describe these forms as mural hypertrophy, respectively with or without dilatation of the chamber involved. Be that as it may, this descriptive approach correlates well with the commonest clinically identified causes of the hypertrophy, namely increased pressure or increased volume.

Hypertrophy due to pressure loading

The morphology in this setting is that of so-called concentric hypertrophy, in which the thickness of the wall increases without concomitant enlargement of the affected chamber (Fig. 3.6). As indicated, such a response is encountered in patients with adaptive hypertrophy of the ventricle due to an increased pressure load. The commonest conditions producing such pressure loading of the left ventricle include systemic hypertension, aortic coarctation, and aortic valvar stenosis. Pressure loading of the right ventricle may be the consequence of pulmonary valvar stenosis, disease of the left side of the heart (with left heart failure), or pulmonary disease causing an increase in pulmonary vascular resistance.

In the concentric hypertrophy induced by pressure loading, in which there is no dilatation of the chamber, the degree of myocytic hypertrophy differs in the various layers of the myocardium, although the overall effect is to produce an increase in wall thickness. The increased thickness counteracts the elevated systolic pressures and compensates, according to the law of Laplace, for a potentially high stress of the wall during peak systole (Fig. 3.7).

The increase in cellular volume is accompanied by hyperplasia of myofibrillar units. Eventually, a reduction occurs in the ratio of the volume of mitochondria to myofibrils. The extent of the perimitochondrial volume, which normally is just

Laplace's law

$$\text{Tension} = \frac{\text{pressure} \times \text{radius}}{2 \times \text{wall thickness}}$$

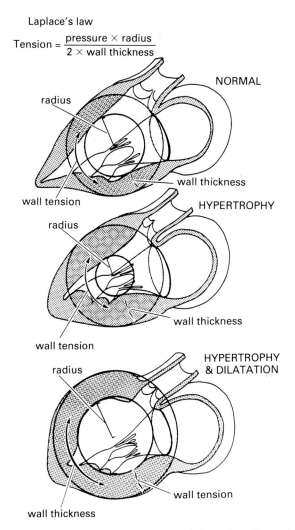

Fig. 3.7 Drawing illustrating Laplace's law as it applies to the heart. The normal anatomy (upper) is related to left ventricular hypertrophy with (lower) and without (middle) chamber dilatation.

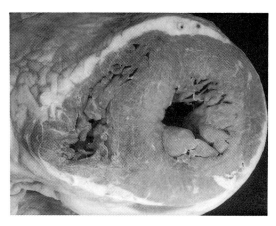

Fig. 3.8 Volume load hypertrophy. Cross-section of the heart showing marked left ventricular hypertrophy accompanied by mild dilatation of the left ventricular chamber.

sufficient to ensure that adenosine triphosphate reaches the contractile proteins, may thus become the limiting factor in myocardial adaptation. The capillary bed also increases concomitantly with the increase in size of the myocytes.

Hypertrophy due to volume loading

When hypertrophy of the wall is associated with an increased volume of the chamber the result is so-called eccentric hypertrophy, the effect being that the overall ratio between volume and wall thickness of the affected chamber remains unaltered (Fig. 3.8). This is in contrast to the so-called concentric variant due to pressure loading, in which the ratio of volume to thickness decreases. The eccentric arrangement is seen, therefore, in adaptive hypertrophy of the left ventricle due to increased volume load. Volume loading is one of the adaptations occurring in response to exercise, particularly in dynamic forms of conditioning as seen in athletes undertaking endurance events such as long-distance running, cycling or swimming. Examples of pathological conditions that cause hypertrophy of the left ventricle due to volume loading are aortic and mitral regurgitation. Volume loading of the right ventricle can occur due to pulmonary or tricuspid valvar insufficiency; it may also eventually follow malfunction of the left side of the heart.

As discussed, the hypertrophy induced is said to be eccentric, in that the usual hypertrophy occurs concomitantly with enlargement of the affected chamber and an increase in the length of the myocytes.[10] The myocytic lengthening counteracts the increased wall stress during end-diastole, thus accommodating the increased volume of blood. The integrity of all components of the extracellular matrix is essential to prevent lateral slippage of the myocytes and spatial disorganization of the myocardium. The fractional volumes of mitochondria and myofibrils remain almost constant, this fact constituting the morphological counterpart of the normal or improved contractile properties of the myocardium.

Eccentric hypertrophy occurring as a consequence of moderate exercise is associated with expansion of the capillary network in proportion to the increased mass of muscle. Strenuous exercise, in contrast, may be inadequately compensated for by the concomitant growth of capillaries, thus jeopardizing the supply of oxygen to the myocardium. Increased wall tension in this context is itself an energy-consuming process. Hence, hypertrophy as the consequence of an excessive volume load may lead to a state in which the myocardium is more susceptible to ischaemia than would be expected from the extent of mural hypertrophy alone.

Reactive hypertrophy

The classic example of reactive myocardial remodelling is seen after myocardial infarction (Fig. 3.9). In these circumstances, part of the myocardium is replaced by scar tissue. There is then compensatory hypertrophy of the viable myocardium, probably proportional to the amount of loss of myocardial cells in the infarcted zone. The ability to undergo hypertrophy, however, is still largely determined by the effect of the underlying vascular obstructive disease. In general, myocytes will increase in diameter and the ratio of the volume of mitochondria to myofibrils remains constant in proportion to cell growth.[10] Depending on the extent of loss of myocardial cells, the ventricle may undergo chronic volume overload and subsequent lengthening of myocytes may occur. Moreover, the compensatory response of the capillary vasculature to infarction lags behind the adaptive growth of the myocytes. Hence, the hypertrophied ventricle is more subject to further ischaemic episodes after an initial infarction.

DILATATION

Dilatation of a cardiac chamber is an increase in its volume. Sudden increases in volume load usually lead to instant dilatation. Chronic dilatation may be related to hypertrophy occurring in response to a volume load, producing the so-called eccentric response (see above), or to heart failure (Fig. 3.10). Depending on the cause, dilatation may resolve or persist, either as compensated adjustment or as part of chronic volume overload with impairment of haemodynamics.

COMPLICATIONS OF MYOCARDIAL REMODELLING

When hypertrophy of the myocardium and dilatation of the cardiac chambers occur as adaptive

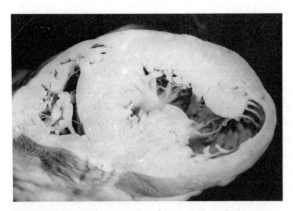

Fig. 3.9 Reactive hypertrophy. Cross-section of a heart showing left ventricular hypertrophy consequent upon myocardial infarction with aneurysm formation in the left ventricular lateral wall.

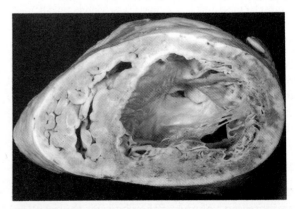

Fig. 3.10 Cross-section of a heart showing chronic dilatation in a patient with chronic heart failure (due to recurrent myocardial infarcts).

mechanisms, they may set the scene for secondary complications. Dilatation of a ventricular chamber, whether acute or chronic, may initiate dysfunction of the papillary muscles and, hence, atrioventricular valvar regurgitation. The latter condition in itself may cause further remodelling of the ventricle as evidenced by enlargement due to augmented volume load.

Hypertrophy, whether concentric or eccentric, may affect the ventricular geometry. This becomes particularly pronounced in cases of marked right ventricular hypertrophy with concomitant dilatation. In this circumstance, the interventricular septum assumes an almost straight configuration. It is not yet known whether this has functional implications. The reverse situation, extreme hypertrophy of the left ventricle with bulging of the septum into the right ventricle (formerly known as Bernstein's disease) may be a cause of right ventricular impairment.

The most important consequences of these compensatory mechanisms relate to impairment of myocardial perfusion. Marked increase in the volume load of the left ventricle, with overt chamber dilatation and myocardial hypertrophy, may affect the transmural perfusion pressure, thus leading to impaired oxygenation of the subendo-

cardial myocardial layers. This phenomenon is particularly prevalent when volume overload and dilatation coexist with obstructive coronary arterial disease (Fig. 3.11). Hence, compensated hypertrophy secondary to a chronic volume overload may ultimately be complicated by myocardial necrosis due to myocardial ischaemia. Once induced, this process will further aggravate the impairment of myocardial perfusion by further dilatation of the ventricle. This will allow an increased end-diastolic left ventricular volume and produce a concomitant increase in pressure (Fig. 3.11). Such hypertrophy occurring secondary to volume overload is not always compensated for by an adequate adaptation of the microvasculature. The sequence of events discussed above is more likely to occur with strenuous exercise.

THE HEART IN TRAINED SPORTSMEN

It is well established that one of the consequences of the long-term conditioning needed by highly trained competitive athletes is enlargement of the heart. This enlargement is due to hypertrophy of the ventricular walls. In endurance sports, such as

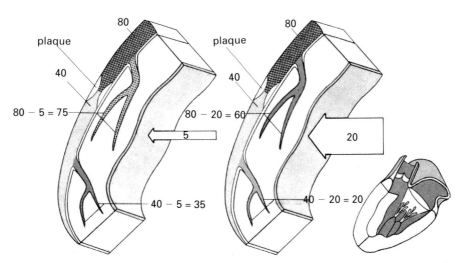

Fig. 3.11 Schematic drawing illustrating the effect of transmural myocardial perfusion in case of obstructive coronary artery disease (plaque) in hearts with (right) and without (left) chamber dilatation due to a volume overload. The figures are intraluminal pressures in mmHg.
(From Becker A E, Hart en vaten. In: Hoedemaeker Ph J, Bosman F T, Meijer C J L M, Becker A E, eds. Pathologie, 2nd ed. Utrecht: Wetenschappelijke Uitgeverij Bunge, 1991; Ch.6, Fig.6.2. With permission of the publisher.)

marathon running, the strain of the prolonged exercise also invokes an increased volume load and, hence, eccentric hypertrophy. As already discussed, the hypertrophy seen under such conditions is symmetrical. Occasionally, an asymmetrical pattern may ensue. The absolute thickening of the septum in these circumstances, however, is minimal; the ratio of the thickness of the septum to the free wall remains below 1:3. This suggests disproportionate septal thickening rather than asymmetrical septal hypertrophy occurring as a manifestation of hypertrophic cardiomyopathy, although the latter possibility should always be carefully evaluated and excluded.

It remains speculative whether the type of exercise is important with respect to the changes in cardiac structure. It has been demonstrated that athletes participating in dynamic endurance sports are exposed primarily to conditions producing a volume overload and, as a result, develop eccentric hypertrophy. On the other hand, athletes involved in sports that are primarily static, such as weightlifting, are conditioned primarily to produce hypertrophy in consequence of an increased pressure load. It is endurance athletes, therefore, who are more prone to secondary myocardial complications, at least when additional pathological circumstances such as obstructive coronary arterial disease are present. Indeed, sudden death in competitive athletes is almost always caused by additional cardiovascular abnormalities which may have been unnoticed clinically. Nevertheless, sudden death may occur in athletes in whom no additional abnormalities can be detected other than chamber enlargement and myocardial hypertrophy without obstructive coronary arterial disease. In some of these instances, the heart shows extensive fibrosis and, occasionally, circumscribed scars, indicating previous clinically unrecognized infarction. In other cases, there is no detectable abnormality and the mechanisms underlying such sudden deaths remain unclear.

THE AGEING HEART

The increased longevity in the western world has led to an increased interest in geriatric cardiology, and the consequent remodelling induced simply by ageing. The myocardium of the elderly may be expected to show atrophy, unless other circumstances prevail to induce compensatory changes. Systemic hypertension is a frequent disorder, and a substantial number of elderly patients have myocardial hypertrophy on that basis. With increasing age, moreover, major abnormalities frequently occur in the fibrous tissues making up the cardiac skeleton, including the cardiac valves. In elderly patients, therefore, morphological abnormalities of the valves, particularly the aortic and mitral valves, are the rule rather than the exception.

In a significant proportion of patients these alterations are functionally important, although not necessarily clinically manifest. It is not infrequent at autopsy to detect severe isolated calcific aortic stenosis accompanied by marked myocardial hypertrophy. This condition can cause sudden death in an elderly patient in whom the valvar abnormality was never detected clinically. Likewise, calcification of the atrioventricular junction may induce mitral valvar regurgitation and hypertrophy of the left ventricle as a consequence of the volume overload that, in the presence of obstructive coronary arterial disease, may lead to myocardial ischaemia, infarction and death. At a cellular level, it is still uncertain whether the adaptive phenomena of ageing are equal to those that occur in children or adults. Investigations of such features may provide a better understanding of the pathophysiology of geriatric patients.

REFERENCES

1. Becker AE, Anderson RH. Cardiac pathology. An integrated text and colour atlas. London: Gower, 1983.
2. Robinson TF, Factor SM, Sonnenblick EH. The heart as a suction pump. Sci Am 1986; 254: 84–91.
3. Becker AE. Myocardial remodeling and its complications. In: Hurst JW, Anderson RH, Becker AE, Wilcox BR, eds. Atlas of the heart. New York: Gower, 1988: 2.1–2.7.
4. Cummins P, Lambert SJ. Myosin transitions in the

bovine human heart. A developmental and anatomical study of heavy and light chain subunits in the atrium and ventricle. Circ Res 1986; 58: 846–858.

5. Schwartz K, Lecarpentier Y, Martin JL, Lompre AM, Mercadier JJ, Swynghedauw B. Myosin isoenzymic distribution correlates with speed of myocardial contraction. J Mol Cell Cardiol 1981; 13: 1071–1075.

6. Kissling G, Rupp H, Malloy L, Jacob R. Alterations in cardiac oxygen consumption under chronic pressure overload. Significance of the isoenzyme pattern of myosin. Basic Res Cardiol 1982; 77: 255–270.

7. Robinson TF, Geraci MA, Sonnenblick EH, Factor SM. Coiled perimysial fibers of papillary muscle in rat heart: morphology, distribution and changes in configuration. Circ Res 1988; 63: 577 – 592.

8. Factor SM, Flomenbaum M, Zhao MJ, Eng C, Robinson TF. The effects of acutely increased ventricular cavity pressure on intrinsic myocardial connective tissue. J Am Coll Cardiol 1988; 12: 1582–1589.

9. Becker AE, Caruso G. Congenital heart disease — a morphologist's view on myocardial dysfunction. In: Becker AE, Losekoot G, Marcelletti C, Anderson RH, eds. Paediatric cardiology. Edinburgh: Churchill Livingstone, 1981; 3: 307–323.

10. Anversa P, Ricci R, Olivetti G. Quantitative structural analysis of the myocardium during physiologic growth and induced cardiac hypertrophy: a review. J Am Coll Cardiol 1986; 7: 1140–1149.

11. Maron BJ, Epstein SE. Symposium on the athlete heart. J Am Coll Cardiol 1986; 7: 189–243.

Congenital Heart Disease

SECTION 2

Congenital Heart Disease

Sequential segmental analysis

INTRODUCTION

It is often thought that the study of congenitally malformed hearts is difficult. It is also taught that a knowledge of cardiac development aids in their interpretation. We would take issue with both these contentions. It is our belief that examination of a congenitally malformed heart is a simple procedure provided the approach is made in a simple and straightforward fashion, but we accept that this reflects our own considerable biases. Nonetheless, we hold that interpretation should be based upon the anatomy as it is observed and need owe nothing to concepts of embryogenesis. At best, such concepts are more or less speculative. In this chapter, therefore, we will describe our simple approach to the study of congenitally malformed hearts.

The concept starts with the premise that normality must be proved rather than assumed. In terms of normality, we are concerned with the morphology of the cardiac chambers and great arteries, the way they are interconnected and the relations of the various cardiac structures to each other. The arrangement of the heart itself is considered relative to its position within the thorax and relative to the arrangement of the organs in the rest of the body. When analysing the different components of the heart itself, we consider three basic cardiac segments. These are the atrial chambers (including their venous connexions), the ventricular mass, and the arterial trunks (Fig. 4.1). The system of looking at how these segments are interconnected is called sequential segmental analysis.[1-3] This approach itself is derived from the system of segmental

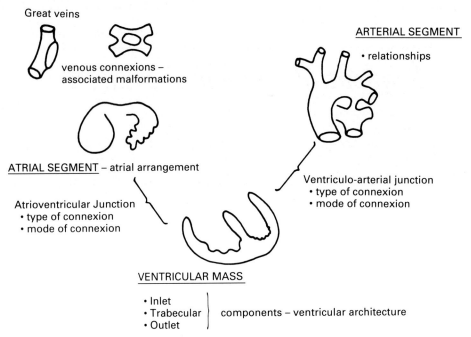

Great veins

venous connexions –
associated malformations

ARTERIAL SEGMENT

• relationships

ATRIAL SEGMENT – atrial arrangement

Atrioventricular Junction
• type of connexion
• mode of connexion

Ventriculo-arterial junction
• type of connexion
• mode of connexion

VENTRICULAR MASS

• Inlet
• Trabecular   } components – ventricular architecture
• Outlet

Fig. 4.1 For the purposes of analysis of congenital malformations, the heart is considered as being made up of atrial, ventricular and arterial segments. Following description of atrial arrangement, the junctions between the segments are dissected in terms of type and mode of connexion. Anomalies of venous connexion are considered as associated malformations.

analysis developed independently by Van Praagh and his colleagues[4,5] and by de la Cruz and Nadal-Ginard.[6] The segmental approaches emphasized the intrinsic anatomy of each of the cardiac segments, being mostly concerned with the topological arrangement of the structures within each segment. Topology of any given structure is the arrangement of its topography within space. Topographical relationships can be changed by simple rotation. Such rotation does not change the relationships of the components of the given structure to each other. It is this intrinsic architecture which we describe in terms of topology. Initially, the segmental approaches[4-6] were much less concerned with connexions. When we came to apply such a system, although we were also concerned with the arrangement within each segment, it seemed to us that connexions were paramount. Following the precedent of Kirklin and his colleagues,[7] we emphasized the segmental connexions while taking careful note of the topology of each segment.[3] Indeed, without

knowledge of the arrangement of the different components of each segment, it is not possible to determine the segmental connexions. The basic approach to analysis of any heart, therefore, must first be to determine the spatial arrangement of the atrial chambers. To do this, it is self-evidently essential to distinguish the nature of each individual atrium. Thereafter, it is necessary to discover how the atriums are connected to the ventricular mass. This makes it equally necessary to establish how many chambers there are within the ventricular mass, to determine their morphological nature and to find out whether each ventricle is connected to an atrial chamber. Thereafter, a similar process conducted at the ventriculo–arterial junction will determine how many arterial trunks are present and whether the trunk or trunks are connected to one or more ventricles. While making these observations, careful note will have been taken of the arrangement of valves guarding the atrioventricular and ventriculo–arterial junctions respectively.

When this process is complete, the basic route of blood through the heart will have been established. A careful catalogue should then be made of any and all associated malformations present within the heart and great vessels. These anomalies may be the consequence of abnormal connexions of the great veins, defects between the various chambers or arterial trunks, or stenotic or regurgitant lesions along the systemic or pulmonary pathways. The various cardiac anomalies are then considered within the setting of the heart itself. This is because the heart may be abnormally positioned relative to the other thoracic organs. Alternatively, there may be anomalous arrangement of either the thoracic or abdominal organs in association with cardiac malformations. When a patient with suspected congenital heart disease is approached in this fashion, no lesion should prove impossible to diagnose, since the diagnosis depends only on description and owes nothing to prior experience. All that is required in terms of prior knowledge is the ability to distinguish a morphologically right atrium from a left atrium, a morphologically right ventricle from a left ventricle and a left or right ventricle from a solitary and indeterminate ventricle, and an aorta from a pulmonary trunk and each from a common or solitary arterial trunk.

It is the ability to distinguish the different chambers or arteries from one another in each segment of the heart which is the cornerstone of understanding. These distinctions are based on knowledge of their structure in the normal heart. Unfortunately, the most obvious features of the different components of the normal heart are not always the most reliable indicators of the given structure in a malformed heart. For example, the most obvious marker of the left atrium is the connexions of the pulmonary veins. This feature is of little value in identifying the left atrium when there is totally anomalous pulmonary venous connexion (the lesion in which all the pulmonary veins connect to a site other than the morphologically left atrium). Similarly, the morphology of the atrioventricular or arterial valves is of little value in determining ventricular morphology in a ventricle composed only of the apical trabecular component and having neither an inlet nor an outlet component. These facts point to a most important principle in the study of malformed hearts. This had been dubbed the 'morphological method'.[8,9] It states that structures should, in the final analysis, be identified according to their most constant components. Other features may be used to aid identification when they are present. The variable features should not be the ultimate arbiter. The overall features of the various cardiac chambers have been described in Chapter 1. In the context of the atriums, it is the appendages which are most constantly present and which have the most characteristic structure. Within the ventricles, it is the apical trabecular component which fulfills this pivotal role. The arterial trunks, however, are recognized according to their pattern of branching, since they have no constant intrinsic features. With these ground rules established, we are now in a position to describe the process of sequential segmental analysis.

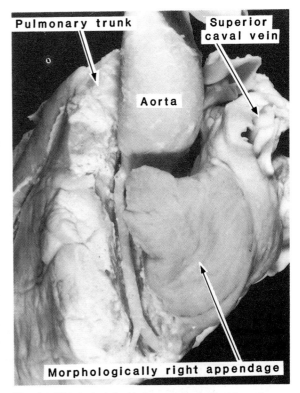

Fig. 4.2 This is the left-sided morphologically right atrium from an otherwise normal heart arranged in mirror-image fashion.

THE OVERALL APPROACH

The essence of analysis is to progress sequentially through the cardiac segments, noting the presence of normality or abnormality at each stage and cataloguing the existence of all anomalies. In ascertaining the normal, note is taken of the morphology of each segment, the relationships and topology of its component parts and their connexions with the adjacent segments. The findings are then synthesized in terms of the arrangement of the heart itself within the thorax and the organization of the remainder of the organs of the body. Normality is never assumed, it is proven. In this way, abnormality should always be observed when present since it is positively sought. The first step is the determination of atrial arrangement ('situs'). There follows an analysis of the atrioventricular and ventriculo–arterial junctions. Finally, the catalogue is made of the associated malformations. The associated lesions will receive full coverage in subsequent chapters.

In this introduction we are concerned with the basic principles of analysis together with a description of the conventions used to account for the malpositioned heart.

Determination of atrial arrangement

It is the appendages which are the arbiters of morphological rightness or leftness of the atrial chambers. All hearts we have seen thus far have possessed two atriums (albeit that one atrium may, on occasion, be divided — see Ch. 6). Each atrium, with very rare exceptions,[10] always possesses an appendage, which is of right or left morphology. It may be thought that this is not the case. Thus, in hearts with grossly malformed atriums, such as in the so-called visceral hetero-taxic syndrome, the feasibility of always being able to distinguish the appendages according to right-ness or leftness may be in doubt. We have recently shown that, in a large series of malformed hearts, all appendages are indeed recognizable irrespec-

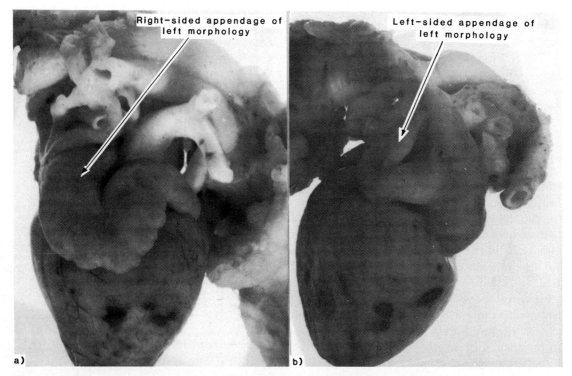

Right-sided appendage of left morphology

Left-sided appendage of left morphology

a) b)

Fig. 4.3 a,b These atriums have appendages of like morphology but are essentially mirror-images of each other. This arrangement is termed isomerism, in this case of left type.

tive of the degree of congenital heart disease present.[11] No problem is encountered in identifying the greater majority with usual arrangement ('solitus'). Neither should there be any difficulty in noting cases with mirror-image arrangement ('inversus' — Fig. 4.2). The appendages are also recognizable as having the same morphology on both sides (Fig. 4.3). The findings of this investigation[11] confirmed our opinion that the appendages could accurately be used for the determination of atrial arrangement. They demonstrate that there are only four possible atrial arrangements (Fig. 4.4). Two of these can be said to be lateralized, namely the usual and mirror-image arrangements which have a morphologically right appendage to one side and a left to the other. The other two arrangements are isomeric, having appendages of either morphologically right or left type on both sides. Almost always the rest of the organs will be arranged in harmony with the atrial appendages. It is helpful confirmation for the pathologist, therefore, to observe the bronchial arrangement. The possibilities are again two lateralized and two isomeric variants (Fig. 4.5). The abdominal organs almost certainly will be arranged in usual or mirror-image format when there are lateralized atrial chambers. They will most frequently exhibit heterotaxy in the setting of isomerism. In the latter respect, absence of the spleen (asplenia) accompanies right isomerism in the majority of cases, while multiple spleens (polysplenia) are usually found with left isomerism. The latter associations are by no means universal. Nor are the bronchi always arranged in harmony with the atrial appendages.[12] In the final analysis, therefore, it must be the morphology of the atrial appendages which is used to decide the atrial arrangement. A word of caution is in order concerning the nature of atrial isomerism. It should not be presumed that the terms right or left isomerism mean that the entirety of both atriums is in the form of the normal right or left atrial chambers. The venous components of the atriums do not exhibit isomerism; it is the appendages which show mirror-image symmetry (see Ch. 16).

Analysis of the atrioventricular junction

In order to determine the complete morphology of the atrioventricular junction, we need to know the arrangement of the atrial chambers together with the anatomy of the ventricular mass. We ascertain, therefore, the way in which the atrial myocardium is or is not connected to the ventricular myocardium. In this respect, the junctions are analysed in terms of right and left components. The two junctions may be guarded by one valve, but such a valve is only deemed common if it guards both junctions. The fashion in which the atrial tissues are or are not connected to the ventricular muscle masses is termed the type of atrioventricular connexion. The morphology of the valves guarding the two junctions, or one junction when the other is absent, is independent of the type of connexion and is described as the mode of connexion.

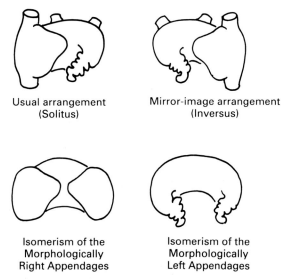

Usual arrangement
(Solitus)

Mirror-image arrangement
(Inversus)

Isomerism of the
Morphologically
Right Appendages

Isomerism of the
Morphologically
Left Appendages

Fig. 4.4 This diagram shows the four possible arrangements of atrial chambers which have either morphologically right or left appendages. The venous connexions have deliberately been excluded from the isomeric arrangement since these are independent variables in each heart — only the appendages are isomeric.

Type of atrioventricular connexion

There are six types of atrioventricular connexion. These are divided into two groups of three. The first group accounts for the arrangements whereby

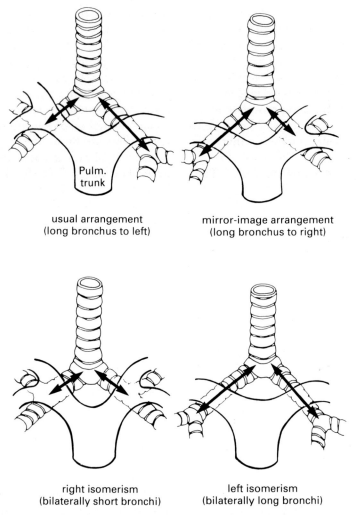

usual arrangement
(long bronchus to left)

mirror-image arrangement
(long bronchus to right)

right isomerism
(bilaterally short bronchi)

left isomerism
(bilaterally long bronchi)

Fig. 4.5 There are four possible patterns of bronchial arrangement based on the concept that the morphologically left bronchus is longer than the right.

each atrium connects to its own ventricle. Collectively, these are biventricular atrioventricular connexions. Specifically, they are the concordant, discordant and ambiguous variants. The concordant and discordant connexions exist when each one of the lateralized atriums connects harmoniously or disharmoniously with a ventricle (Fig. 4.6). These two types of connexion can exist only in the setting of usual or mirror-image atriums. This is because, when isomeric atriums each connect to their own ventricle, half the arrangement must be concordant and the other half discordant, irrespective of the topological

anatomy of the atriums and ventricles (Fig. 4.7). The biventricular connexion of isomeric atriums to the ventricular mass is, therefore, ambiguous. To describe fully the morphology of ambiguous and biventricular connexions, note must also be taken of the pattern of ventricular topology. The concept of atrial topology is relatively easy to understand. A heart with usual arrangement of its atriums can never be converted into one with mirror-image arrangement simply by turning the heart in space. To change usual arrangement into the mirror-image variant, it would be necessary physically to separate the two chambers and re-

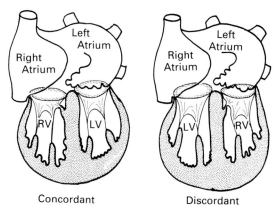

Concordant   Discordant

Fig. 4.6 Hearts with usual or mirror-image atrial chambers, each connected to a separate ventricle, must have concordant or discordant atrioventricular connexions. This shows the connexions in the setting of usual atrial arrangement.

assemble their component parts. So it is with the ventricles in all hearts having biventricular atrioventricular connexions. If one considers the ventricular mass in the normally constructed heart, then the topological arrangement can be conceptualized in terms of the way that the palmar surface of one's hands can be placed upon the septal surface of the right ventricle with the thumb in the inlet, the wrist in the apical component and the fingers in the outlet (Fig. 4.8). When attempted in this fashion, it is only the right hand which can be placed in the normal right ventricle. Similarly, it is only the left hand which can be placed upon the septal surface of the right ventricle in the ventricular mass of the otherwise

normal individual with complete mirror-image arrangement of his heart and organs (complete situs inversus). These are truly topological patterns since, like the atrial arrangements, they cannot be changed one into the other simply by turning or rotating the ventricular mass in space. The ventricular topological patterns exist irrespective of the relationships of the ventricles. If one examines the topology of the ventricular mass in individuals with discordant atrioventricular connexion, then, almost without exception, one finds that patients with usual atrial arrangement have left-hand pattern ventricular topology while those with mirror-image atrial chambers almost always have right-hand ventricular topology. Note must be taken of the caveat 'almost without exception' as it is known that these are not universal associations in hearts with lateralized atrial chambers. Hearts are described[13,14] with usual atrial arrangement and discordant atrioventricular connexions but with right-hand rather than the anticipated left-hand pattern of ventricular topology. Rare cases have also been described[14] where usual atrial arrangement was accompanied by left-hand ventricular topology despite the presence of concordant atrioventricular connexions. In these very rare instances, it is necessary to account for the unexpected topological arrangement of the ventricle in addition to describing the types of atrioventricular connexions. Unless specified in this fashion, the topology can be inferred from the known connexion. When there is an ambiguous

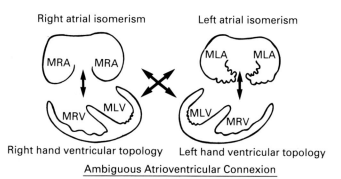

Fig. 4.7 When isomeric atrial chambers are each connected to a separate ventricle, the connexion is biventricular but ambiguous. This can exist with either right or left atrial isomerism, and with either right-hand or left-hand ventricular topology.

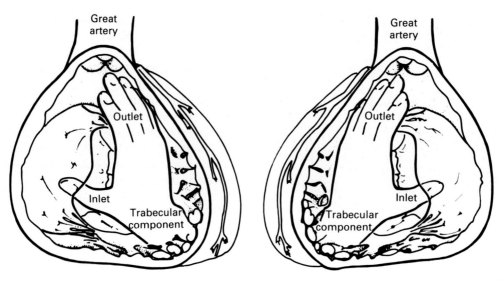

Fig. 4.8 The two possible topological arrangements of the ventricular mass can be conceptualized in terms of the way in which the palmar surface of the right hand can be applied to the septal surface of the right ventricle. This gives right-hand and left-hand patterns.

biventricular connexion, however, it is always necessary additionally to specify the topological pattern. This is because, as shown in Figure 4.7, the biventricular connexion associated with isomeric atriums is appropriately described as ambiguous irrespective of the topological pattern of the ventricular mass.

The second set of atrioventricular connexions produces the arrangement whereby the atrial chambers are connected to only one ventricle, in other words they are univentricular. The three connexions producing this arrangement are double inlet and absence of the right or left connexion. Double inlet ventricle exists when both segments of atrial myocardium, that is, those belonging to the right-sided and left-sided atriums, are connected to the same ventricle (Fig. 4.9). As such, the connexion can exist with any one of the atrial arrangements. The ventricle to which the atriums are connected can be of either left, right or indeterminate morphology depending upon the nature of its apical trabecular component. An atrioventricular connexion is absent when the involved atrium has a completely muscular floor and exhibits not even a rudiment of the atrioventricular junction. The atrial floor is then separated from the ventricular mass by the

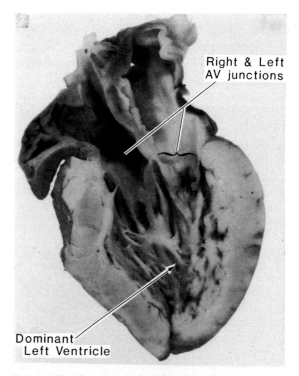

Fig. 4.9 The 'four chamber' section shows the atrioventricular connexion of double inlet, in which both right and left atrioventricular (AV) junctions are connected to the same ventricle, in this heart of left morphology.

fibrofatty tissue of the atrioventricular groove (Fig. 4.10). The right atrioventricular connexion can be absent when the left-sided atrium is connected to a left, right or solitary and indeterminate ventricle (Fig. 4.11). Similarly, the left atrioventricular connexion can be absent (Fig. 4.12) where the right atrium is connected to a right, left or solitary and indeterminate ventricle. These hearts with absence of one atrioventricular connexion produce one variant of atrioventricular valve atresia. They are to be distinguished from those having an imperforate valve.

Of all the hearts unified by their univentricular atrioventricular connexion, very few possess only one chamber within that ventricular mass despite the fact that they are often described as single ventricles. Instead, the majority of hearts unified in this fashion possess two ventricles, albeit that one is almost always dominant and the other incomplete and rudimentary. Size of a ventricle must be described separately from its component make-up. In this respect, it has been possible in all the hearts we have encountered with two chambers in the ventricular mass to account for the formation of the ventricles, no matter how malformed, simply in terms of the sharing of the inlets and outlets between the apical trabecular components. Hearts with dominant ventricles always possess incomplete ventricles of complementary pattern. The incomplete ventricles may be exceedingly small and difficult to find in a clinical setting, but they should always be identified when the pathologist has the heart in his hands. Knowledge of their anticipated position is helpful when attempting to locate them. Incomplete right ventricles are always located anterosuperiorly relative to the dominant ventricle ('on the shoulders' of the ventricular mass) while incomplete left ventricles are postero-inferior ('in the hip pocket'). Either type of incomplete ventricle can be right-sided or left-sided. Some describe this position of the incomplete ventricle in terms of the topological pattern, but the essence of topological arrangement is that it cannot be changed simply by rotation of the heart in space. This is not the case with hearts having univentricular connexion to a dominant left ventricle. In these hearts, the incomplete right ventricle can be moved from right-sided to left-sided position (presumed right-hand to left-hand topology) simply by rotating the ventricular mass. For this reason, and for its greater immediacy and simplicity, we prefer to describe the location of incomplete ventricles in terms of their right-sided or left-sided position.

Mode of atrioventricular connexion

When both atriums are connected to the ventricular mass (in other words, in hearts with concordant, discordant, ambiguous and double inlet atrioventricular connexions) then the two atrioventricular junctions can be guarded by two separate valves or by a common atrioventricular valve (Fig. 4.13). One of two valves can be imperforate irrespective of the type of connexion. An imperforate valve produces another variant of atrioventricular valve atresia but is to be distinguished from absence of an atrioventricular connexion. The connexion must be formed in order to have an imperforate valve. One of two valves, or rarely both, may straddle the ventricular

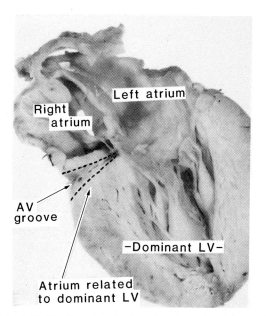

Fig. 4.10 The 'four chamber' section shows the anatomy of classical tricuspid atresia. There is complete absence of the right atrioventricular (AV) connexion, the muscular floor of the right atrium being separated from the ventricular mass by the atrioventricular groove. The left atrium is connected to a dominant left ventricle (LV), the rudimentary and incomplete right ventricle not being seen in this section.

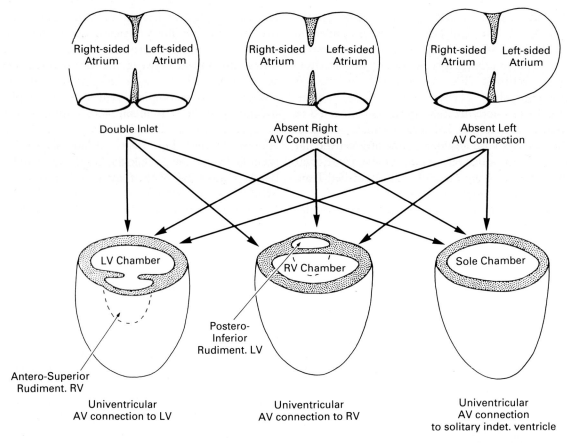

Fig. 4.11 The atrioventricular (AV) connexions producing the situation where only one ventricle is connected to the atrial chambers (univentricular arrangement) can exist because of double inlet, absent right or absent left connexion (upper panels). This can be found with any atrial arrangement and with the atriums connected to a morphologically right (RV), left (LV) or solitary and indeterminate (indet.) ventricle (lower panels). Note that only the indeterminate ventricular pattern produces 'univentricular hearts'. This diagram does not account for variability in terms of right/left relationships of dominant and incomplete ventricles or ventriculo–arterial connexions.

septum. In this respect, we distinguish between the terms straddling and overriding. We use 'straddling' to account for the arrangement in which the tension apparatus of a valve is attached in both ventricles. When a valve straddles in this fashion, then usually its atrioventricular junction is also connected to both ventricles. The biventricular connexion of an atrioventricular junction is called overriding. The two features do not always co-exist. Straddling defined in this way can be found in isolation, as can overriding. The feature of overriding is important since the precise degree of override will also determine the type of atrioventricular connexion present. Hearts with overriding atrioventricular junctions are intermediate between biventricular and univentricular connexions. Like Kirklin and his colleagues,[7] we prefer to avoid intermediate categories. We judge the precise connexion in the presence of an overriding atrioventricular junction according to its connexion to the ventricles. The valve is assigned to the ventricle connected to the greater part of its junction and the connexion determined accordingly. This approach is called the '50% Rule'.

Common valves are defined as ones draining both atrial chambers to the ventricular mass. Such valves may rarely be imperforate in their right or left components. More usually they straddle and override in the sense that these terms were defined above. Indeed, common valves will straddle and override by definition in all hearts with biventric-

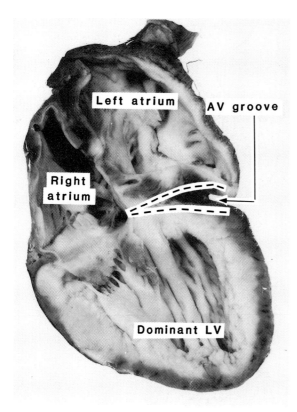

Fig. 4.12 This 'four chamber' section shows absence of the left atrioventricular (AV) connexion, again with the other atrium (in this heart the right) connected to a dominant left ventricle (LV).

ular atrioventricular connexions. But, in hearts with double inlet ventricle, a common valve can be exclusively connected to the dominant ventricle. In this circumstance it will neither override nor straddle. As with one of two valves, there is a spectrum of abnormality in hearts having common valves with biventricular or univentricular atrioventricular connexions. The dividing point between the two is made on the basis of a '75% Rule'.

The modes of connexion are strictly limited in hearts having absence of one atrioventricular connexion. Such hearts of necessity possess a solitary atrioventricular valve. The solitary valve most usually is exclusively connected to the dominant ventricle. Rarely it may straddle and/or override. In the latter circumstance, both ventricles will be incomplete since neither will possess its full complement of component parts. The connexion produced will be uniatrial but biventricular. The decision as to which ventricle is dominant will then be made according to size. When such a valve straddles, its orifice may be divided into separate components for each ventricle. This should not be interpreted as indicating the presence of two valves.

Ventricular relationships

When discussing the significance of ventricular topology, we indicated that the criterion for existence of the right-hand and left-hand patterns was that one could not be changed into the other simply by rotating the heart or moving it in space. This does not imply that the relationships of the ventricles to each other and to the orthogonal planes of the body are insignificant. We tend to put less emphasis on relations, preferring to emphasize the central role of connexions in determining the route of flow of blood through the heart. At the same time, we do not ignore the way in which the ventricles relate to one another. Indeed, we have indicated how, in the setting of a univentricular atrioventricular connexion, we prefer simply to describe the relationships of dominant and incomplete ventricles as an important feature in categorization. The relationships of the ventricles in hearts with biventricular atrioventricular connexions become vital in diagnosis and description when they are not as anticipated for the given connexion and ventricular topology. For example, in hearts with usual atrial arrangement and a concordant atrioventricular connexion, it would be most unexpected for the morphologically right ventricle not to be right-sided and relatively antero-inferior to the morphologically left ventricle. Yet, on rare occasions, the morphologically right ventricle in hearts with these connexions and topologies can be left-sided. Similarly, in hearts with usual atrial arrangement, discordant atrioventricular connexion and left-hand topology, the morphologically right ventricle can be found in right-sided rather than its expected left-sided position. These unexpected ventricular relationships, which are the result of rotation of the ventricular mass along its long axis,

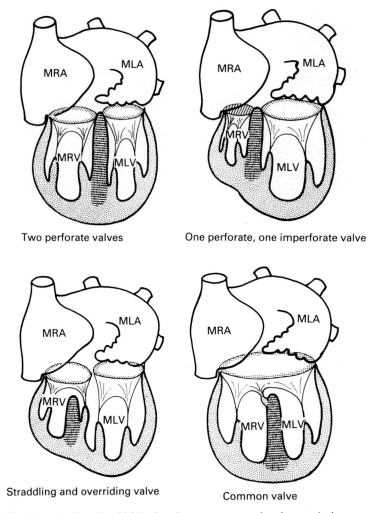

Two perforate valves

One perforate, one imperforate valve

Straddling and overriding valve

Common valve

Fig. 4.13 Any heart in which both atriums are connected to the ventricular mass (concordant, discordant, ambiguous or double inlet connexions) can be found with two valves or a common valve. Either of two valves can be imperforate or, when a septum is present, straddle and/or override. These possibilities are termed the modes of connexion.

produce the so-called 'criss-cross' arrangement.[15] The essence of the criss-cross heart is the finding of unexpected ventricular relationships for the given connexion. Usually the ventricular topology is still as anticipated for the connexion. A criss-cross arrangement was also present in the hearts in which ventricular topology was not as expected for the given atrioventricular connexion.[13,14] In these latter cases, the topology as well as the relationship was disharmonious with the connexion. These cases serve to illustrate the point that, to describe all hearts accurately, it is necessary to note separately (and with mutually exclusive terms) the connexions, the topological arrangement and the relationships of the different cardiac chambers. The so-called 'supero-inferior' (or 'upstairs-downstairs') ventricular relationship is a less extreme form of unexpected chamber locations. In these instances the ventricular mass is tilted along its long axis in one or other direction so that the ventricles are arranged in layered rather than upright fashion.

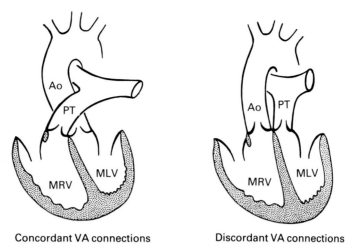

Fig. 4.14 The nature of concordant ventriculo–arterial connexions is shown in this diagram in the setting of the usual arterial relationships. The same connexions can be found with abnormal relationships.

Analysis of the ventriculo–arterial junction

The steps involved in analysis of the atrioventricular junction can be summarized in terms of the type and mode of connexion together with knowledge of the ventricular topology and chamber relationships (see above). The same basic steps are observed at the ventriculo–arterial junction, looking at the type and mode of connexion again but this time supplemented by considerations of infundibular morphology and the relationships of the arterial trunks.

Type of ventriculo–arterial connexion

To determine the type of ventriculo–arterial connexion, it is necessary to know the ventricular morphology and the number and arrangement of the arterial trunks. There are four possibilities. The first two exist when each of two ventricles gives rise to its own arterial trunk (Fig. 4.14). This can be when the arterial trunks, aortic and pulmonary, arise either from the appropriate ventricle (concordant ventriculo–arterial connexions) or from an inappropriate ventricle (discordant connexions). The third pattern exists when both great arteries are connected to the same or to a solitary ventricle (Fig. 4.15). This is termed double outlet and can self-evidently occur from the morphologically right or left ventricle or from a solitary and indeterminate ventricle. The final

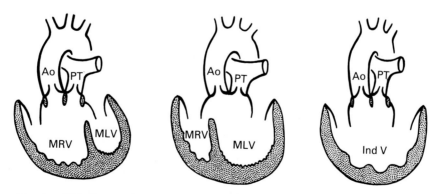

Fig. 4.15 This diagram shows the three options for a double outlet ventriculo–arterial connexion. They can be found with various combinations amongst the other cardiac segments.

pattern exists when only a single arterial trunk can be found in connexions, potential or actual, with the ventricular mass. This pattern, called single outlet of the heart, can itself have one of four variants; these are for the single vessel to be a common trunk, a pulmonary trunk in the setting of aortic atresia, an aortic trunk in the presence of pulmonary atresia, or a solitary arterial trunk when there is absence of the central pulmonary arteries (Fig. 4.16). When there is a single outlet, the solitary trunk usually overrides the ventricular

septum when there are two ventricles, but less commonly it may be exclusively connected to one or other ventricle irrespective of the morphological nature of that ventricle. When there is a solitary ventricle then, of necessity, the trunk will be exclusively connected to it. These patterns of ventricular origin must always be specified.

Mode of ventriculo–arterial connexion

Since the arterial valves possess no tension

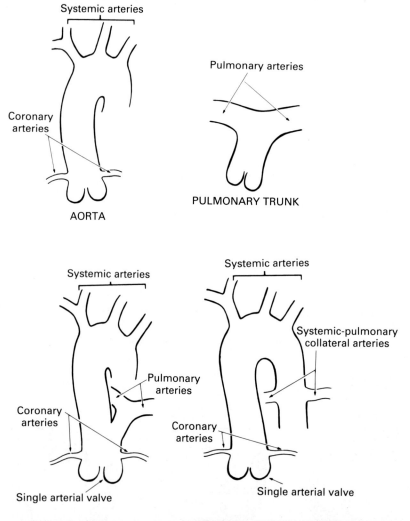

Fig. 4.16 The nature of the arterial trunks is decided according to their branching pattern. In addition to the possibilities of aortic, pulmonary and common trunks, one pattern, existing in the absence of intrapericardial pulmonary arteries, is best described as a solitary trunk.

apparatus, unlike the atrioventricular valves, they are unable to straddle. All the other modes of connexion, however, can occur also at the ventriculo–arterial junction. Thus, there may be a common arterial valve which, nonetheless, can exist only in the presence of a common arterial trunk. Either the aortic or the pulmonary valve can be imperforate. Such imperforate arterial valves can be found in association with concordant, discordant or double outlet connexions. They produce one type of arterial valve atresia, but this is to be distinguished from the other type found with single outlet of the heart. The distinguishing feature is that there must be a potential ventriculo–arterial connexion present in order to confirm an imperforate valve, or muscular atresia with a blind-ending trunk connected to the underlying ventricle (see Ch. 10). The diagnosis of single outlet via an aortic or a pulmonary trunk is made only when it is not possible to trace the atretic arterial trunk to a ventricular origin. The other mode of connexion is overriding of an arterial valve. Overriding has already been referred to in the setting of single outlet, where the ventricular origin of the solitary trunk must be described to provide complete categorization of

the connexion. When one of two arterial valves, or rarely both, overrides the septum, then, as with overriding atrioventricular valves, the precise morphology of the overriding junction determines the connexion present. This is decided using the '50% Rule'. The mechanics of determining the degree of override depend upon projecting the chord subtended by the ventricular septum onto the circle of the overriding valve (Fig. 4.17). The inclination of the ventricular septum has no bearing on the decision-making process. When the '50% Rule' is applied in the setting of double outlet ventricle, it is possible to broaden the definition of the condition to more than half of both arterial valves connected to the same ventricle (see Ch. 21).

Infundibular morphology

Considerable significance has been assigned previously to the muscular or fibrous arrangement of the subarterial ventricular outflow tracts. Indeed, the presence of a given infundibular arrangement has been taken as the criterion for a ventriculo–arterial connexion. For example, many continue to require the existence of a bilat-

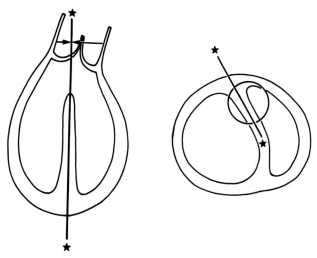

Fig. 4.17 The degree of override of an arterial valve is not decided according to the inclination of the long axis of the septum (left-hand panel). Instead, it depends on the proportion of the leaflets attached within the two ventricles. This is estimated by constructing the chord subtended by the ventricular septum relative to the circle of the orifice of the arterial valve (right-hand panel).

erally complete infundibulum (bilateral conus) before diagnosing the presence of double outlet right ventricle. This convention makes no sense, since discordant, or even concordant, ventriculo–arterial connexions can be found in the presence of bilaterally complete infundibular structures. We take note of infundibular morphology, but we do not afford it a role beyond its significance in the determination of the connexion. The infundibular morphology simply exerts a weak modifying effect on the way the great arteries are connected to the underlying ventricles. There are four patterns which, within the physical possibilities, can exist with any connexion. There may be a complete ring of outlet musculature supporting the pulmonary valve while there is fibrous continuity between the aortic and the atrioventricular valves. This is the most common arrangement and is that found in the normal heart. Secondly, the complete infundibulum may support the aortic valve while the pulmonary valve is in fibrous continuity with the atrioventricular junction. This is the arrangement seen most frequently in hearts with discordant ventriculo–arterial connexions. Thirdly, there may be complete muscular cones supporting both the aortic and pulmonary valves (Fig. 4.18). This is the pattern found most frequently in double outlet right ventricle. Fourthly, both arterial valves may be in fibrous continuity with the atrioventricular junction. This, the least frequent pattern, is usually seen in association with double outlet left ventricle. None of these patterns is found exclusively in the setting of one connexion. Infundibular morphology is independent of the ventriculo–arterial connexion.

Arterial relationships

As with infundibular morphology, so in the past has the relationship of the great arteries been taken as an indication of the ventriculo–arterial connexion. There is as little justification for this convention as for that concerning the bilateral

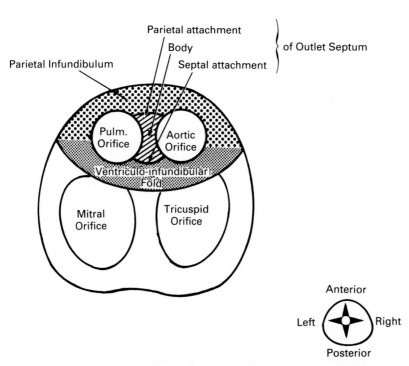

Fig. 4.18 This shows the idealized complete infundibular structures supporting both the aortic and pulmonary valves. More often one or other, or rarely both, infundibula are incomplete because of attenuation of part of the ventriculo-infundibular fold. The outlet septum may also be lacking.

infundibulum. Arterial relationships are independent of both the ventriculo–arterial connexion and the infundibular morphology. There are two aspects to be considered. The first is the interrelationships of the aortic and pulmonary valves relative to the right–left and antero-posterior coordinates of the body. The second is the relationships of the ascending portions of the arterial trunks one to the other. The pulmonary trunk usually spirals round the aorta, but, in many hearts, particularly those with abnormal ventriculo–arterial connexions, the arterial trunks arise in parallel fashion. Usually, the aorta arches superiorly to the pulmonary trunk but even this arrangement is not invariable since cases have been seen where the right pulmonary trunk passes to the lung above the aortic arch.

Associated malformations

The steps described in the preceding paragraphs will simply have set the scene in permitting the investigator to assess the basic make-up of the congenitally malformed heart. In the majority of instances, all the various examinations will have yielded normal findings. The essence of the malformation in such cases will come with identification of the associated malformation or

malformations. These lesions will then become *the* diagnosis of an otherwise normal heart. Their morphology will be described in detail in the subsequent chapters. Even when the segmental arrangement of a malformed heart is itself abnormal, the diagnosis is incomplete until a full search has been made for all potential associated lesions. Sequential segmental analysis, therefore, is but the opening move in examination of suspected congenital heart disease, but a step without which a definitive diagnosis cannot be achieved. Pursuing this approach, observation of a malpositioned heart should not be ignored, but is very much a step towards the end of the diagnostic process. Finding of the heart in an abnormal location is not a diagnosis in itself other than one of malposition. The unusually positioned heart may be entirely normal. Alternatively, it may be grossly malformed. Malposition, therefore, is an indicator of the necessity for careful sequential segmental analysis. When describing the malpositioned heart, we describe separately its location within the chest — left-sided, right-sided or central — and the direction of its apex, to the left or to the right. Such simple description avoids the need to construct formidable and daunting definitions for dextrocardia and similar terms.

REFERENCES

1. Shinebourne EA, Macartney FJ, Anderson RH. Sequential chamber localization — logical approach to diagnosis in congenital heart disease. Br Heart J 1976; 38: 327–340.
2. Tynan MJ, Becker AE, Macartney FJ, Quero-Jimenez M, Shinebourne EA, Anderson RH. Nomenclature and classification of congenital heart disease. Br Heart J 1979; 41: 544–553.
3. Anderson RH, Becker AE, Freedom RM et al. Sequential segmental analysis of congenital heart disease. Ped Cardiol 1984; 5: 281–288.
4. Van Praagh R, Van Praagh S, Vlad P, Keith JD. Anatomic types of congenital dextrocardia. Diagnostic and embryologic implications. Am J Cardiol 1964; 13: 510–531.
5. Van Praagh R. The segmental approach to diagnosis in congenital heart disease. In: Birth defects: Original Article Series. Baltimore: Williams & Wilkins, 1972; 8: 4–23.
6. De la Cruz MV, Nadal-Ginard B. Rules for the diagnosis of visceral situs, truncoconal morphologies and ventricular inversions. Am Heart J 1972; 84: 19–32.
7. Kirklin JW, Pacifico AD, Bargeron IM, Soto B. Cardiac repair in anatomically corrected malposition of the great arteries. Circulation 1973; 48: 153–159.
8. Lev M. Pathologic diagnosis of positional variations in cardiac chambers in congenital heart disease. Lab Invest 1954; 3: 71–82.
9. Van Praagh R, David I, Wright GB, Van Praagh S. Large RV plus small LV is not single RV. Circulation 1980; 61: 1057–1058.
10. Gerlis LM, Dickinson DF, Fagan DG. An unusual type of anomalous pulmonary venous drainage associated with a complex left heart hypoplasia and a variety of divided left atrium ('cor triatriatum'). Int J Cardiol 1985; 7: 245–250.
11. Macartney FJ, Zuberbuhler JR, Anderson RH. Morphological considerations pertaining to recognition of atrial isomerism. Consequences for sequential chamber localisation. Br Heart J 1980; 44: 657–667.
12. Caruso G, Becker AE. How to determine atrial situs? Considerations initiated by 3 cases of absent spleen with a discordant anatomy between bronchi and atria. Br Heart J 1979; 41: 559–567.
13. Weinberg PM, Van Praagh R, Wagner HR, Cuaso CC. New form of criss-cross atrioventricular relation: an

expanded view of the meaning of D and L-loops. Abstract book of World Congress of Paediatric Cardiology, London 1980. 1980; 319.

14. Anderson RH, Smith A, Wilkinson JL. Disharmony between atrioventricular connexions and segmental combinations — unusual variants of 'criss cross' hearts. J Amer Coll Cardiol 1987; 10: 1274–1277.

15. Anderson RH. Criss-cross hearts revisited. Ped Cardiol 1982; 3: 305–313.

Anomalies of venous connexions

INTRODUCTION

Anomalous systemic or pulmonary venous connexions can exist in isolation. They can also complicate other lesions: when they do so it is almost always as part of one or other of the syndromes of atrial isomerism. These characteristic patterns and combinations will be described in the next chapter. In this chapter we are concerned with describing the anatomy of the individual malformations, since the sum of these morphologies accounts for most of the anatomical features seen in hearts with isomeric atrial appendages.

ANOMALOUS SYSTEMIC VENOUS CONNEXIONS

As described in Chapter 1, the superior and inferior caval veins in the normal heart, along with the coronary sinus, have a characteristic arrangement within the morphologically right atrium. Cases are described with totally anomalous connexion of all these venous structures to the 'left atrium'.[1] We have seen lesions approximating to this pattern only in the presence of atrial isomerism. Indeed, in hearts with usual or mirror-image atrial arrangement, it is rare for more than one of these venous channels to be anomalously formed or connected. It is most convenient, therefore, to describe the malformations of each channel, recognizing that, in rare cases, such anomalies may co-exist even in the absence of isomerism.

Anomalies of the superior caval vein

The commonest anomaly of venous drainage involving the superior caval vein is when the flow from the left side of the head and the left arm, instead of being channelled through an anastomotic vessel to the right superior caval vein, drains instead directly to the right atrium through a persistent left superior caval vein.[2] Almost always, such an anomalous channel enters the right atrium through the orifice of an enlarged coronary sinus. To this extent, therefore, the lesion could be considered as an anomaly of the coronary sinus. It has a characteristic morphology. The venous channel descends through the mediastinum and reaches the heart in the angle between the left atrial appendage and the left pulmonary veins. The caval vein then runs down the back of the left atrium to enter the left atrioventricular groove and continues through this groove to empty into the coronary sinus (Fig. 5.1). This is the site in the normal heart of the oblique ligament and vein of Marshall (oblique vein of the left atrium) (Fig. 5.2). The

anomalous channel represents persistence of the left horn of the embryonic sinus venosus, this horn involuting during normal development to become the coronary sinus.[3] When found in this pattern, the anomaly is of no functional significance since the systemic venous blood continues to return to the morphologically right atrium. It may produce problems for the cardiac surgeon and, on occasions, the surgeon may wish to divide the persistent left vein. It is then important to establish whether or not an anastomotic channel connects the persistent left with the usual right superior caval vein (Fig. 5.3). If such a communication is absent, ligation of the left-sided venous channel can be disastrous. In some circumstances, the left caval vein may be the only channel draining blood from the head and both arms. This is when the usual right superior caval vein is absent. Associated sometimes with sudden cardiac death, absence of the right superior caval vein might be thought to disturb the arrangement of the sinus node. An histological study of several cases, however, showed the node to be located within the terminal groove even when the right

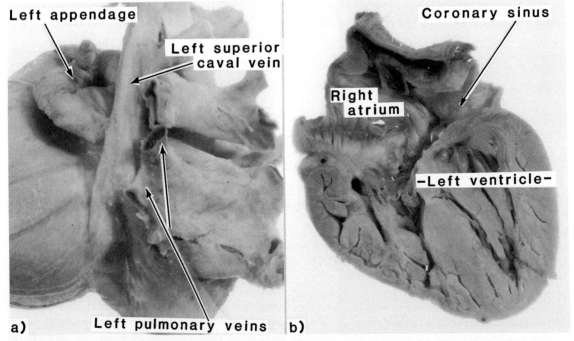

a) **b)**

Fig. 5.1 a,b These illustrations show the posterior aspect (**a**) and a 'four chamber' section (**b**) of a persistent left superior caval vein draining to the right atrium through an enlarged coronary sinus.

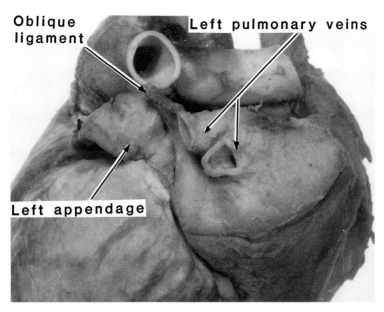

Fig. 5.2 This heart, viewed from its posterior aspect, shows the cord-like remnant of the left superior caval vein known as the oblique ligament of Marshall.

superior caval vein was absent.[4] Rarely, a persistent left superior caval vein can be connected to the roof of the left atrium between appendage and pulmonary veins rather than to the coronary sinus. This anomaly is associated with 'unroofing' of the usual course of such a vein between the left atrium and the coronary sinus. The orifice of the coronary sinus then persists as an interatrial communication (see Ch. 6). This morphological pattern must be distinguished from bilateral connexions of superior caval veins in the setting of right atrial isomerism. In the latter, the connexion of the left-sided venous channel is to a morphologically right atrium.

It is pertinent at this point to mention the venous connexion described as a 'laevo-atrial cardinal vein'.[5] This rare venous structure is found in association with mitral atresia and an intact atrial septum: it then provides the only route of exit for the pulmonary venous return. The vein runs from the roof of the left atrium, from the anticipated site of a left superior caval vein connecting to the left atrium, and connects to the left brachiocephalic vein. The venous content of the laevo-atrial vein is then returned to the right atrium through the usual right-sided superior

caval vein. The channel can be interpreted in terms of persistence of a left superior caval vein connected to the left atrium.

Other reports describe rare anomalies affecting the superior caval vein. The right superior caval vein has been seen connecting to the morphologically left atrium.[6] It has also been described as connecting with both the morphologically right and left atrial chambers through separate orifices in the presence of an intact atrial septum.[7] We have not encountered such lesions. Aneurysmal dilatation of the superior caval vein is recognized as being an acquired lesion of the heart and is rarely seen in children.[8]

Anomalies of the inferior caval vein

The majority of congenital defects involving anomalous formation or connexion of the inferior caval vein are an integral constituent of atrial isomerism. Rarely, anomalous formation of this vein is found in individuals with usual or mirror-image atrial arrangement. The commonest lesion is interruption of the abdominal portion of the caval vein with continuation through either the azygos or the hemiazygos venous structures.

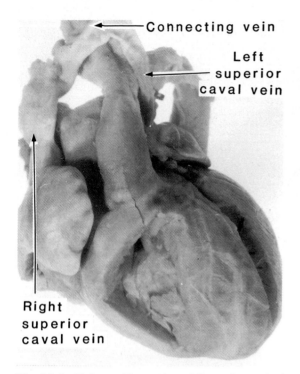

Fig. 5.3 In this heart with a persistent left superior caval vein, there is also a large anastomotic channel from the left side to the normal superior caval vein.

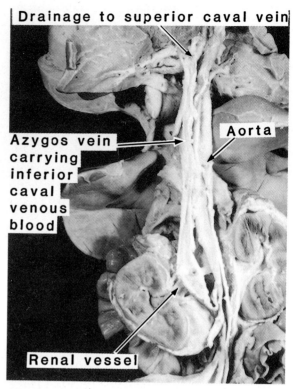

Fig. 5.4 The venous return from the lower body in this patient with left atrial isomerism passes through the azygos system of veins to the left-sided superior caval vein. Note that the azygos continuation of the inferior caval vein runs posteriorly to and adjacent with the aorta.

Described simply as 'azygos continuation' (Fig. 5.4); it is important when finding such a malformation always to exclude the existence of left atrial isomerism. As will be described (see Ch. 16), this is a simple matter for the pathologist, who can examine the morphology of the atrial appendages. It is less easy for the clinician, who is usually dependent on inference in order to recognize the presence of isomerism. A clinical technique in such cases is to examine ultrasonically the connexions of the hepatic veins.[9] The rationale for using this procedure was a belief that, when azygos continuation was associated with an isomeric body arrangement, the hepatic veins would connect bilaterally to the atrial chambers, whereas, in the case of usual or mirror-image arrangements, they would connect to the morphologically right atrium through a suprahepatic venous confluence. It is now known, from examination of a large series of hearts with left atrial isomerism, that this is not the case. It may be found that the hearts with left isomerism

have such a suprahepatic venous confluence (see Ch. 16). Distinction of isomerism in the presence of an azygos continuation, therefore, requires other means such as the identification of bronchial morphology[10] or, for the pathologist, direct examination of the atrial appendages. When there is interruption of the inferior caval vein with azygos continuation, all the systemic venous return reaches the morphologically right atrium through a superior caval vein. With azygos continuation, this is the right-sided vein. When there is hemiazygos continuation, the inferior caval venous blood can be returned through a persistent left superior caval vein.

There are several reports which describe anomalous connexion of the inferior caval vein to the morphologically left atrium.[11-13] Doubt has recently been cast upon such descriptions,[14] which mostly are based upon clinical demonstra-

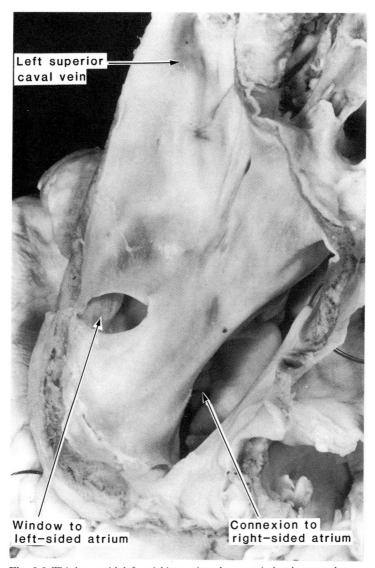

Fig. 5.5 This heart with left atrial isomerism shows a window between the enlarged coronary sinus draining a left superior caval vein and the left-sided atrium.

tion of the presumed anomalous connexion. We endorse this doubt. In our experience, what appeared to be connexion of the inferior caval vein to the morphologically left atrium proved, on closer examination, to be persistence of the Eustachian valve which directed the venous channel into the left atrium through an atrial septal defect within the oval fossa. In other circumstances, the inferior caval vein can achieve a biatrial connexion through an inferior sinus

venosus atrial communication. Apart from such cases, and cases of left atrial isomerism (in which the inferior caval vein can connect bilaterally in the absence of a morphologically right atrium), we have never seen or read a well-documented example or report of connexion of the inferior caval vein to the morphologically left atrium.

A range of anomalous formations of the inferior caval vein may be found within the abdomen; all are well accounted for in terms of

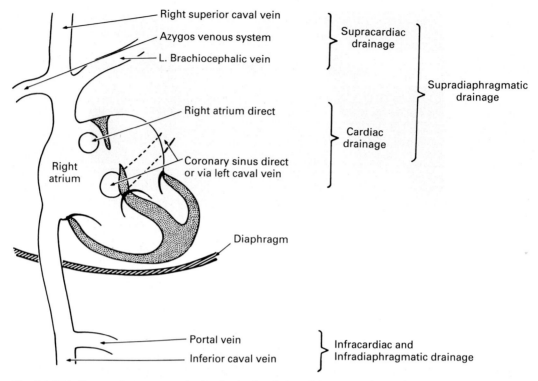

Fig. 5.6 This diagram shows a categorization for the description of the potential sites of anomalous pulmonary venous connexion.

the heterogeneous embryological origin of the vein.

Lesions of the coronary sinus

The most frequent morphological anomaly of the coronary sinus is persistence of a left superior caval vein which drains through the orifice of the sinus (Fig. 5.1). In these circumstances, the origin of the sinus is enlarged. It was suggested that the lesion disturbed the architecture of the atrioventricular node[15] but this was not confirmed on subsequent investigation.[4] Various degrees of 'unroofing' of the coronary sinus (Fig. 5.5) can produce windows into the left atrium and provide the potential for interatrial shunting.[16] The extreme form of this lesion is the interatrial communication at the mouth of the sinus (see Ch. 6). Coronary sinus windows can rarely occur, however, when there is no persistent left superior caval vein and when the atrial septum is intact.[17,18] An extensive Thebesian valve may

produce obstruction to flow from the coronary sinus and, in some circumstances, it can totally occlude the orifice (atresia). In these circumstances, the venous return from the heart reaches the right atrium through the Thebesian veins, which may be dilated. Dilatation of these veins is also encountered when the coronary sinus is hypoplastic. Other rare reported anomalies of the coronary sinus include connexion of hepatic veins to the sinus, fistulous connexions between the sinus and the coronary arteries[17] and connexion of the sinus to the inferior caval vein.[19]

ANOMALIES OF PULMONARY VENOUS CONNEXION

When describing anomalies of the pulmonary veins, it is important to distinguish between anomalous connexion and anomalous drainage. Anomalous connexion exists when one or more of the pulmonary veins connect to a site other than

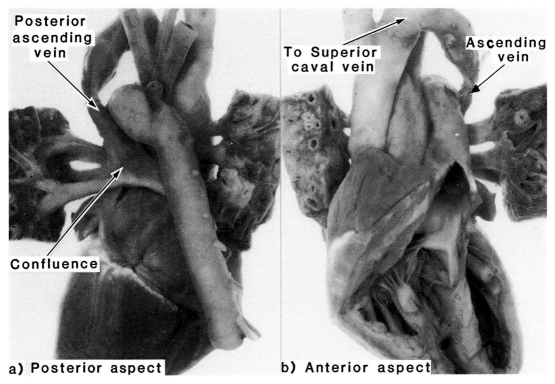

Fig. 5.7 a,b The posterior (**a**) and anterior (**b**) aspects of a heart with totally anomalous pulmonary venous connexion to the superior caval vein. Note the stenotic area where the channel passes round the aortic arch.

the morphologically left atrium. As described in Chapter 1, there is a very characteristic pattern for normal connexion of the pulmonary veins to the left atrium. In this respect, connexion of the pulmonary veins to a left-sided morphologically right atrium, as can occur in right atrial isomerism, should be considered an anomalous cardiac connexion in morphological terms. Anomalous drainage of the pulmonary veins, in contrast, can be found when the pulmonary venous connexions are normal. The best example of this is seen in the setting of a laevo-atrial cardinal vein and mitral atresia. The pulmonary veins are connected to the left atrium but, because the atrial septum is intact and the mitral valve atretic, the venous blood drains into the superior caval venous system and thence to the right atrium.

In this section, we are concerned with description of anomalous connexions; these can be complete or partial. Completely anomalous connexion is usually described as 'total'. Partially

anomalous connexions can involve a solitary vein, all the venous connexions from one lung, or all of the connexions from one lung and most from the other, a solitary vein retaining a normal connexion to the morphologically left atrium. This indicates that, at every autopsy, the pathologist should check carefully the connexions of each pulmonary vein. Anomalous connexion of solitary pulmonary veins is said to occur as often as once among 200 autopsies.[20,21] In an extensive study of anomalous connexions, seven-tenths of the cases involved partially anomalous connexions.[22] That this has not been our recent experience may reflect the fact that we are now dealing with material from centres concerned with treatment by surgical repair. Partially anomalous connexions of the pulmonary veins may be of no functional significance. When seen in association with the sinus venosus atrial septal defect, they are of considerable surgical significance (see Ch. 6). Partially anomalous connexion is also important in the setting of the 'scimitar syndrome'. Taken

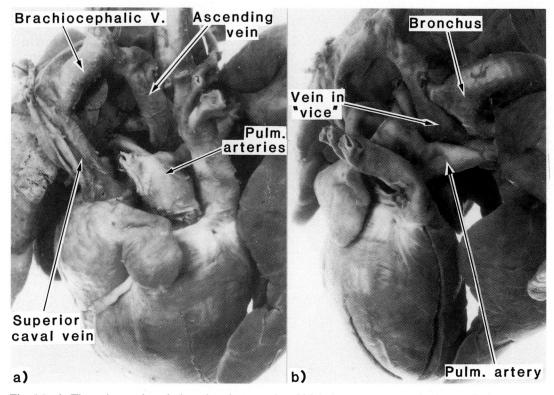

Fig. 5.8 a,b These pictures show the bronchopulmonary vice which is the commonest mechanism producing obstruction in supracardiac totally anomalous pulmonary venous connexion. The trachea is reflected forwards in (**b**).

overall, totally anomalous pulmonary venous connexion is more significant (see below).

Totally anomalous pulmonary venous connexion

The term 'totally anomalous' indicates that all the pulmonary veins are connected to a site other than the morphologically left atrium. Totally anomalous connexion is an essential component of right atrial isomerism, in which the morphologically left appendage is totally lacking (see Ch. 16). In this section, we are concerned with totally anomalous pulmonary venous connexion in the setting of usual or mirror-image atrial arrangement. The anatomical features of note are the site of anomalous connexion, the presence or absence of obstruction within the pulmonary venous pathways, the effect on the rest of the heart, and the effect upon the pulmonary vasculature.

Site of anomalous connexion and obstruction

The anomalously connecting veins can be connected to any adjacent systemic venous channel, either within the thorax or within the abdomen. The connexion to the systemic site can function for the entire venous return (confluent anomalous connexion), or individual pulmonary veins can connect anomalously to different sites. The latter pattern is described as 'mixed' anomalous connexion. Taken overall, the patterns are sufficiently constant to permit categorization (Fig. 5.6). The anomalous connexion can first be divided into supradiaphragmatic and infradiaphragmatic forms. The infradiaphragmatic variant is also infracardiac. The variant with anomalous connexion above and within the thorax can be further divided into supracardiac and cardiac patterns.

Supracardiac pulmonary venous connexion is the commonest anomalous pattern, in which

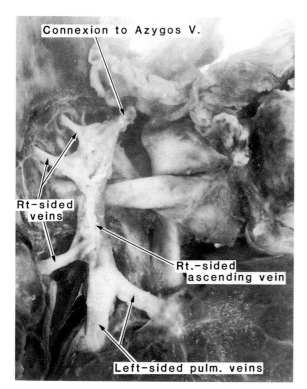

Connexion to Azygos V.

Rt-sided veins

Rt.-sided ascending vein

Left-sided pulm. veins

Fig. 5.9 In this rare variant of supracardiac totally anomalous pulmonary venous connexion, the confluence crosses the midline inferiorly and ascends on the right to drain into the azygos vein.

pulmonary veins join in a confluence immediately behind the left atrium and a venous channel usually ascends to the left and joins the left brachiocephalic vein (Fig. 5.7). The venous return then reaches the right atrium through the superior caval vein. This arrangement gives a characteristic radiographic appearance known as the 'snowman' heart. The upper part of the radiographic image is the venous pathway while the lower part is the heart itself. A characteristic feature of any form of totally anomalous pulmonary venous connexion is the ease with which the heart can be deflected surgically or at autopsy from its pericardial cradle. This is an important pathological marker for the condition. Obstruction occurs with some frequency in the 'snowman' variant, and is due usually to trapping of the venous channel between the pulmonary artery and the bronchus (Fig. 5.8). This arrangement has been graphically characterized as the

'bronchopulmonary vice'.[23] Although supracardiac connexion involves a left-sided ascending channel in most instances, rarely the anomalous venous confluence may cross the midline and ascend within the right paravertebral gutter, picking up the right pulmonary veins as it ascends before joining the azygos vein (Fig. 5.9). This pattern can also exist with the right-sided channel embedded within the substance of the right lung.[24] Obstruction is much rarer with this variant.

Cardiac connexion is almost always to the coronary sinus. All four pulmonary veins may come separately into the sinus but usually there is a short confluence and a common channel behind the left atrium (Fig. 5.10). The anomalous connexion results in gross enlargement of the orifice of the sinus, and an extensive common wall is to be found between the sinus and the remnant of the left atrium. Observation of this feature led to the ingenious suggestion[25] that this particular variant could best be repaired by removal of the common wall and closure of the mouth of the coronary sinus, this procedure restoring, more or less, the anatomy of the normal heart. If cases are seen by the pathologist subsequent to such a repair, care must be taken to see whether the operation had spared the site of the atrioventricular node and was performed without producing residual stenosis. Congenital stenosis in this form of connexion is exceedingly rare, but has been reported as the consequence of a persistent Thebesian valve.[26] Totally anomalous connexion of the pulmonary veins can also be directly to the right atrium but this is much rarer. Taken overall, connexion directly to the heart is the rarest form of totally anomalous return.

Infracardiac and infradiaphragmatic pulmonary venous connexion is usually to the portal venous system (Fig. 5.11a) or directly to the venous duct (Fig. 5.11b). Rarely it is to the inferior caval vein. When the connexion is to the portal system then patency of the venous duct determines the natural history of the condition. While the duct remains open, the pulmonary venous return will achieve a relatively unobstructed pathway to the heart. As soon as the venous duct closes, all the pulmonary flow must pass through the sinusoids of the liver before

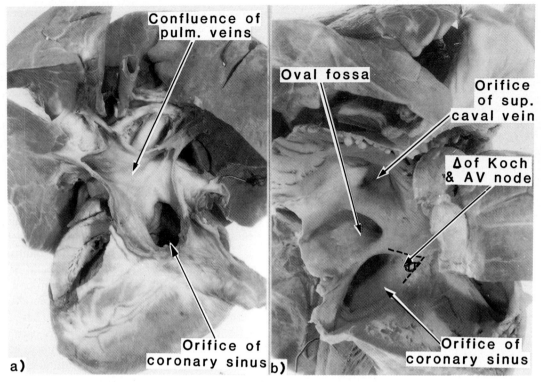

Fig. 5.10 a,b These figures show totally anomalous connexion of the pulmonary veins to the coronary sinus; (**a**) shows a dissection from the posterior aspect while (**b**) shows the enlarged orifice of the sinus and the site of the atrioventricular node.

reaching the right atrium. Severe obstruction can also occur as a consequence of the anatomical anomaly itself. In the most extreme example of this type that we have seen, the descending channel split into a leash of veins which then anastomosed with the gastric veins. Mixed totally anomalous connexion can involve any of the sites of anomalous connexion but most usually is a combination of cardiac and supracardiac connexions.

Effect upon the heart

The major effect of totally anomalous pulmonary venous connexion is that all the venous return, systemic and pulmonary, is to the morphologically right atrium. Because of this, the right heart chambers and the pulmonary trunk are much larger than their left-sided counterparts. It often seems that the left ventricle is hypoplastic but it is difficult for the pathologist to judge whether this is true hypoplasia or a relative feature due to the right-sided overload — most likely it is the latter.[27] Because all the venous return is to the right atrium, the circulation is dependent upon flow of blood through the atrial septum. The oval fossa, therefore, is usually widely patent, although it is rare to find a true deficiency of the floor. In contrast, the finding of an intact, or virtually intact, atrial septum is a significant feature. In most cases, the anomalous connexion of the pulmonary veins is the only lesion within the heart. Anomalous connexion can co-exist with other lesions. Sometimes, as with complete transposition, it is beneficial in the natural history of the associated condition. As already indicated, in other instances the anomalous pulmonary venous connexion is an integral part of a complex of lesions. Right atrial isomerism is the prime example of this but anomalous connexion of the right pulmonary veins is a very common accompaniment of the sinus venosus interatrial commu-

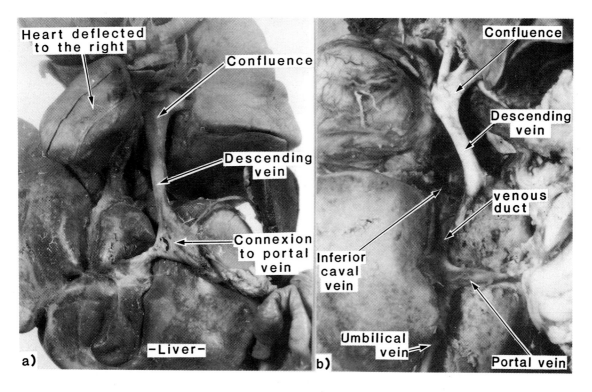

Fig. 5.11 a,b These two cases with infradiaphragmatic totally anomalous pulmonary venous connexion show the descending vein connected (**a**) to the portal vein and (**b**) to the venous duct.

nication. The anomalous connexion which is part of the 'scimitar syndrome' is discussed below.

Effect upon the lungs

The anomalous route of venous circulation imposing an increased load on the right heart has a major effect upon the structure of the pulmonary vasculature. Changes are to be found even in neonates.[27,28] The muscularity of the pulmonary arteries is increased and the degree increases further with age, even in those with low pulmonary flow. The pulmonary veins are also muscularized. Studies of large numbers of specimens permit the calculation of an index of pulmonary vascular disease.[29] The index is higher in cases with obstructed pulmonary venous flow. Multiple anastomoses develop between the pulmonary and bronchial veins. The evidence indicates that most of these changes are already present during fetal life, so the excellent results of surgery in most cases indicate that such changes are not inimical to survival.

The 'scimitar syndrome'

When first used,[30] the term 'scimitar syndrome' was applied to a radiographic finding in a familial disease characterized by a right-sided heart with partially anomalous pulmonary venous connexion. The anomalous connexion was to the inferior caval vein and the shadow produced was likened to the curve of a Turkish sword. Since then, it has become evident that similar features may be present in a range of cases, not all of which represent familial disease and not all exhibiting all features of the original cases. The heart is usually right-sided because of hypoplasia of the right lung. Part of the lung is often sequestrated in terms of its bronchial supply and usually there is also an anomalous pulmonary arterial supply through systemic collateral arteries derived

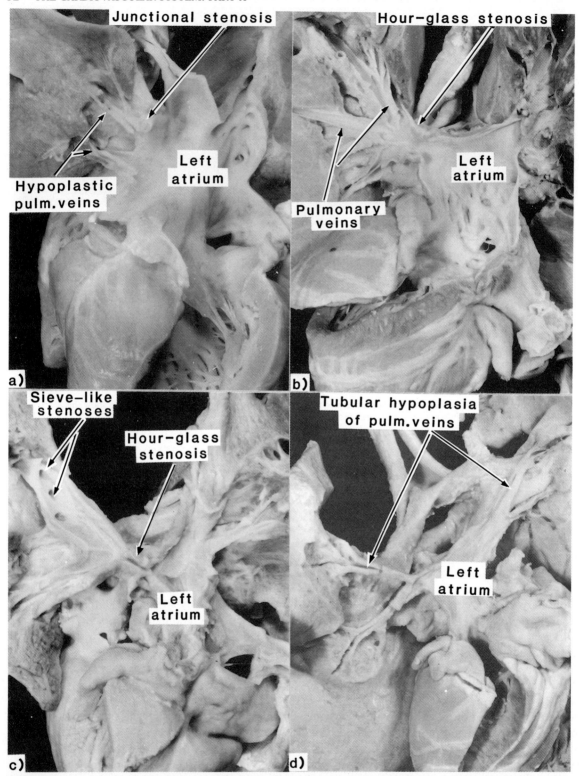

Fig. 5.12 a–d These illustrations show variants in the morphology of pulmonary venous stenosis. In (**a**), the veins are hypoplastic with stenotic areas at their junction with the left atrium. The veins are normal with junctional stenosis in (**b**), while (**c**) shows a junctional hour-glass stenosis along with sieve-like stenosis of individual veins. The worst variant is seen in (**d**), where all the veins show tubular hypoplasia.

from the descending aorta. The venous return is also anomalous in most cases, often for the entire right lung but sometimes for only part of it. The anomalous pulmonary venous connexion pierces the diaphragm and terminates in the inferior caval vein. Documentation of these changes is largely clinical. Study of a large number of cases shows that any individual case must be described specifically in terms of bronchial, venous and arterial supply of the affected lung.[31]

Other lesions of the pulmonary veins

Atresia of the common pulmonary vein is a severe malformation which is incompatible with life unless relieved by urgent surgery. In the absence of co-existing anomalous pathways (which would be comparable, if present, to the laevo-atrial cardinal vein) the pulmonary venous return is through bronchopulmonary venous anastomoses.

Stenosis of the pulmonary veins has a very poor prognosis.[32] Individual veins can be stenosed[33] but more usually the condition affects all veins. The stenoses can be tubular (Fig. 5.12a), usually with extension into the lung, or discrete. Discrete stenoses tend to be formed at the point of junction of the veins with the left atrium (Fig. 5.12b). In one case that we have seen, the stenoses were in the form of a sieve-like connexion between multiple small veins and a venous confluence (Fig. 5.12c). The morphology of these various stenoses suggests that only the discrete variant is amenable to surgical correction. In the series we studied,[34] the only example of this operable type was in an infant with the hypoplastic left heart syndrome. Obstruction of individual pulmonary veins can also complicate cases with totally anomalous pulmonary venous connexion.

Aneurysmal dilatation of pulmonary veins also occurs (pulmonary varix) and usually affects individual veins, most often the upper right one. It has been seen in a child of 7 years; it can rupture and cause death.[35]

REFERENCES

1. Pearl WR, Spicer MJ. Total anomalous systemic venous return. South Med J 1980; 73: 259–261.
2. Winter FS. Persistent left superior vena cava: survey of world literature and report of 30 additional cases. Angiology 1954; 5: 90–132.
3. Fischer DR, Zuberbuhler JR. Anomalous systemic venous return. In: Anderson RH, Macartney FJ, Shinebourne EA, Tynan M, eds. Paediatric cardiology, vol. I. Edinburgh: Churchill Livingstone, 1987; 497–508.
4. Lenox CC, Hashida Y, Anderson RH, Hubbard JD. Conduction tissue anomalies in absence of the right superior caval vein. Int J Cardiol 1981; 8: 251–260.
5. Lucas RV, Lester RG, Lillehei CW, Edwards JE. Mitral atresia with levoatriocardinal vein. A form of congenital pulmonary venous obstruction. Am J Cardiol 1962; 9: 607–613.
6. Kirsch WM, Carlsson E, Hartmann AF. A case of anomalous drainage of the superior vena cava into the left atrium. J Thorac Cardiovasc Surg 1961; 41: 550–556.
7. Shapiro EP, Al-Sadir J, Campbell NPS, Thilenius OG, Anagnostopoulos CE, Hays P. Drainage of right superior vena cava into both atria. Review of the literature and description of a case presenting with polycythemia and paradoxical embolization. Circulation 1981; 63: 712–717.
8. Franken EA. Idiopathic dilatation of the superior vena cava. Pediatrics 1972; 49: 297–299.
9. Huhta JC, Smallhorn JF, Macartney FJ. Two dimensional echocardiographic diagnosis of situs. Br Heart J 1982; 48: 97–108.
10. Deanfield J, Leanage R, Stroobant J, Chrispin AR, Taylor JFN, Macartney FJ. Use of high kilovoltage filtered beam radiographs for detection of bronchial situs in infants and young children. Br Heart J 1980; 44: 577–583.
11. Gardner DL, Cole L. Long-term survival with inferior vena cava draining into the left atrium. Br Heart J 1955; 17: 93–97.
12. Meadows WR. Isolated anomalous connection of a great vein to the left atrium. Circulation 1961; 24: 669–676.
13. Kim YS, Serrato M, Long DM, Hastreiter AR. Left atrial inferior vena cava with atrial septal defect. Ann Thorac Surg 1971; 11: 165–170.
14. Van Praagh R, Van Praagh S. Does connection of the IVC with the LA exist? Letter to the Editor. Ped Cardiol 1987; 8: 151.
15. Anderson RH, Latham RA. The cellular architecture of the human atrioventricular node, with a note on its morphology in the presence of a left superior vena cava. J Anat 1971; 109: 443–455.
16. Rose AG, Beckman CB, Edwards JE. Communication between coronary sinus and left atrium. Br Heart J 1974; 36: 182–185.
17. Mantini E, Grondin CM, Lillehei CW, Edwards JE. Congenital anomalies involving the coronary sinus. Circulation 1966; 33: 317–327.
18. Allmendinger P, Dear WE, Cooley DA. Atrial septal defect with communication through the coronary sinus. Ann Thorac Surg 1874; 17: 193–196.

19. Sherman FE. An atlas of congenital heart disease. Philadelphia: Lea & Febiger, 1963; 69.
20. Hughes CW, Rumore PC. Anomalous pulmonary veins. Arch Pathol 1944; 37: 364–366.
21. Healey JE. An anatomic survey of anomalous pulmonary veins: their clinical significance. J Thorac Surg 1952; 23: 433–444.
22. Snellen HA, Van Ingen HC, Hoefsmit ECM. Patterns of anomalous pulmonary venous drainage. Circulation 1968; 38: 45–63.
23. DeLisle G, Ando M, Calder AL et al. Total anomalous pulmonary venous connection: report of 93 autopsied cases with emphasis on diagnostic and surgical considerations. Am Heart J 1976; 91: 99–122.
24. Brenner JI, Bharati S, Berman MA, Lev M. Rare type of intrapulmonary drainage of one lung by the other with total anomalous pulmonary venous return. J Amer Coll Cardiol 1983; 2: 1174–1177.
25. Van Praagh R, Harken AH, Delisle G, Ando M, Gross RE. Total anomalous pulmonary venous drainage to the coronary sinus. A revised procedure for its correction. J Thorac Cardiovasc Surg 1972; 64: 132–135.
26. Arciniegas E, Henry JG, Green EW. Stenosis of the coronary sinus ostium. An unusual site of obstruction in total anomalous pulmonary venous drainage. J Thorac Cardiovasc Surg 1980; 79: 303–305.
27. Haworth SG, Reid L. Structural study of pulmonary circulation and of heart in total anomalous pulmonary venous return in early infancy. Br Heart J 1977; 38: 80–92.
28. Haworth SG. Total anomalous pulmonary venous return. Prenatal damage to pulmonary vascular bed and extrapulmonary veins. Br Heart J 1982; 48: 513–524.
29. Newfeld EA, Wilson A, Paul MH, Reisch JS. Pulmonary vascular disease in total anomalous pulmonary venous drainage. Circulation 1980; 61: 103–109.
30. Neill CA, Ferencz C, Sabiston DC, Sheldon H. The familial occurrence of hypoplastic right lung with systemic arterial supply and venous drainage 'scimitar syndrome'. Johns Hopkins Med J 1960; 107: 1–15.
31. Clements BS, Warner JO, Shinebourne EA. Congenital bronchopulmonary vascular malformations: clinical application of a simple anatomical approach in 25 cases. Thorax 1987; 42: 409–416.
32. Bini RM, Cleveland DC, Ceballos R, Bargeron LM Jr, Pacifico AD, Kirklin JW. Congenital pulmonary vein stenosis. Am J Cardiol 1984; 54: 369–375.
33. Nakib A, Moller JH, Kanjuh VI, Edwards JE. Anomalies of the pulmonary veins. Am J Cardiol 1967; 20: 77–90.
34. Fong LV, Anderson RH, Park SC, Zuberbuhler JR. Morphologic features of stenosis of the pulmonary veins. Am J Cardiol 1988; 62: 1136–1138.
35. Klinck GH Jr, Hunt HD. Pulmonary varix with spontaneous rupture and death: report of a case. Arch Pathol 1933; 15: 227–237.

Lesions of the atrial chambers

INTRODUCTION

In this chapter, we will concentrate on those lesions which provide the anatomical potential for shunting between the atriums and are, most accurately, described as interatrial communications. We will also consider lesions of the atriums themselves, such as prominence of the so-called venous valves in the right atrium, juxtaposition of the appendages, and the lesion most frequently described as 'cor triatriatum', but reality no more than a partition within the morphologically left atrium.

INTERATRIAL COMMUNICATIONS

The term interatrial communications rather than atrial septal defect is used for a specific reason. All those lesions which produce the anatomical potential for shunting between the atrial chambers[1] are not necessarily within the confines of the atrial septum. Thus, the so-called ostium primum atrial septal defect is, in reality, a deficiency at the site of the atrioventricular septum.[2] This lesion, therefore, will be considered in the next chapter. In this chapter, we are concerned with those lesions confined within the oval fossa (true atrial septal defects) and with the so-called sinus venosus and coronary sinus defects. As will be explained, the last two lesions permit unequivocal interatrial shunting but are outside the confines of the atrial septum. Crucial to an understanding of the defects to be discussed in this section is knowledge of the confines of the normal atrial septum.

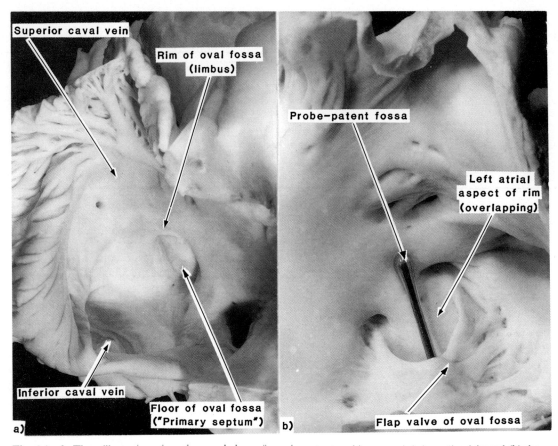

Fig. 6.1 a,b These illustrations show the morphology of a probe-patent oval foramen; (**a**) shows the right and (**b**) the left atrial aspects. A probe has been passed across the foramen in (**b**).

The normal atrial septum

There is a potential deficiency within the atrial septum of the normal heart because, during fetal life, the richly oxygenated placental blood returns to the right atrium through the umbilical vein. This blood needs to reach the left atrium in order to enter the left ventricle, the aorta and thence to reach, in particular, the brain. To do this, it must cross the atrial septum. The communication permitting this transfer is located opposite the orifice of the inferior caval vein and is so arranged that, during fetal life, the raised right atrial pressure promotes the required shunt from right to left atrial chambers. After birth, when left atrial pressure is higher than right, the anatomical arrangement permits mechanical closure of the communication. The septal communication,

known as the oval foramen, is arranged with a flange on the right atrial surface and a flap valve within the left atrium (Fig. 6.1). The flange is often described as the 'septum secundum', but, in reality, is simply an infolding of the atrial roof. The greater part of the septum is made up of the floor of the oval fossa. During fetal life, this is a hinged flap with an upper margin which floats freely. This upper edge in most adult hearts is firmly fused to the right atrial flange, producing both mechanical and haemodynamic closure of the septum. In from one-quarter to one-third of normal hearts, however, the upper edge of the flap valve is not fused with the flange.[3] This arrangement, called a probe-patent oval foramen, produces mechanical closure of the septum as long as the right atrial pressure is higher than the left. In its presence, if the pressure in the left

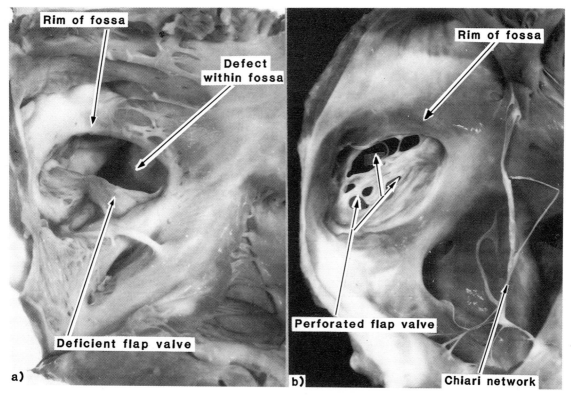

Fig. 6.2 a,b These hearts have (**a**) a deficiency and (**b**) perforation of the flap valve of the oval fossa. Both result in an atrial septal defect.

atrium exceeds that in the right atrium, there will be the potential for interatrial shunting. The probe-patent atrial septum, nonetheless, is not usually considered as a septal defect.

Defects within the oval fossa

Defects within the oval fossa are the true atrial septal defects. They are also the commonest variety of interatrial communication. They exist either because the flap valve of the septum is of insufficient size to overlap the right atrial flange (Fig. 6.2a) or because the valve itself is perforated or otherwise deficient (Fig. 6.2b). Sometimes the entire floor of the fossa is missing. If the flange is effaced in these circumstances, the interatrial communication may become sufficiently large to warrant the term 'common atrium'. More usually, such common atrial chambers are seen in the setting of an atrioventricular septal defect, partic-

ularly when there is co-existing atrial isomerism. A deficiency within the oval fossa must be distinguished from probe patency (see above). When the flap valve is too small, or perforated, the potential for shunting across the septum will exist irrespective of the pressures in the atrial chambers. As explained above, shunting through a probe-patent septum can take place only when the left atrial pressure exceeds the right, which is a very rare occurrence. The location of defects within the oval fossa can vary to a limited degree. Most are found superiorly because of deficiency of the top edge of the flap valve. The most important variant is one in which the septal deficiency extends into the mouth of the inferior caval vein. This permits the caval vein to override the septal flange and communicate, in part, directly with the left atrium. Such an arrangement should be distinguished from an inferior sinus venosus defect. If found, it should not be described as left atrial origin of the caval vein. The surgeon must

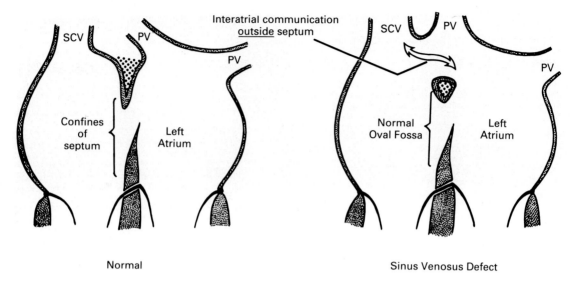

Fig. 6.3 These diagrams show how bi-atrial connexions of the superior caval and pulmonary veins produce a so-called 'sinus venosus' interatrial communication which is outside the confines of the normal atrial septum.

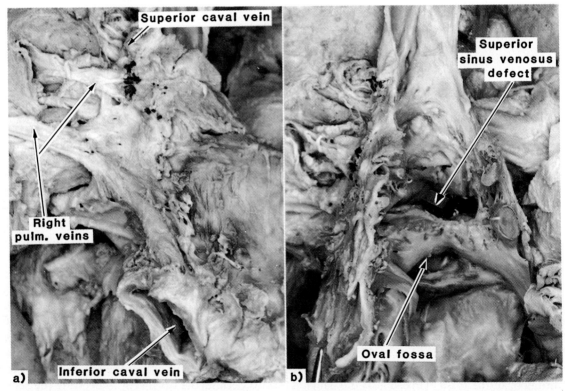

Fig. 6.4 a,b These illustrations show (**a**) the anomalous connexions of the right pulmonary veins and (**b**) an interatrial communication outside the oval fossa in a superior sinus venosus defect.

also be aware of the precise morphology of such connexions so that he may avoid closing the defect in such a way as to leave the inferior caval vein draining to the left atrium.[4]

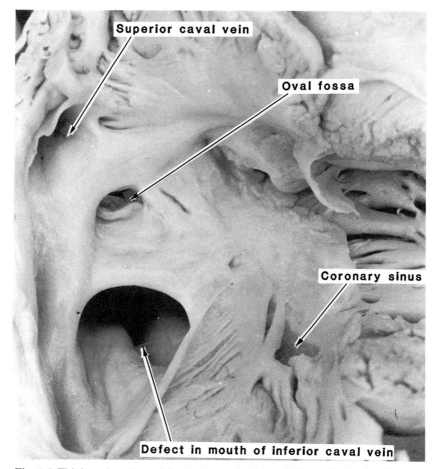

Superior caval vein

Oval fossa

Coronary sinus

Defect in mouth of inferior caval vein

Fig. 6.5 This heart has a large defect in the mouth of the inferior caval vein which is outside the confines of the normal atrial septum. This is a so-called inferior sinus venosus defect.

The sinus venosus defects

Knowledge of the correct morphology of the so-called 'sinus venosus' defects is grounded in the fact that they are outside the confines of the atrial septum. They cannot be produced simply as a consequence of some deficiency of part of the septal mechanics. It needs some other abnormal venous connexion to create an extra-septal tunnel and provide a conduit between the right and left atriums (Fig. 6.3). That conduit is provided by bi-atrial connexion of either the superior or inferior caval vein, often in association with anomalous connexion of the right pulmonary veins. The superior sinus venosus defect, with anomalous connexion of the superior caval vein, is by far the commoner arrangement. This produces an inter-atrial communication cephalad to the superior rim of the oval fossa. The fossa itself may be intact or may exhibit a true atrial septal defect. The defect thus produced by the caval venous overriding does not distort the location or morphology of the sinus node (Fig. 6.4). Owing to the association of anomalous pulmonary and systemic venous connexions, however, it is often difficult for the surgeon to close such a defect without producing either superior caval or pulmonary venous obstruction. Often, therefore, the surgical procedure will include placement of a gusset to enlarge the superior caval channel. Such an incision may place the artery to the sinus node very much at risk, and, if the surgeon is unaware

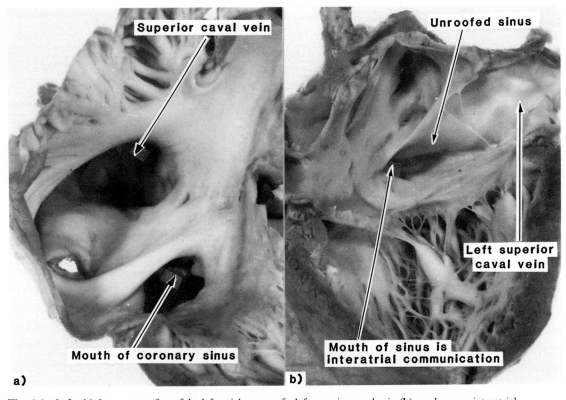

Fig. 6.6 a,b In this heart, unroofing of the left atrial course of a left superior caval vein (**b**) produces an interatrial communication at the mouth of the coronary sinus (**a**).

of the extent of the sinus node, may produce nodal damage. Such damage is almost certainly the cause of the postoperative arrhythmias reported by some, but by no means all, centres subsequent to the closure of superior sinus venosus defects.[5] The inferior sinus venosus defect, which is much less common, is found in the mouth of the inferior caval vein as a consequence of connexion of this vein, in part, to the left atrium (Fig. 6.5). As discussed, it must be distinguished from the oval fossa defect which extends into the mouth of the caval vein (see above). Like the superior sinus venosus defect, the inferior sinus venosus defect is often associated with anomalous connexion of the right pulmonary veins.

The coronary sinus defect

By far the rarest interatrial communication is that found at the site of the orifice of the coronary sinus.[6] This hole represents the mouth of the coronary sinus. It almost always co-exists with anomalous connexion of a persistent left superior caval vein to the roof of the left atrium (Fig. 6.6). The defect then can be considered simply as the extreme form of unroofing of the coronary sinus. Lesser forms of this lesion exist in the shape of windows of varying size between the coronary sinus and the left atrium.[7] An interatrial communication at the site of the coronary sinus can rarely be found in the absence of a persistent left superior caval vein. The coronary veins themselves in this setting drain directly to the cavities of the atrial chambers and the coronary sinus, as such, is lacking.

OTHER ATRIAL MALFORMATIONS

Apart from exceedingly rare conditions, such as aneurysms of the atrial wall or dilatation of the

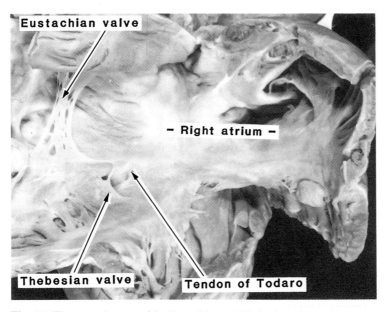

Fig. 6.7 The normal extent of the Eustachian and Thebesian valves at the mouths of the inferior caval vein and the coronary sinus, respectively. Note that the commissure of the two valves buries itself into the sinus septum as the tendon of Todaro.

atrial appendages, the significant atrial lesions are undue prominence of the valves of the embryonic venous sinus, juxtaposition of the atrial appendages, and division of the left atrium (cor triatriatum).

Undue prominence of the valves of the venous sinus

It is well recognized that the right atrium is derived from two components.[8] One is the primitive atrial segment of the heart tube, the other is the venous sinus (sinus venosus). Early in development, well-formed flaps or valves are seen between the two components. These valves are simply inflections of the adjacent walls of the two segments. For the larger part, the flaps regress during infancy, leaving only small folds which guard the entrances of the inferior caval vein and coronary sinus to the right atrium. These structures are known as the Thebesian and Eustachian valves, respectively (Fig. 6.7). In some hearts, more extensive remnants of the embryonic valves persist which are not always of functional significance. Usually they persist as fenestrated

networks (Chiari nets) which extend from the terminal crest to be attached superiorly to the 'septum spurium'. In rare circumstances, the valves can persist as more solid sheets and can then produce obstruction to flow through the right side of the heart.[9,10] Very rarely, such structures can be discovered in otherwise normally connected hearts and produce obstruction to flow through the right heart chambers.[11] Removal of the windsock-like lesion is then curative (Fig. 6.8). More usually, the restrictive sheets are found in hearts in which there is already obstruction or atresia along the right-sided flow pathways.[12] The typical setting for these lesions, which are then often described as 'cor triatriatum dexter', is in pulmonary atresia with an intact ventricular septum (Fig. 6.9a) or in tricuspid atresia (Fig. 6.9b). Although it is often suggested that the prominence of these remnants of the valves of the embryonic venous sinus is causative of the associated lesions, it is just as likely that the valves themselves persist because of the presence of the obstructive lesions. The function of these valves during embryonic life is to direct the richly oxygenated inferior caval venous flow across the

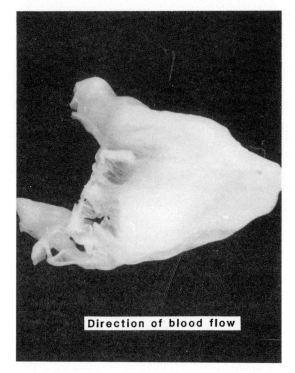

Fig. 6.8 This windsock-like structure is an aneurysmal malformation formed from the venous valves which was removed surgically from an infant with obstructed flow across the tricuspid valve.

atrial septum and into the left-sided heart chambers. When, in extrauterine life, there is atresia along the right-sided pathways (pulmonary or tricuspid atresia), there is no incentive for the venous valves to regress.

Juxtaposition of the atrial appendages

In the normal situation, the appendages of the atrial chambers are situated one on either side of the arterial pedicle. In some circumstances, usually in the presence of complex associated lesions but occasionally with simple lesions such as an atrial septal defect, both appendages are found on the same side of the arterial pedicle. In the individual with usual atrial arrangement, it is the right appendage which is most frequently juxtaposed in such a way that it comes to lie within the transverse sinus so that its tip is to the left of the great arteries (Fig. 6.10a). This arrangement is known as left juxtaposition.[13] It is a harbinger of abnormal ventriculo–arterial connexions, usually discordant or double outlet right ventricle, and it is often found with the aorta in left-sided position. Left juxtaposition is also frequently found with tricuspid atresia. Whatever the associated lesions,

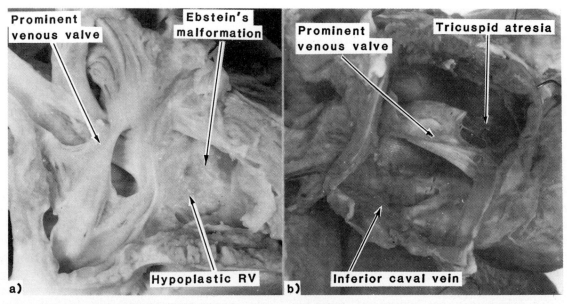

Fig. 6.9 a,b These illustrations show unduly prominent venous valves dividing the right atrium in the setting (a) of pulmonary atresia with intact ventricular septum and (b) of tricuspid atresia.

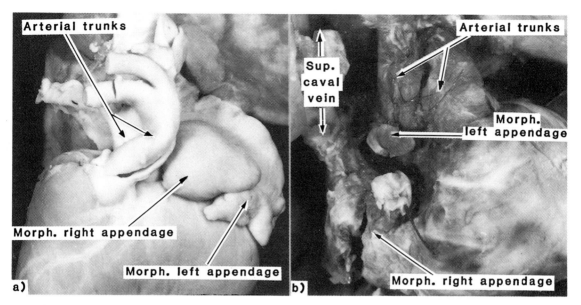

Fig. 6.10 a,b These illustrations show (**a**) left-sided and (**b**) right-sided juxtaposition of the atrial appendages (Morph. = morphologically).

the juxtaposition tends to distort the location of the sinus node by virtue of the abnormal orientation of the terminal groove.[14] In some instances the appendage may be partially juxtaposed. Either partial or complete juxtaposition also distorts the internal architecture of the right atrium in such a way that the orifice of the appendage occupies the anticipated site of the oval fossa, the latter being squashed and deviated postero-inferiorly. Much more rarely, the left atrial appendage may be distorted so that it comes to extend through the transverse sinus to assume a right-sided position.[15] Such right juxtaposition (Fig. 6.10b) tends to occur with much simpler lesions, such as atrial septal defect, but can also be found in the setting of complex lesions. Right juxtaposition can also be found with mirror-image atrial arrangement, when it is simply the mirror-image of the commoner left variant and is associated with similar lesions. It can also be seen with atrial isomerism when both appendages are of like morphology. The associated lesions then reflect the presence of isomerism.

Division of the left atrium

As mentioned above, persistence of the valves of

the embryonic venous sinus is often described as 'cor triatriatum dexter'. When used in isolation, the term 'cor triatriatum' almost always refers to division of the left atrium. Several patterns exist in which the left atrial chamber is divided, often in association with anomalous pulmonary venous connexions or other lesions.[16] The greater majority of cases, nonetheless, are of a pattern which can be considered as the 'classic' lesion.[17] In this variant (Fig. 6.11), an oblique partition separates a proximal atrial chamber, to which are connected the pulmonary veins, from a distal chamber in free communication with the vestibule of the mitral valve and the mouth of the atrial appendage. Most frequently, the oval fossa (which may be deficient, probe-patent or intact) is in actual or potential communication with the distal chamber. Cases are well described, however, in which the fossa is in communication with the distal chamber. The severity of the lesion depends upon the size of the orifice between the divided components of the left atrium. This communication is usually seen in the part of the shelf where it joins inferiorly with the atrial septum and, in cases coming to autopsy, is usually of pin-hole size. A divided left atrium is seen most

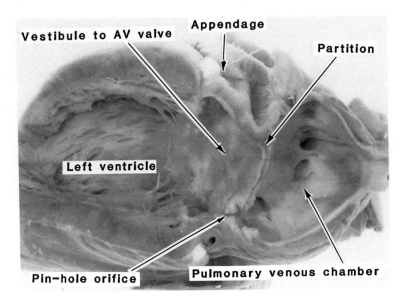

Fig. 6.11 This heart has a fibromuscular partition dividing the left atrium into a pulmonary venous compartment and another component leading to the mitral valve which is in communication with the left appendage.

frequently as an isolated lesion but it can co-exist with any other defect. Notable associations are with atrioventricular septal defect or totally anomalous pulmonary venous connexion, where the presence of the obstructive shelf may be masked clinically.

REFERENCES

1. Bedford DE, Sellors TH, Somerville W, Belcher JR, Besterman EMM. Atrial septal defect and its surgical treatment. Lancet 1957; 1: 1255–1261.
2. Becker AE, Anderson RH. Atrioventricular septal defects. What's in a name? J Thorac Cardiovasc Surg 1982; 83: 461–469.
3. Hagen PT, Scholz DG, Edwards WD. Incidence and size of patent foramen ovale during the first decades of life: an autopsy study of 965 normal hearts. Mayo Clin Proc 1984; 59: 1489–1494.
4. Hartung HW, Rolfs F, Klein HH, de Vivie ER. Iatrogenic transposition of vena cava inferior to the left atrium, a rare complication in surgical repair of atrial septum secundum defect. Abstract. J Thorac Cardiovasc Surg 1987; 35: I: 76–77.
5. Clark EB, Roland JA, Varghese PJ, Neill CA, Haller JA. Should the sinus venosus type ASD be closed? A review of the atrial conduction defects and surgical results in twenty eight children. Abstract. Am J Cardiol 1975; 35: 127.
6. Raghib G, Ruttenberg HD, Anderson RC, Amplatz K, Adams PJr, Edwards JE. Termination of left superior vena cava in left atrium, atrial septal defect, and absence of coronary sinus. A developmental complex. Circulation 1965; 31: 906–918.
7. Rose AG, Beckman CB, Edwards JE. Communication between coronary sinus and left atrium. Br Heart J 1974; 36: 182–185.
8. Wenink ACG. Embryology of the heart. In: Anderson RH, Macartney FJ, Shinebourne EA, Tynan M, eds. Paediatric cardiology, vol. II. Edinburgh: Churchill Livingstone, 1987; 83–108.
9. Hansing CE, Young WP, Rowe CC. Cor triatriatum dexter. Persistent right sinus venous valve. Am J Cardiol 1972; 30: 559–564.
10. Doucette J, Knoblich R. Persistent right valve of the sinus venosus. Arch Pathol 1963; 75: 105–112.
11. Jones RN, Niles NR. Spinnaker formation of the sinus venosus valve. Circulation 1968; 38: 468–473.
12. Trento A, Zuberbuhler JR, Anderson RH, Park SC, Siewers RD. Divided right atrium (prominence of the Eustachian and Thebesian valves). J Thorac Cardiovasc Surg 1988; 96: 457–463.
13. Melhuish BPP, Van Praagh R. Juxtaposition of the atrial appendages. A sign of severe cyanotic congenital heart disease. Br Heart J 1968; 30: 269–284.
14. Anderson RH, Smith A, Wilkinson JL. Right juxtaposition of the auricular appendages. Eur J Cardiol 1976; 4: 495–503.
15. Ho SY, Monro JL, Anderson RH. The disposition of the sinus node in left-sided juxtaposition of the atrial appendage. Br Heart J 1979; 41: 129–132.

16. Thilenius OG, Bharati S, Lev M. Subdivided left atrium: an expanded concept of cor triatriatum sinistrum. Am J Cardiol 1976; 37: 743–752.

17. Van Praagh R, Corsini I. Cor triatriatum: pathologic anatomy and a consideration of morphogenesis based on 13 postmortem cases and a study of normal development of the pulmonary vein and atrial septum in 83 human embryos. Am Heart J 1969; 78: 379–405.

Atrioventricular septal defect

INTRODUCTION

There is a group of cardiac malformations characterized by complete absence of normal atrioventricular septal structures (see Ch. 1). The justification for grouping together these hearts has long been recognized[1–3] but the individual malformations have been described in differing ways. Obstacles to their understanding have, in our opinion, been constructed through the slavish application of questionable embryological concepts in the interpretation of their morphology. Understanding of morphology depends upon knowledge of the effect of the absence of normal atrioventricular septation. The description that we prefer for the group, therefore, is atrioventricular septal defect.[4] Not included in this group is the hole which exists at the site of the membranous atrioventricular septum in a heart with otherwise normal atrioventricular septation (the Gerbode defect), even though it is an atrioventricular septal defect in the strictest sense. This is because atrioventricular septation in such hearts is otherwise normal.[5] Also excluded are lesions such as isolated cleft of the mitral valve or straddling tricuspid valve which also have normal atrioventricular septation.[6] Following our concept, we shall describe a group of lesions having a characteristic morphology which readily permits their distinction from hearts with normal atrioventricular septation. First we describe the consequences of deficient septation, indicating particularly how this feature distorts the normal anatomy. Thereafter we give an account of the features which differentiate the various subsets of atrioventricular septal defect.

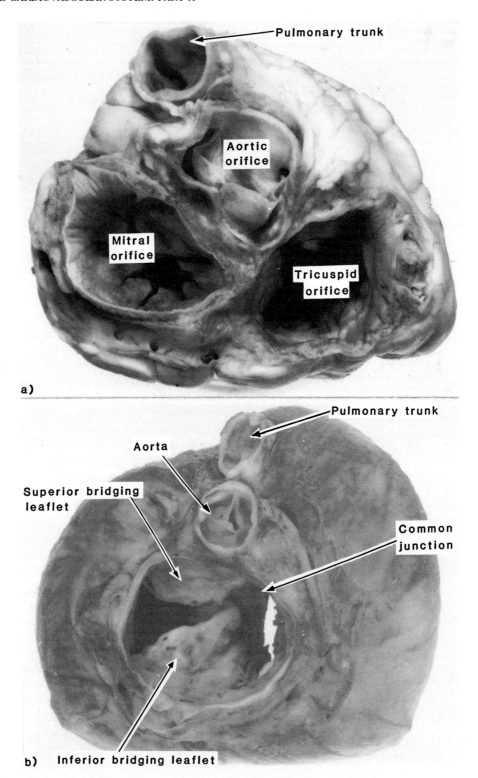

Fig. 7.1 a,b These dissections of the short axis of (**a**) a normal heart and (**b**) an atrioventricular septal defect with a common valve orifice demonstrate the fundamental effect on the atrioventricular junction of deficient atrioventricular septation. The hearts are viewed from the atrial aspect.

THE ANATOMICAL HALLMARKS

Absence of normal atrioventricular septation distorts the anatomy of the atrioventricular junction in at least four distinct ways. Firstly, it produces a common atrioventricular junction with so-called 'unwedging' of the aortic valve. Secondly, absence of normal septation results in formation of a common atrioventricular valve with five leaflets. Thirdly, the unwedged aorta sits above a distinctly narrowed left ventricular outflow tract. Fourthly, there is gross disproportion between the inlet and outlet dimensions of the left ventricular septal surface. Each of these features warrants separate consideration.

The common atrioventricular junction

The arrangement of the atrioventricular junction relative to the aortic valve in the normal heart can be likened to a trefoil (Fig. 7.1a). Absence of the atrioventricular septal structures distorts totally this arrangement. The atrioventricular junction is disposed in an oval arrangement encircling both right and left atrioventricular orifices. The effect is to produce a common atrioventricular orifice guarded by a common valve (Fig. 7.1b). The aortic valve is situated on top of this common junction, producing an arrangement akin to the body (the junction) and the head (the aorta) of a snowman when viewed from above.

The common atrioventricular valve

The common valve guarding the common junction differs from the normal mitral and tricuspid valves, particularly from the mitral valve. This is largely because two of the leaflets are anchored in both right and left ventricles — in other words they are bridging leaflets located in superior and inferior position (Fig. 7.2). This changes the arrangement of the left atrioventricular valve to the extent that it bears scant resemblance to the normal mitral valve. The distinguishing feature of the normal mitral valve is the arrangement of its mural and aortic leaflets. The mural leaflet is long and shallow, occupying two-thirds of the annular circumference of the

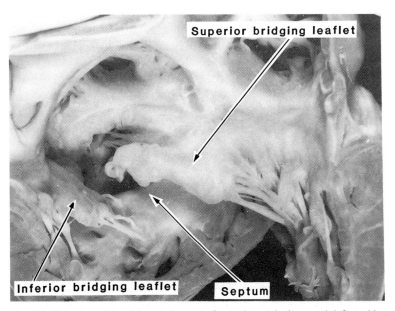

Fig. 7.2 This view of the right-sided aspect of an atrioventricular septal defect with a common valvar orifice shows the morphology of the two leaflets which bridge the ventricular septum, having cordal attachments within both ventricles. The leaflets are found in superior and inferior location when the heart is in the anatomical position.

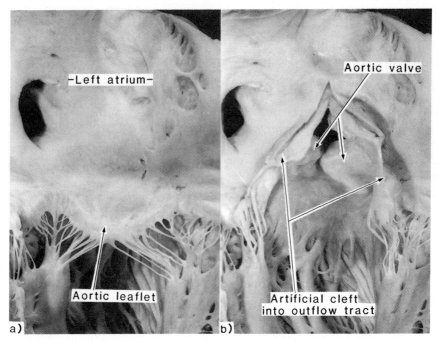

Fig. 7.3 a,b This dissection of the normal heart shows the effect of cleaving the aortic leaflet of the normal mitral valve. Panel (**a**) shows the intact valve. As shown in panel (**b**), the cleft runs into the subaortic outflow tract.

atrioventricular orifice. The aortic leaflet is deeper but shorter, occupying the remaining third of the circumference. An artificial cleavage plane through this leaflet leads into the subaortic outflow tract (Fig. 7.3). The left valve in atrioventricular septal defects, in contrast, possesses three leaflets. The mural leaflet is short, guarding a third (or less) of the left junction. The remainder of the junction is guarded by the left ventricular components of the bridging leaflets (Fig. 7.2). The space between these leaflets has usually been described as a 'cleft' in the 'anterior leaflet of the mitral valve'. In reality, it is a naturally occurring space between the left ventricular components of the bridging leaflets — a commissure (junction) between the leaflets. The left atrioventricular valve in atrioventricular septal defects (Fig. 7.4), therefore, is a three-leaflet structure.[7,8] It bears no resemblance to a 'cleft mitral valve' and is better not described as such. 'Left' valve is both simple and accurate. The difference in leaflet morphology of the common valve is reflected in the anatomy of the support

mechanism within the ventricular mass. The right-sided papillary muscles are essentially the same as their counterparts in the normal heart. The muscles in the left ventricle are markedly different, being found one above the other rather than obliquely situated as in the normal heart (Fig. 7.5).

The subaortic outflow tract

In the normal heart, this tract is interposed between the aortic leaflet of the mitral valve and the septum. It is this arrangement which permits clefts in the mitral valve to open into the outflow tract (Fig. 7.3). In atrioventricular septal defect, the left junction is a component part of the overall junction common to both atrial chambers. The subaortic outflow tract, of necessity, can no longer be situated between this valve and the septum. Instead, it is located anteriorly within the ventricle, being squashed between the junction and the parietal ventricular wall (Fig. 7.4). The extent of the outflow tract, in terms of length

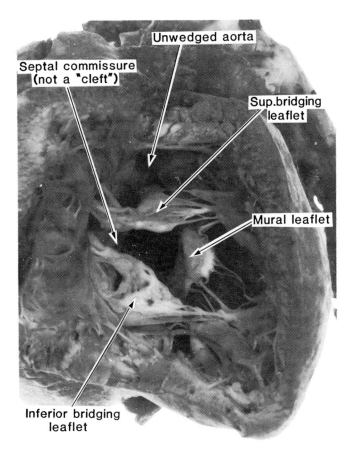

Fig. 7.4 This illustration of the left valve in an atrioventricular septal defect with separate right and left valvar orifices (ostium primum defect) shows the trifoliate arrangement of the leaflets. The structure so often described as a 'cleft' in the anterior leaflet of a mitral valve is, in reality, the space between the left ventricular components of the two leaflets which bridge the ventricular septum.

rather than breadth, depends upon the attachment of the superior bridging leaflet relative to the ventricular septal crest (Fig. 7.6). The outflow tract is much shorter in the presence of a common valve orifice than when there are separate right and left orifices.

Inlet–outlet septal disproportion

In the normal heart, the ratio of inlet and outlet dimensions is more or less unity. In hearts with deficient atrioventricular septation, the outlet dimension is significantly longer than the inlet. In general, the inlet–outlet discrepancy is the same for all atrioventricular septal defects in that, if the valve leaflets are removed from the septum, there is no way of distinguishing whether the heart initially had a common valve orifice or fell into the group of 'primum' defects (Fig. 7.7). When account is taken of the degree of deficiency of the ventricular septum, however, there is greater septal deficiency in the group of hearts with a common atrioventricular orifice.[9]

THE COMMON FEATURES OF ATRIOVENTRICULAR SEPTAL DEFECTS

In the next section, we describe the features which permit categorization of the different forms of

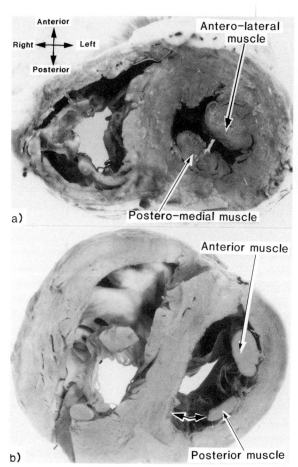

Fig. 7.5 a,b These views of the ventricular aspect of the short axis of (**a**) a normal heart and (**b**) an atrioventricular septal defect show the different orientation of the left ventricular papillary muscles in the setting of deficient atrioventricular septation.

atrioventricular septal defect. Two features, however, are common to all defects, namely the disposition of the conduction tissues and the basic arrangement of the left ventricular outflow tract.

The atrioventricular conduction axis

The atrioventricular conduction axis in the normal heart is carried on the atrial surface of the muscular atrioventricular septum and penetrates through the membranous atrioventricular septum to reach the subaortic outflow tract. Deficient atrioventricular septation distorts this arrange-

ment.[10,11] The ventricular component of the axis is carried on the crest of the ventricular septum but, by virtue of the anterior location of the subaortic outflow tract, is not related to the latter structure. The bundle branches are disposed across the scooped-out part of the septum. There is then a long non-branching bundle which ascends the inlet septum and penetrates into the atrial tissues at the crux of the heart. From the atrial aspect, this is marked by a nodal triangle (Fig. 7.8) which is distinct from the triangle of Koch. The triangle of Koch (Ch. 1) occupies its regular position within the lower extent of the atrial septum and does not house the atrioventricular node. The nodal triangle is formed by the postero-inferior leading edge of the atrial septum, the atrioventricular junction and the mouth of the coronary sinus.

The subaortic outflow tract

One of the anatomical features common to all atrioventricular septal defects is the relatively narrow subaortic outflow tract. As described above, this feature reflects the unwedged position of the aortic valve. Clinical information indicates that the narrowed tract does not, in itself, produce obstruction to left ventricular outflow, but any lesion which further narrows the tract very rapidly produces overt obstruction.[12,13] Malformations producing such obstruction include tissue tags derived from adjacent valvar or fibrous tissues, a septal bulge, anomalous attachment of the tension apparatus of the left atrioventricular valve or a fibrous subaortic shelf. The outflow tract is much more susceptible to such stenosis when there are separate right and left atrioventricular orifices. This is because the tethering of the superior bridging leaflet to the septum increases the length of the outflow tract (Fig. 7.6).

DIFFERENT TYPES OF ATRIOVENTRICULAR SEPTAL DEFECT

Although atrioventricular septal defects present almost similar anatomical appearances, they can differ markedly in their clinical manifestations.

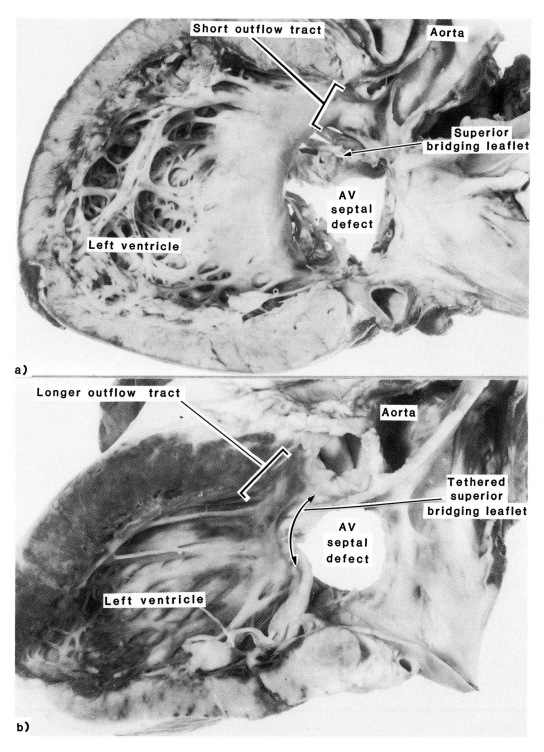

Fig. 7.6 a,b These two specimens, one with a common valvar orifice (**a**) and the other (**b**) with separate right and left orifices (ostium primum defect), show how the length of the left ventricular outflow tract is dependent upon the attachment of the superior bridging leaflet. When this is firmly attached to the ventricular septum (as in panel **b**), the outflow tract is much longer than with a floating leaflet (panel **a**).

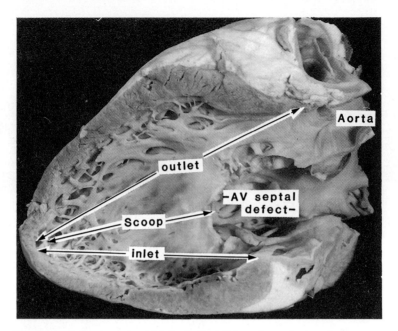

Fig. 7.7 This specimen, in which the leaflets of the atrioventricular valve have been removed from the ventricular mass, illustrates the fundamental inlet–outlet septal disproportion of hearts with deficient atrioventricular septation.

There are other important anatomical differences within the ostensibly similar group which account for this clinical variability. These concern the morphology of the bridging leaflets of the common atrioventricular valve and their relation to the septal structures.

Common versus separate atrioventricular orifices

The most fundamental difference is whether the common atrioventricular junction is guarded by a common valve or by a valve supported by a common junction but divided into right and left orifices. This depends upon the relation of the bridging leaflets one to another. A common atrioventricular orifice requires the bridging leaflets to be discrete structures restricted to the superior and inferior quadrants of the atrioventricular orifice (Fig. 7.9a). This variant is often called a 'complete' defect but it is better simply to call it one with a common valvar orifice. The counterpart to this arrangement is when the facing surfaces of the bridging leaflets are themselves joined by a tongue of valve tissue running along the crest of the ventricular septum. Although not necessarily fused to the septal crest (see below), the presence of this tongue joining the bridging leaflets means that the common junction is guarded by separate right and left atrioventricular valvar orifices (Fig. 7.9b). This variant with separate valves has been described as the 'partial' type of atrioventricular septal defect, and as an 'ostium primum defect', but it is preferable simply to describe the separate right and left atrioventricular orifices.

The potential for physiological shunting of blood through the septal defect

The real key to the clinical presentation of these malformations is the potential for physiological shunting of blood through the atrioventricular septal defect which can then be compounded by additional deficiencies of the atrial or ventric-

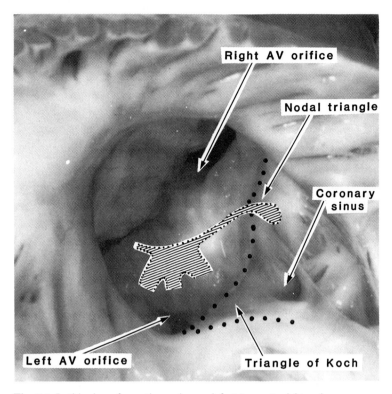

Fig. 7.8 In this view of an ostium primum defect (separate right and left atrioventricular [AV] orifices) viewed from the right atrium in surgical orientation, the location of the conduction axis (hatched area) has been superimposed on the anatomical structures. Note that the node is contained within a nodal triangle (dots) rather than the regular triangle of Koch and that the axis is hidden beneath the inferior bridging leaflet.

ular septum or by the presence of an arterial duct. Here we are concerned with shunting through the atrioventricular septal defect itself. The potential for shunting relates to the way the bridging leaflets are attached to the septal structures. The feature of the so-called 'primum' defect is that the bridging leaflets of the common valve, along with the connecting tongue, are depressed into the ventricular mass and fused to the crest of the ventricular septum (Fig. 7.9b). This means that the shunting through the atrioventricular septal defect is confined to the atrial level, albeit that most of the shunt occurs below the level of the atrioventricular junction. When the bridging leaflets are separate structures (common orifice), the leaflets themselves almost always 'float' to various degrees, being unattached

to the adjacent atrial and ventricular septal structures. When they float in this fashion, the potential exists for shunt at both atrial and ventricular levels. The extent of shunting will depend upon the degree of tethering of the bridging leaflets (the ventricular communication) along with the size of the orifice between the atrial aspect of the leaflets and the lower edge of the atrial septum (the atrial communication—see Fig. 7.9a). The potential for ventricular as well as atrial shunting can also exist in hearts with separate orifices if the connecting tongue and the bridging leaflets are not firmly fused to the underlying ventricular septum (Fig. 7.10).

There is then one additional arrangement of the bridging leaflets which affects the potential for shunting through the atrioventricular septal

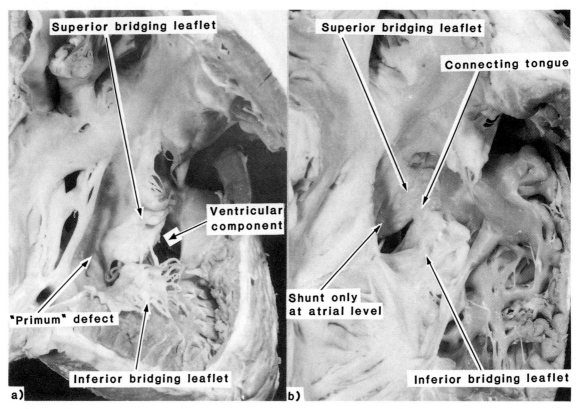

Fig. 7.9 a,b These hearts, viewed from the right side, show that the basic difference between a heart with a common valvar orifice (**a**) and one with separate right and left orifices (ostium primum, panel **b**) is the presence of a connecting tongue of leaflet tissue between the bridging leaflets in the latter lesion.

defect. We have described attachment of the bridging leaflets to the atrial septum and the arrangement by which they float, but there is also the situation where the leaflets are attached to the underside of the atrial septum (Fig. 7.11). This arrangement confines the potential for shunting to ventricular level and produces a ventricular septal defect due to deficient atrioventricular septation. Hearts of this type have all the morphological stigmas of atrioventricular septal defects, which are to be distinguished from large perimembranous ventricular septal defects opening to the inlet of the right ventricle and from defects associated with straddling tricuspid valves. The hearts of the latter group, although often described as 'ventricular septal defect of atrioventricular type' have none of the anatomical features of atrioventricular septal defects. It follows that the major differentiating features of atrioventric-

ular septal defects can be accounted for by describing separately the arrangement of the leaflets of the atrioventricular valve (common orifice or separate orifices) and the potential for shunting through the defect (at atrial, ventricular or atrioventricular levels). When described in this fashion, there is no need further to complicate categorization by the introduction of 'transitional'[2] or 'intermediate' variants.

The morphology of the bridging leaflets

Rastelli and his colleagues[14] have written extensively concerning the arrangement of the superior bridging leaflet and its significance for surgical repair. Analysis of the entire spectrum of atrioventricular septal defects, however, suggests that the Rastelli approach can be expanded.[15] Rastelli

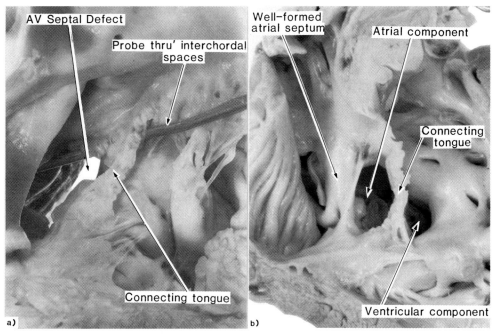

Fig. 7.10 a,b These two hearts, both with separate right and left valvar orifices, show that ventricular shunting can occur with this valvar arrangement when the bridging leaflets are not fused to the crest of the ventricular septum. The communication is minimal in the heart shown in panel (**a**) (probe through intercordal spaces) but is large in the specimen seen in panel (**b**).

and his colleagues[14] noted that the arrangement of the superior bridging leaflet itself could be considered a variable in defects with a common orifice. They identified three variants (types A, B and C) which we interpret as a spectrum of anatomy having its starting point in the lesions with separate right and left atrioventricular orifices. If the 'septal' leaflet of the right valve is studied in hearts with separate orifices, a minority of cases will reveal formation of discrete free-standing leaflets (Fig. 7.12a). Usually, the superior part of the leaflet seems to be absent. Close examination then shows that the superior leaflet and the connecting tongue are turned in as they cross the septum to achieve a linear attachment along the right ventricular surface of the septum (Fig. 7.12b). It is then a short step from this arrangement to recognize the variant described by Rastelli and his colleagues[14] as their 'type A'. In this pattern, there is a common valvar orifice and the superior leaflet barely crosses the septum (Fig. 7.13). It is attached to

the septum by multiple short cords which limit the interventricular communication beneath the leaflet. The end of the leaflet, nonetheless, is tethered to the medial papillary muscle within the right ventricle. The division between the superior bridging and the anterosuperior leaflets is a commissure directly comparable with the anteroseptal commissure of the normal tricuspid valve.[16] The other morphological characteristics noted by Rastelli and his colleagues (their types B and C) are readily accounted for in terms of increasing commitment of the superior leaflet to the right ventricle (Fig. 7.14). As the superior leaflet bridges more into the right ventricle, so the papillary muscle supporting its junction with the antero-superior leaflet moves down the surface of the septomarginal trabeculation until, in the extreme form, the bridging part of the superior leaflet is supported by a large anterior papillary muscle and the anterosuperior leaflet is markedly reduced in size. In effect, the extent of the antero-

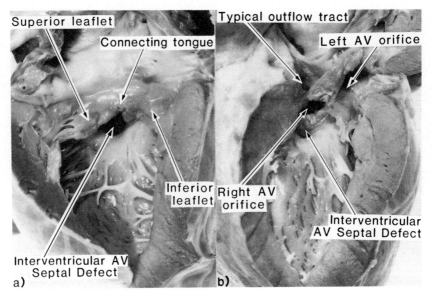

Fig. 7.11 a,b In this atrioventricular septal defect with separate right and left valvar orifices, the bridging leaflets are firmly fused to the underside of the atrial septum. As seen from the left atrium (panel **a**), the effect of this arrangement is to obliterate the 'ostium primum' defect. As shown from the left ventricle (panel **b**), shunting through the atrioventricular (AV) septal defect then occurs only at ventricular level. The effect of this morphology is to produce an isolated ventricular shunt in the setting of an atrioventricular septal defect.

superior leaflet within the right ventricle is inversely related to the extent of bridging of the superior leaflet. It is a general rule that the more the superior leaflet bridges the less well is it tethered to the septum. Variation is also to be found in the arrangement of the inferior bridging leaflet.[16] The important feature in this respect is the extent of bridging into the left ventricle. Here there is an inverse relationship between the extent of bridging and the size of the left ventricular mural leaflet. The inferior leaflet also shows variability in its tethering. It may be firmly attached by a raphe as it crosses the septum or by multiple short cords, or it may float freely.[16] This variability is independent of the arrangement of the superior leaflet.

ASSOCIATED MALFORMATIONS

So far, we have been concerned with the basic

morphology of atrioventricular septal defects. In any individual case, associated lesions in other parts of the heart must be anticipated. Some lesions are sufficiently frequent to be considered an integral part of the malformation — as, for example, a particular association with atrial isomerism. An atrioventricular septal defect is also the most frequent cardiovascular anomaly found in Down's syndrome. We are more concerned here with other lesions of the heart in patients with usual atrial arrangement. Deficiency of the atrial septum has already been mentioned and most examples of 'common atrium' will be seen in association with an atrioventricular septal defect. Malformations of the left ventricular outflow tract have also been discussed in some depth. The major lesions to be considered now are those affecting the atrioventricular valves, the sharing of the atrioventricular junction between the atrial and ventricular chambers, and the morphology of the ventricular outflow tracts.

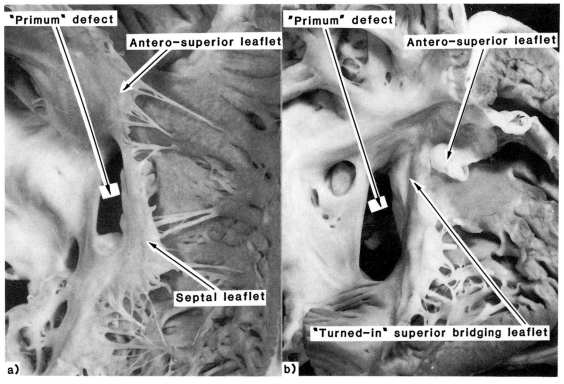

Fig. 7.12 a,b These hearts, viewed from the right side, both have an atrioventricular septal defect with separate right and left valvar orifices (ostium primum). They show the different morphology of the right-sided valve. In panel (**a**), there is a discrete septal leaflet fused by a midline raphe to the underlying septum. In panel (**b**), the connecting tongue and superior bridging leaflet are themselves attached firmly to the septal crest, so that there is no formation of free-standing leaflet tissue superiorly along the septum.

Lesions of the atrioventricular valves

The major malformations in this category are multiple orifices and anomalies of the papillary muscles. The lesion with separate right and left atrioventricular valves (the 'primum' defect) can be considered as a dual orifice in a common atrioventricular valve. Dual orifices are also found in the left valve as associated anomalies and, sometimes, in the right. They are produced by the same mechanism which converts a common orifice into separate right and left orifices. A tongue of leaflet tissue extends to connect the facing surfaces of two adjacent leaflets, at the same time dividing the orifice (Fig. 7.15). This arrangement is usually associated with distortion of the supporting papillary muscles, but the muscles themselves can be anomalously formed.

The most severe example of this is seen in the so-called 'parachute' lesion[17] affecting the left valve in such a way that a solitary muscle supports the leaflet tissue, usually in association with a diminutive or absent mural leaflet (Fig. 7.16). The extreme form of this anomaly results in an imperforate left component of the atrioventricular valve and, usually, gross hypoplasia of the left ventricle.

Commitment of the atrioventricular junction

In most examples, the atrioventricular junction is shared in more or less equal fashion between the atrial and ventricular chambers — the so-called balanced defect.[18] In some cases there is dominance of one or other side of the heart. Right

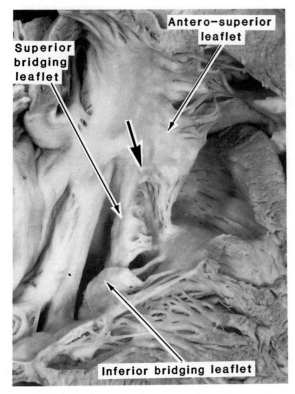

Fig. 7.13 This view of an atrioventricular septal defect with a common valvar orifice and minimal bridging of the superior leaflet shows marked similarity to the 'primum' defect illustrated in Fig. 7.12b except that there is no fusion between the bridging leaflets and there are intercordal spaces between the superior bridging leaflet and the septum. The commissure between the superior bridging leaflet and the antero-superior leaflet of the right ventricle (short arrow) is supported on the infundibular aspect by the medial papillary muscle.

ventricular dominance with hypoplasia of the left ventricle (Fig. 7.17) carries a particularly poor prognosis, since almost always this variant is associated also with coarctation or interruption of the aortic arch. If series of hearts are studied, a progression can be made between right ventricular dominance and the presence of double inlet right ventricle. A similar progression can be noted between left ventricular dominance and double inlet left ventricle. Malalignment between the septal structures in this setting produces an abnormal location of the atrioventricular conduction axis. Malalignment of the septal structures is also important in the context of unequal sharing of the atrioventricular junction between the atrial chambers. When the atrial septum is eccentrically positioned, one or other atrium connects to both ventricles, the other atrium then communicating with the rest of the heart through the 'ostium primum' defect (Fig. 7.18). Some authors call this arrangement 'double outlet atrium'.[19]

Malformation of the outflow tracts

In most examples of atrioventricular septal defect, the ventriculo–arterial connexions are concordant and the right ventricular outflow tract is unobstructed. Obstruction to the left ventricular outflow, potential and real, is well recognized and has been described above. Right ventricular outflow obstruction can also occur as an associated lesion, most often in tetralogy of Fallot. This frequently co-exists with shunting through the atrioventricular septal defect at ventricular level, but can be found with the more typical defects. Usually there is a common atrioventricular orifice and the superior leaflet exhibits extreme bridging and is free-floating. Double outlet right ventricle also occurs with some frequency, particularly in association with atrial isomerism, with or without a bilateral infundibulum. This combination is found most frequently with a free-floating superior bridging leaflet.

NATURAL HISTORY AS AFFECTED BY SURGERY

Unlike ventricular septal defect, it is very rare for an atrioventricular septal defect spontaneously to diminish in size or to close, but we have seen one heart which had all the morphological stigmata of an atrioventricular septal defect yet had intact septal structures.[20] The morphological findings suggested that a defect permitting an interatrial communication had closed during fetal development. We have also seen a heart in which a defect permitting an interatrial communication was virtually closed by formation of tissue tags from the bridging leaflets and the connecting tongue (Fig. 7.19). Formation of 'pouch lesions' from the superior bridging leaflets in cases with separate

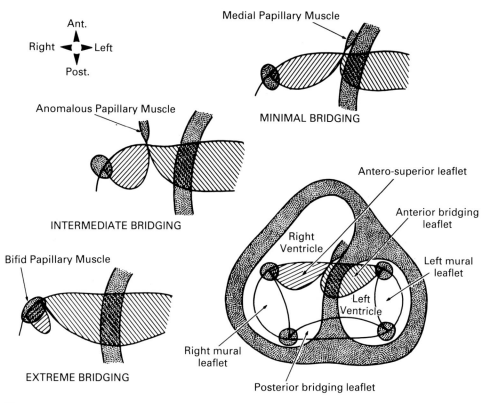

Fig. 7.14 This diagram, illustrating the ventricular aspect of the short axis seen from beneath, shows the continuation of the spectrum of bridging of the superior leaflet demonstrated in Figs 7.12 and 7.13. This is the morphology described by Rastelli and his colleagues[14] in terms of types A–C. An example of the so-called type C, with extreme bridging, is seen in Fig. 7.2.

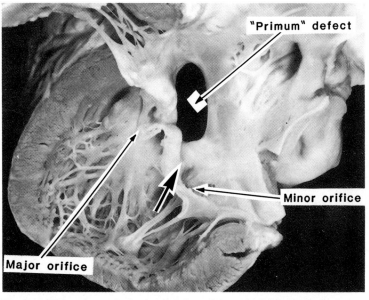

Fig. 7.15 This atrioventricular septal defect, with separate right and left valve orifices, has dual orifices in the left valve by virtue of a tongue of leaflet tissue (short arrow) connecting the inferior and mural leaflets.

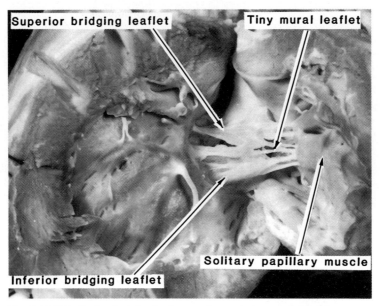

Fig. 7.16 This diminutive left valve in an atrioventricular septal defect is supported by a solitary papillary muscle, the so-called 'parachute' deformity. Note the small size of the mural leaflet.

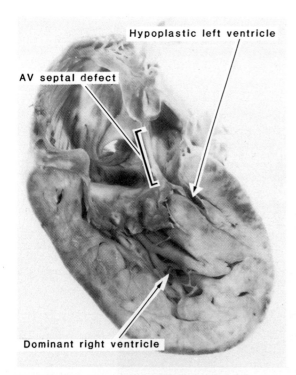

Fig. 7.17 This simulated 'four chamber' section shows an atrioventricular septal defect with separate right and left valve orifices and marked right ventricular dominance.

orifices is well recognized, but rarely to the extent that they virtually close the defect. Important features in the natural history of the lesion are the development of atrioventricular conduction disturbances and regurgitation through the left atrioventricular valve. Both of these mechanisms can occur simply with increasing age and may be arrested by surgery. The conduction problems are due to fibrosis within the long non-branching bundle and it remains to be proved that they can be circumvented by early surgical repair. Regurgitation through the left valve can certainly be prevented or alleviated by surgery. Equally, the process can be made worse by surgery. The key to success is recognition of the basically trifoliate valvar anatomy. The other major feature determining natural history is the state of the pulmonary vasculature. Unless the defect is relieved by surgical measures, irreversible pulmonary vascular disease occurs in a significant proportion of patients with a common atrioventricular orifice during the first year of life. A recent study showed significant changes already to be present during the period from 7–12 months of age.[21] It remains unresolved

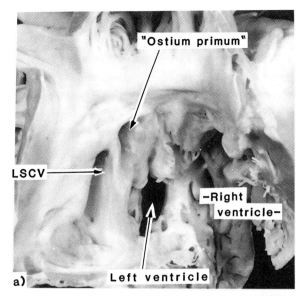

a)

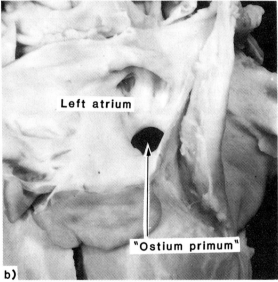

b)

Fig. 7.18 a,b This atrioventricular septal defect is characterized by marked malalignment between the atrial septum and the ventricular septum. The atrial septum connects to virtually the left parietal border of the junction (note also the persistent left superior caval vein [LSCV] draining to the coronary sinus). The right atrium, in consequence, drains to both ventricles (panel **a**) while the left atrium exits through the ostium primum (panel **b**).

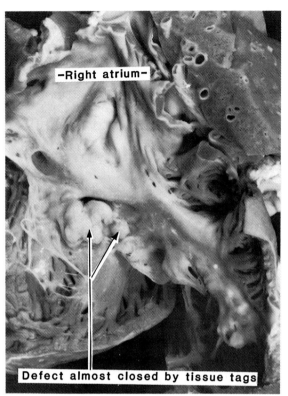

Fig. 7.19 In this atrioventricular septal defect with separate right and left valve orifices, the defect is virtually blocked by tissue tags derived from the bridging leaflets.

whether patients with Down's syndrome have a more reactive pulmonary vasculature, but patients with this syndrome show the most severe lesions.

REFERENCES

1. Bedford DE, Sellors TH, Somerville W, Belcher JR, Besterman EMM. Atrial septal defect and its surgical treatment. Lancet 1957; 1: 1255–1261.
2. Wakai CS, Edwards JE. Pathologic study of persistent common atrioventricular canal. Am Heart J 1958; 56: 779–794.
3. Campbell M, Missen GAK. Endocardial cushion defects: common atrioventricular canal and ostium primum. Br Heart J 1957; 19: 403–418.
4. Becker AE, Anderson RH. Atrioventricular septal defects. What's in a name? J Thorac Cardiovasc Surg 1982; 83: 461–469.
5. Di Segni E, Edwards JE. Cleft anterior leaflet of the mitral valve with intact septa. A study of 20 cases. Am J Cardiol 1983; 51: 919–926.
6. Neufeld HN, Titus JL, Dushane JW, Burchell HB, Edwards JE. Isolated ventricular septal defect of the persistent common atrioventricular canal type. Circulation 1961; 23: 685–696.
7. Peacock TB. Malformation of the heart consisting in an imperfection of the auricular and ventricular septa. Trans Pathol Soc (London) 1846; 1: 61–62.
8. Carpentier A. Surgical anatomy and management of the mitral component of atrioventricular canal defects. In: Anderson RH, Shinebourne EA, eds. Paediatric cardiology. Edinburgh: Churchill Livingstone, 1978; 477–486.
9. Anderson RH, Ebels TJ, Zuberbuhler JR, Silverman NH. Anatomical and echocardiographic features of the left valve in atrioventricular septal defect. In: Anderson RH, Neches WH, Park SC, Zuberbuhler JR eds. Perspectives in pediatric cardiology, vol. 1. New York: Futura, 1988; 299–310.
10. Lev M. The architecture of the conduction system in congenital heart disease. I. Common atrioventricular orifice. Arch Pathol 1958; 65: 174–191.
11. Thiene G, Wenink ACG, Frescura C, Wilkinson JL, Gallucci V, Ho SY, Anderson RH. The surgical anatomy of the conduction tissues in atrioventricular defects. J Thorac Cardiovasc Surg 1981; 82: 928–937.
12. Piccoli GP, Ho SY, Wilkinson JL, Macartney FJ, Gerlis LM, Anderson RH. Left sided obstructive lesions in atrioventricular septal defects. J Thorac Cardiovasc Surg 1982; 83: 453–460.
13. Lappen RS, Muster AJ, Idriss FS et al. Masked subaortic stenosis in ostium primum atrial septal defect: recognition and treatment. Am J Cardiol 1983; 52: 336–340.
14. Rastelli GC, Kirklin JW, Titus JL. Anatomic observations on complete form of persistent common atrioventricular canal with special reference to atrioventricular valves. Mayo Clin Proc 1966; 41: 296–308.
15. Penkoske PA, Neches WH, Anderson RH, Zuberbuhler JR. Further observations on the morphology of atrioventricular septal defects. J Thorac Cardiovasc Surg 1985; 90: 611–622.
16. Anderson RH, Zuberbuhler JR, Penkoske PA, Neches WH. Of clefts, commissures and things. J Thorac Cardiovasc Surg 1985; 90: 605–610.
17. David I, Castaneda AR, Van Praagh R. Potentially parachute mitral valve in common atrioventricular canal. J Thorac Cardiovasc Surg 1982; 84: 178–186.
18. Bharati S, Lev M. The spectrum of common atrioventricular orifice (canal). Am Heart J 1973; 86: 553–561.
19. Van Mierop LHS. Pathology and pathogenesis of endocardial cushion defects. Surgical implications. In: David JC, ed. Second Henry Ford Hospital International Symposium on Cardiac Surgery. New York: Appleton-Century-Crofts, 1977; 201–207.
20. Silverman NH, Ho SY, Anderson RH, Smith A, Wilkinson JL. Atrioventricular septal defect with intact atrial and ventricular septal structures. Int J Cardiol 1984; 5: 567–572.
21. Frescura C, Thiene G, Franceschini E, Talenti E, Mazzucco A. Pulmonary vascular disease in infants with complete atrioventricular septal defect. Int J Cardiol 1987; 15: 91–100.

Ventricular septal defect

INTRODUCTION

Communications between the ventricular chambers are the commonest congenital cardiac lesions which will confront the pathologist either in isolation or as part of a more complex malformation. When found as an associated lesion, they can be an integral part of the circulatory pathways (as in double outlet or double inlet ventricle, common arterial trunk, or atrioventricular or arterial valve atresia) or they can be complicating lesions (as in complete or corrected transposition). The particular morphology of the defects as they exist in these various settings will be described at the appropriate points. In this chapter, we will be concerned with the categorization and description of otherwise 'isolated' defects. The principles used for description and categorization, nonetheless, are applicable in all circumstances and will be used (when writing of them) throughout this section of the book.

CATEGORIZATION

Several features can be used to catalogue ventricular septal defects. Some authorities use a system based upon embryology. We do not. Even those who depart from morphological premises, however, find ample room for disagreement. This is because they choose different features as their primary criterion. All of these features are important and, when pertinent, all should be described. It is not our place as morphologists to grade their practical value. Instead, we prefer simply to describe the various features. The features which warrant description are size, location within the septum, the morphological nature of the boundaries, the relationship to atrioventricular and arterial valves, the relationship to the atrioventricular conduction axis, and the relationship to structures which may have promoted spontaneous closure during life. All of these features can readily be described in simple and unambiguous terms. At the same time, some 'shorthand' terms are now well established in the vocabulary (or jargon) of ventricular septal defects. When using these terms, we will describe our understanding of them and then use them in our understood fashion.

SIZE OF DEFECT

The size of a ventricular septal defect is crucial in determining the prevailing haemodynamics and the chances of spontaneous closure. In clinical terms, defects are considered restrictive when the shunt through them is insufficient to equalize ventricular pressures. They are described as non-restrictive when the ventricular pressures are equal. The pathologist will not always have the benefit of knowing the measured pressures within the ventricles during life so must grade the dimensions as best he can. Measuring the area or diameter of the defect is probably best, but this must then be compared with some yardstick such as the size of the heart or, better, the diameter of the aortic root. When there is overriding of an arterial valve, it will be necessary to take note of both right and left ventricular borders of the cone of space enclosed beneath the valvar orifice (see below). At least, the defect can simply be described as small, medium or large.

POSITION OF THE DEFECT WITHIN THE VENTRICULAR SEPTUM

Almost always until now, ventricular septal defects have been described in the setting of the normal ventricular septum. This convention is less than ideal because some defects, when compared with the normal heart, occupy areas which are not usually interventricular.[1] The best

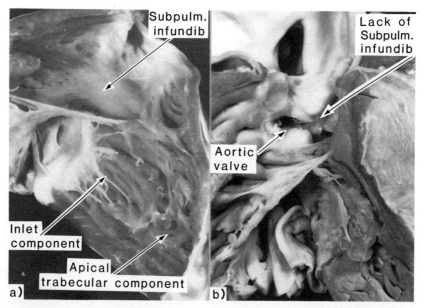

Fig. 8.1 a,b These views of the right ventricular aspect of a normal heart (**a**) and a so-called 'supracristal' defect (**b**) show how the defect occupies the 'septal' aspect of the subpulmonary infundibulum. This part of the 'septum' is, in reality, part of the outer wall of the heart (see Fig. 8.2).

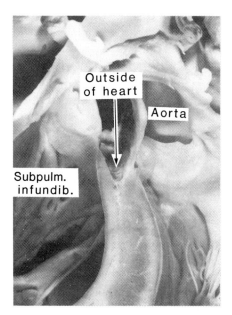

Fig. 8.2 A long axis section of the normal right ventricle showing how both arterial valves are supported on sleeves of subarterial musculature which are not interventricular septal structures. The entire anatomy of this region must be distorted in the setting of a defect between the subaortic and subpulmonary outlet components.

example is the so-called 'supracristal' defect (Fig. 8.1), which has been presumed to result from absence of the outlet component of the ventricular septum. It tends to be conceptualized as occupying the subpulmonary infundibular area of the normal right ventricle. The problem with

this approach[2-4] is that, in the normal heart, most of the subpulmonary infundibulum is not a septal structure (Fig. 8.2). When a defect occupies the site of the normal subpulmonary infundibulum, therefore, the inference can be made, firstly, that the heart containing the defect is dissimilar to the normal heart and, secondly, that development has occurred in an abnormal fashion. Presence of the hole cannot be interpreted simply in terms of arrested development of the normal septum. Other problems can be found in current terminologies because of the dissimilarity between the right and left ventricular aspects of the normal septum. These septal surfaces do not match each other in perfect fashion (in other words, with the right ventricular outlet component directly opposed to its left ventricular counterpart, and so on). This has been demonstrated above with regard to the subpulmonary infundibulum and the lack of an 'outlet septum' in the normal heart (Fig. 8.2). Similar lack of 'matching' is found in the ventricular inlets. Part of the atrioventricular junction of the normal heart is an atrioventricular septal structure. Defects found at this site have their own particular morphology (see Ch. 7). Some of these defects permit only interventricular shunting. In this respect, they are appropriately termed ventricular septal defects. They are also, nonetheless, atrioventricular septal defects and therefore are dealt with in Chapter 7. There are other problems which arise from the non-

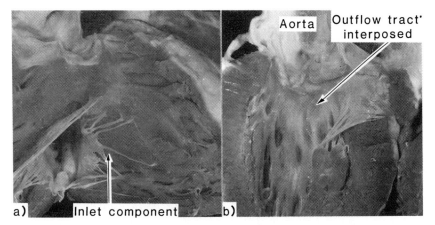

Fig. 8.3 a,b Comparative views of the right (**a**) and left (**b**) ventricular inlet components. Note that the tricuspid valve is directly adherent to the septum while the subaortic outlet intervenes between the mitral valve and the septum.

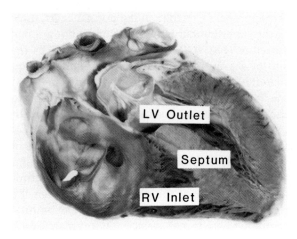

Fig. 8.4 A simulated subcostal section in the paracoronal plane showing how the postero-inferior part of the muscular ventricular septum separates the right ventricular inlet from the left ventricular outlet.

matching arrangement of the ventricular inlet components. The septal leaflet of the morphologically tricuspid valve hugs closely the ventricular inlet septum so that the attachments of its tendinous cords delineate well the right ventricular extent of this septum (Fig. 8.3a). In the left ventricle, however, the mitral valve is largely separated from the septum by the extensive posterior component of the subaortic outflow tract

(Fig. 8.3b). This means that the part of the septum beneath the septal leaflet of the tricuspid valve, perceived from the right ventricle as an inlet septum, separates in reality the right ventricular inlet from the left ventricular outlet (Fig. 8.4). It is more accurate to describe this as an inlet/outlet septum. It is incorrect to speak of defects 'excavating' or 'extending into' an inlet septum. It is better to describe such defects as opening to the inlet of the right ventricle. We must, therefore, choose our terms carefully so that we may accurately describe the position of defects within the septum. This is because, despite the caveats listed above, it remains both advantageous and necessary to account for the location of defects relative to the confines of the normal septum.

When considered in this fashion, it can be said that the majority of ventricular septal defects are found adjacent to that area of septum bordering the inner curvature of the heart, a part which is normally composed of fibrous tissue. The area of fibrous tissue is the so-called membranous septum (Fig. 8.5). This term also has deficiencies. A heart may lack an interventricular membranous septum.[5] In hearts that have one, the structure thus described bears little resemblance to a diaphanous membrane. For better or worse, however, the concept of a 'membranous septum'

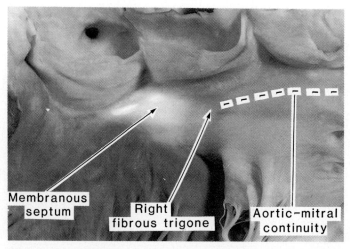

Fig. 8.5 The membranous component of the ventricular septum is shown from its left ventricular aspect. Note how it is directly continuous with the area of fibrous continuity between the aortic and mitral valves.

is firmly embedded within the corpus of cardiological knowledge. It is important, therefore, to know its nature. As described in Chapter 1, the membranous septum is part of the fibrous skeleton of the heart, specifically of that part known as the central fibrous body. It provides an area of continuity between the aortic and tricuspid valves. The area itself, by virtue of its own continuity with the right fibrous trigone, extends so as to be continuous with the aortic leaflet of the mitral valve. More significantly, it is through this membranous septal component of the central fibrous body that the atrioventricular conduction axis runs to pass from right atrium to the crest of the muscular ventricular septum. Most ventricular septal defects are positioned directly adjacent to this 'membranous' area of the septum. It is a mistake, nonetheless, to imagine that the defects result from absence of this particular fibrous septal structure. Part of this 'membranous' septum always persists in hearts with ventricular septal defects, either as an atrioventricular structure or as a fold of fibrous tissue in the margin of the defect. The interventricular communications exist, therefore, because of deficiency of the muscular ventricular septum in the environs of the central fibrous body.

Such defects, when seen from the right ventricle, can occupy different areas of the septum. Some may be centrally placed, extending around the inner heart curvature in the area of valvar fibrous continuity. These may be relatively small (Fig. 8.6a) or extensive. When large, they can occupy a considerable area between the inlet and outlet components of the right ventricle (Fig. 8.6b). They can then be described as confluent. Other defects in this area may be more confined so that they open specifically to the inlet component or to the outlet component of the right ventricle. The 'watershed' between these variants is the location of the medial papillary muscle of the tricuspid valve. Defects opening to the inlet are postero-inferior to this muscle (Fig. 8.7a): they can also be described as 'subtricuspid'. The defect opening to the outlet is antero-superior and cephalad to the medial papillary complex (Fig. 8.7b). It is separated from the pulmonary valve by the persisting component of the subpulmonary infundibulum but is appropriately described as 'subaortic' because of its relationship to the 'wedged' position of the aortic valve within the left ventricle. Often, however, the aortic valve occupies a much more prominent location relative to the defect because it overrides the septum. The outlet component of the septum itself is then much more prominent and is deviated into the right ventricle (Fig. 8.8).

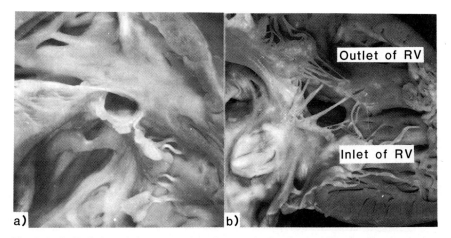

Fig. 8.6 a,b Both these defects are perimembranous in that they are directly adjacent to an area of fibrous continuity between the aortic and tricuspid valves. The defect shown in (**a**), however, is a small defect opening beneath the inner curvature of the heart. In contrast, that shown in (**b**), also beneath the inner curvature, extends to open into both the inlet and outlet components of the right ventricle. Such a defect is termed confluent.

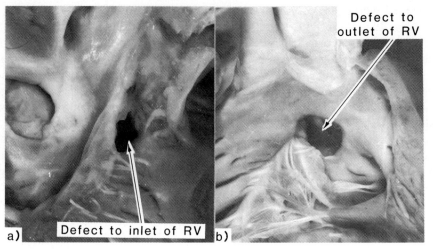

Fig. 8.7 a,b These two defects, both roofed by an area of fibrous continuity between the aortic and tricuspid valves (perimembranous defects), open (**a**) to the inlet and (**b**) to the outlet of the right ventricle.

Moreover, the leaflets of the aortic valve achieve attachments to both right and left ventricular structures, this arrangement being the very basis of 'override'. In the presence of such override, the

nature of the defect becomes more complicated, and may be described as being 'juxta-aortic'. This will be dealt with below.

The common feature of all defects considered thus far is that all are directly adjacent to the central fibrous body, despite the fact that their position within the septum varies markedly. Defects can also occupy similar areas of the septum when they are separated from the central fibrous body. These defects, which are within the substance of the muscular septum, can also open to the inlet of the right ventricle and be subtricuspid (Fig. 8.9). Alternatively, they can be located within the apical trabecular part of the septum, either centrally within this septal component or in its different parts (Fig. 8.10). Defects can be also embedded within the muscular septum yet open to the right ventricular outlet (Fig. 8.11). Such defects cannot be distinguished from those adjacent to the central fibrous body simply by describing their location within the septum. Still another defect is well and accurately described as opening to the outlet of the right ventricle. This particular defect is characterized by fibrous continuity between the facing leaflets of the aortic and pulmonary valves (Fig. 8.12). It is, in this respect, subpulmonary. But then, so is the defect embedded within the septum in which only a tiny muscle rim

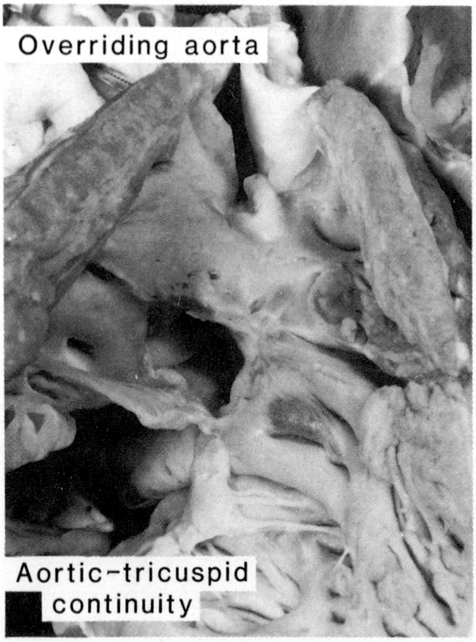

Fig. 8.8 This defect, in which part of the border is made up of fibrous continuity between the aortic and tricuspid valves (perimembranous defect) is also associated with overriding of the aortic valve.

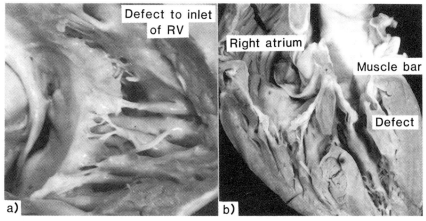

Fig. 8.9 a,b This defect opening into the inlet component of the right ventricle (**a**) is separated by musculature of the inlet septum from the atrioventricular junction (**b**). It is a muscular inlet defect.

interposes between the edge of the defect and the pulmonary valve. Defects cannot adequately be differentiated simply in terms of their position within the septum. Such position is of great importance but equally important is

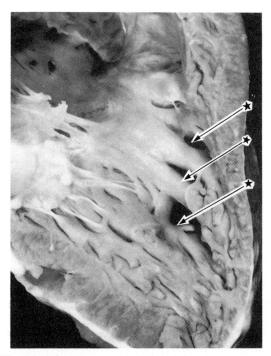

Fig. 8.10 These multiple muscular defects (asterisks), viewed from their right ventricular aspect, occupy the anterior trabecular part of the muscular septum.

the nature of the boundaries of the individual defects.

THE BOUNDARIES OF THE DEFECT

In describing the boundaries of a given defect, the pathologist has the inestimable advantage over the clinician of seeing all its aspects. There are three distinct anatomical patterns, two of which can co-exist.

Defects in part bordered by valvar fibrous continuity predominantly between the atrioventricular valves

The greater majority of defects are directly adjacent to the central fibrous body. Part of their border, therefore, is formed by valvar fibrous continuity. In the normally constructed heart, the continuity will be between the tricuspid, aortic and mitral valves (Fig. 8.13). The precise portion of the border made up of such continuity, and the amount of border contributed by the various valves, will depend upon the position of the defect relative to the septum and according to whether or not there is overriding of the aortic valve. Always, nonetheless, the fibrous tissue forms a direct margin of this kind of defect, which is most simply described as being directly adjacent to the central fibrous body. Initially, however, they were

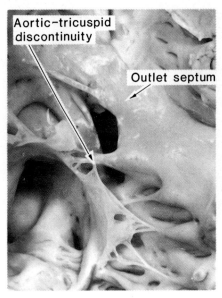

Aortic–tricuspid discontinuity

Outlet septum

Fig. 8.11 This defect with exclusively muscular rims opens to the outlet component of the right ventricle. Note the muscle bundle separating the aortic and tricuspid valves.

described as 'membranous': it has long been suggested that this term is much less than perfect.[6] The defects do not exist simply because of a deficiency of the membranous part of the ventricular septum. When present, they can occupy markedly different parts of the septum. It has now become conventional, therefore, to describe them as being perimembranous, in other words having the membranous part of the septum as part of their perimeter. This convention is both accurate and useful. It has the advantage of grouping together all those defects in which the atrioventricular conduction axis is located postero-inferiorly (Fig. 8.14). The only exception to this rule is in those hearts in which there is malalignment between the ventricular septum and the atrial septum in the presence of overriding and straddling of the tricuspid valve.[7] In those hearts with straddling tricuspid valve, in which the defect is still perimembranous in so far as the edge is directly adjacent to an area of valvar fibrous continuity, the atrioventricular conduction axis penetrates to the atrial tissues at the point where the ventricular septum makes contact with the atrioventricular junction (Fig. 8.15).

Defects in part bordered by valvar fibrous continuity between the arterial valves

Thus far we have described defects in which part of the border is composed of fibrous continuity between the atrioventricular valves, almost always with continuity also with the aortic valve. The second specific type of defect in terms of its margins occurs when there is fibrous continuity between the leaflets of the arterial valves. In perimembranous defects, particularly when they open to the right ventricular outlet, the pulmonary valve is usually supported by a muscular infundibulum of varied dimensions (Fig. 8.16a). In the second type of defect, it is lack of the subpulmonary infundibulum which permits the continuity between the facing leaflets of the arterial valves (Fig. 8.16b). These defects, described most clearly as exhibiting aortic–pulmonary valvar continuity but usually said to be 'doubly committed' and juxta-arterial (or supracristal), always open into the outlet component of the right ventricle. They can possess a muscular postero-inferior rim when the posterior limb of the septomarginal trabeculation fuses with the ventriculo-infundibular fold (Fig. 8.17a). Such a muscle bar protects the atrioventricular conduction axis, the degree of protection afforded being related directly to the dimensions of the bar. Alternatively, the defects can extend so as to be directly adjacent not only to the area of aortic–pulmonary continuity but also to an area of atrioventricular valvar continuity. Such defects (Fig. 8.17b) are both perimembranous and also doubly committed and juxta-arterial. They will have the conduction axis related directly to their postero-inferior rim. In these defects, unified because of aortic–pulmonary valvar continuity, the leaflets of the aortic and pulmonary valves are usually inserted to one another at the same level. This removes the anticipated off-setting of the arterial valves (which is the consequence of the presence of the usually extensive subpulmonary infundibulum). Sometimes a doubly committed juxta-arterial defect can have the aortic and pulmonary leaflets at different levels because of interposition of part of an arterial sinus (usually aortic but possibly pulmonary) as part of the rim (Fig. 8.18). The

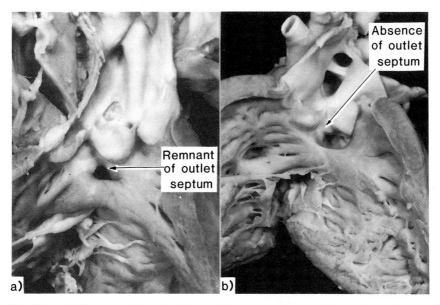

Fig. 8.12 a,b These views from the right ventricle contrast the morphology of a doubly committed defect which is roofed by fibrous continuity between the aortic and pulmonary valves (**b**) from a defect which is immediately beneath both valves yet is roofed by a small rim of outlet septum. The defect shown in (**a**) is a muscular outlet defect.

wall of the sinus in this setting separates the cavity of the ventricle from that of the arterial trunk.

Defects bordered exclusively by ventricular septal musculature

In the third specific type of defect, the margins are made up exclusively by the musculature of the ventricular septum. These are known universally as muscular defects. They can be found within the inlet, apical trabecular or outlet parts of the septum or they can be multiple. They can co-exist with perimembranous or doubly committed and juxta-arterial defects, particularly the muscular defect which opens to the inlet of the right ventricle. Muscular defects will bear a variable relationship to the atrioventricular conduction axis according to their position within the septum (Fig. 8.19). The most important defect in this respect is again the inlet defect. The conduction axis runs anterosuperiorly relative to a muscular inlet defect, whereas it is postero-inferior to a perimembranous defect opening to the inlet of the right ventricle.[8] Taken as a whole, muscular defects give few problems in categorization. The

one exception to this is when there is overriding of an arterial valve. Indeed, the feature of overriding complicates several aspects of description.

OVERRIDING OF ARTERIAL AND ATRIOVENTRICULAR VALVES

When muscular defects are located in the body of the apical trabecular septum, or perimembranous defects are seen with the aortic valve almost exclusively connected to the left ventricle, there is little difficulty in determining and describing the margins of the defect (Fig. 8.10). It is also clear that, in these circumstances, surgical placement of a patch across the defect will 'correct' the malformation. The patch will be secured by the surgeon to the margins of the defect. The situation is more complicated when there is valvar overriding, be it by an arterial or atrioventricular valve.[1] For instance, when there is overriding by the aortic valve (Fig. 8.20), the valve achieves connexions within both the right and the left ventricles. It could be argued that the very presence of a perimembranous or juxta-arterial defect confers

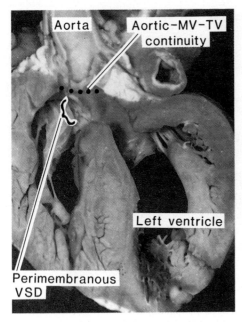

Fig. 8.13 This simulated four chamber section through a perimembranous defect shows how the roof and posterior borders are formed by an area of fibrous continuity between the aortic, mitral and tricuspid valves.

leaflets of the tricuspid or pulmonary valves. The situation is grossly exaggerated when there is overriding. The arterial valve then achieves direct connexion to the ventriculo-infundibular fold and the parietal wall within the right ventricle. As the valve achieves a greater connexion within the right ventricle, problems arise that concern the definitions of the margins of the defect. This is because the overriding creates a cone of space beneath the attachments of the valve leaflets within the right and left ventricles (Fig. 8.21). The inferior border of this cone is linear, being formed by the crest of the ventricular septum. The problem is in defining the precise roof of the defect. The definition chosen depends exclusively upon the view taken by the observer. Some argue that the roof of the defect in these circumstances is the direct extension of a line constructed through the long axis of the muscular ventricular septum. This places the leaflets of the overriding arterial valve as the roof of the defect. Such a roof, of course, would exist only in ventricular diastole, since the leaflets of the arterial valves open during systole to leave the defect, as thus defined, without a roof. The surgeon, furthermore, would never place stitches to the roof when defined in

some degree of right ventricular connexion upon a defect simply because of its relationship to the

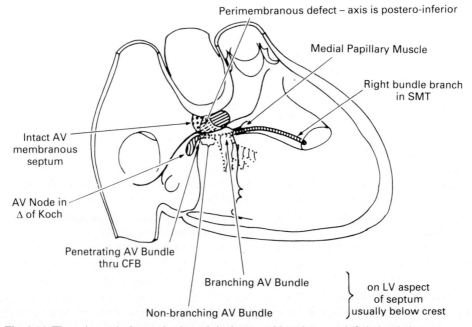

Fig. 8.14 The atrioventricular conduction axis is always positioned postero-inferiorly relative to a perimembranous defect except when there is straddling and overriding of the tricuspid valves (see Fig. 8.15). CFB: central fibrous body. SMT: septomarginal trabecula.

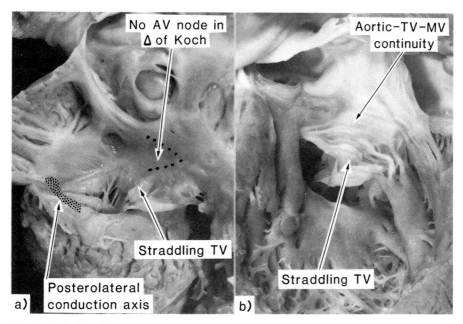

Fig. 8.15 a,b The right (**a**) and left (**b**) aspects of a perimembranous defect associated with straddling and overriding of the tricuspid valve (TV). There is malalignment of the atrial septum relative to the muscular part of the ventricular septum. This produces an unusual posterolateral location of the atrioventricular conduction axis (superimposed in (**a**)).

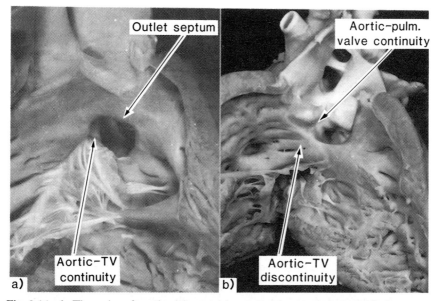

Fig. 8.16 a,b These views from the right ventricle contrast the morphology of defects opening into the subpulmonary outlet which are (**a**) perimembranous and (**b**) doubly committed and directly juxta-arterial. The difference is the presence or absence of the muscular outlet septum together with the 'septal' component of the subpulmonary infundibulum, along with presence or absence of a muscle bar between the aortic and tricuspid valves.

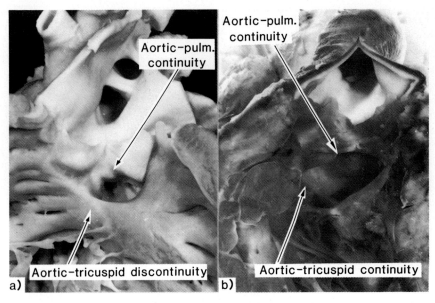

Fig. 8.17 a,b The primary feature of both these defects, which open into the outlet component of the right ventricle, is that they are roofed by fibrous continuity between the aortic and pulmonary valves (doubly committed and juxta-arterial defects). The defect in (**a**), however, is separated by a muscular rim from the tricuspid valve. In contrast, the defect shown in (**b**) extends to be bordered directly by an area of fibrous continuity between the aortic, mitral and tricuspid valves (perimembranous and doubly committed).

this fashion. If considered in this light, a defect bordered by an overriding aortic valve will reasonably be described as juxta-aortic, and a similar convention could be applied to defects overridden by pulmonary or truncal valves.[9] In practice, nonetheless, the border of a defect which is closed in this circumstance is that demarcated by the right ventricular attachments of the valve leaflets. This is the margin which is seen most readily by the pathologist observing the lesion through the right ventricle. When the pathologist considers these right ventricular attachments of the overriding valve, he is able to say whether they are exclusively supported by muscle or whether the aortic leaflets, as seen from the right ventricle, are in fibrous continuity with the tricuspid valve (making the defect perimembranous) or the pulmonary valve (making it doubly committed and juxta-arterial). The pathologist, therefore, viewing the right ventricular margin of the defect found with an overriding valve, may describe it as belonging to any of the three types distinguished in the previous section. There is, of course, yet another margin of the cone of space

found in the presence of overriding valves which has yet to receive consideration, namely the left ventricular margin. When the overriding valve is mostly connected to the left ventricle, this border will be 'taken for granted', and almost always will be formed by an extensive area of fibrous continuity between the aortic and mitral valves (when it is the aorta which overrides). The situation is rather different when the aorta is mostly connected to the right ventricle. Then it may be the left ventricular border of the cone of space which is taken to be *the* defect. Usually, as discussed above, the roof of this margin is composed of fibrous continuity between the mitral and aortic valves. It may, however, be formed by the muscular ventriculo-infundibular fold interposed between these valves, producing a muscular subaortic infundibulum (Fig. 8.22). This arrangement is comparable to that found in double outlet right ventricle, when the left ventricular margin of the subaortic outlet is the interventricular communication. Indeed, when an overriding aortic valve is predominantly connected to the right ventricle, along with

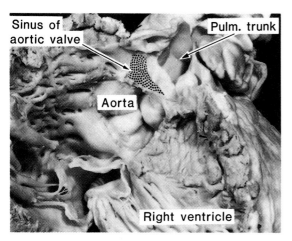

Fig. 8.18 In this doubly committed defect with a muscular postero-inferior rim, there is marked overriding of the septum by the aortic valve. In addition, part of the rim of the defect is formed by the sinus of the aortic valve (dotted area), producing off-setting between the levels of attachment of aortic and pulmonary leaflets at this site.

valves override the septum, it can be important to describe both the right and left ventricular margins of the cone of space beneath the overriding valve leaflets, as well as documenting the extent of the overriding.

The situation is comparable when atrioventricular valves override the septum but is even more complicated in arrangement because, in addition to overriding of the atrioventricular junction, there is usually attachment of the tendinous cords of the valve to both sides of the septum, a feature we describe as 'straddling'.[7] The most important feature of this lesion is the presence of malalignment between the atrial and ventricular septal structures. This will determine the course of the atrioventricular conduction axis (see Fig. 8.15). Straddling and overriding of the tricuspid valve is always found in association with a defect between the ventricular inlets. There is sharing of one of the inlets between the apical trabecular components by virtue of the override. A spectrum of lesions is to be found, therefore, between the extremes of biventricular and double inlet atrioventricular connexions. In contrast, straddling and overriding of the mitral valve occurs in

the pulmonary valve, it makes most sense to consider the ventriculo–arterial connexion as double outlet, irrespective of the state of the subaortic infundibulum.[10] Thus, when arterial

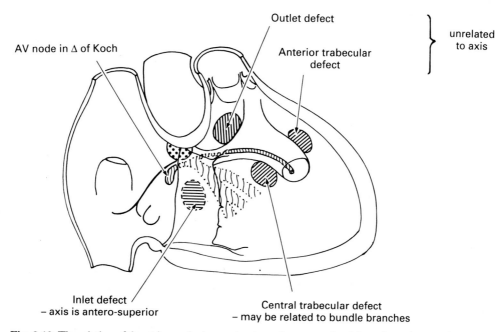

Fig. 8.19 The relation of the atrioventricular conduction axis to muscular defects depends upon the position of the defect within the septum.

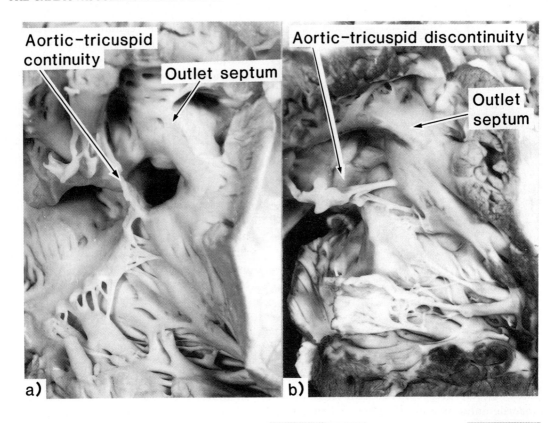

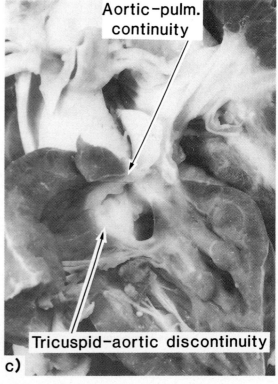

Fig. 8.20 a–c These views from the right ventricular apex show the different morphologies that can co-exist with overriding of the aortic valve. In the heart shown in (**a**), the defect extends to abut on an area of aortic–tricuspid fibrous continuity (perimembranous). In contrast, in the lesion shown in (**b**), a muscular bar separates the aortic and tricuspid valves. The leaflets of the aortic valve in this heart are supported within the right ventricle exclusively by muscle tissue. In the heart seen in (**c**), the anterosuperior margin is formed by fibrous continuity between the aortic and pulmonary valves but a muscle rim interposes between the aortic and tricuspid valves (doubly committed juxta-arterial defect). There is marked malalignment of the outlet septum in the hearts shown in (**a**) and (**b**), producing the typical morphology of the tetralogy of Fallot.

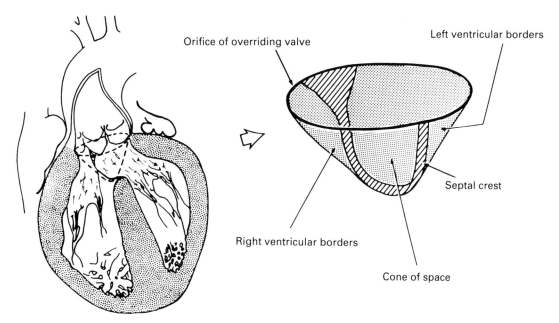

Fig. 8.21 The cone of space which can be conceptualized beneath the leaflets of an overriding aortic valve. All of the area within this cone constitutes a 'septal defect'. For a full description of a given example, it may be necessary to account for both the right and left ventricular borders of this cone.

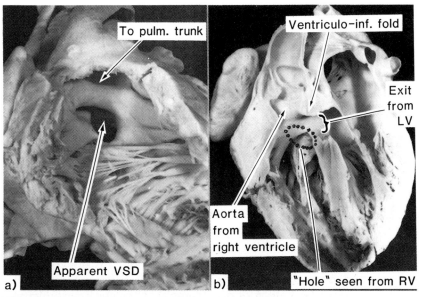

Fig. 8.22 a,b When this heart is viewed from the right ventricle (**a**), there seems to be a muscular outlet defect. Sectioning the heart in four chamber section (**b**), however, shows that there is double outlet ventriculo–arterial connexion and that the ventriculo–infundibular fold produces a restrictive subaortic infundibulum. This illustrates well the two borders of the subaortic cone shown in Fig. 8.21.
Heart photographed and reproduced by kind permission of Dr Eduardo Ruchelli, Children's Hospital of Pittsburgh, Pennsylvania, USA.

relation to a defect opening to the ventricular outlets. Almost always it is found with discordant or double outlet ventriculo–arterial connexion. We have never seen a straddling mitral valve in a heart with concordant ventriculo–arterial connexions.

SPONTANEOUS CLOSURE

The natural history of isolated ventricular septal defects is such that the majority show some tendency to diminish in size while a considerable proportion close completely. It is not possible for the pathologist to determine the proportion which do close, but it is possible to ascertain mechanisms of closure. Often hearts are seen with evidence of previous defects in the muscular septum. The right and left ventricular orifices of the presumed defect are seen, but the septal communication is closed (Fig. 8.23a). More often, evidence is seen of closure or diminution in size of perimembranous defects, but this does not mean that these are the defects that are likeliest to close. The majority of small muscular defects which close never come to the attention of the paediatric pathologist because patients with such defects rarely die in childhood. Perimembranous defects close by two mechanisms. The first is by formation of tags of fibrous tissue from valvar or fibrous structures in the environs of the defect (Fig. 8.23b). Often termed 'aneurysms of the membranous septum', hardly ever are these structures derived from the atrioventricular membranous septum or the remnant of the interventricular membranous septum. Instead, they are derived from the leaflet tissue of the tricuspid valve.[11,12] For that reason, they are best described as tricuspid tissue tags. They are found most frequently when the perimembranous defects are small and adjacent to the inner curvature or else open to the right ventricular inlet. It is exceedingly rare to find such tags when a perimembranous defect opens to the outlet of the right ventricle or when there is overriding of either an arterial or an atrioventricular valve.[13] The other mechanism for closure of a perimembranous defect is by adhesion of the septal leaflet of the tricuspid valve (Fig. 8.23c). This mechanism

can only come into play when the leaflet is adjacent to the defect, so it is those opening to the inlet which are most likely to close. This mechanism can also close muscular inlet defects, although we have never seen evidence of this at autopsy. Whenever defects show evidence of closure (or diminution in size), there is usually formation of fibrous tissue on and around the margins, these processes aiding subsequent complete closure. Some evidence may be seen at autopsy that doubly committed and juxta-arterial defects (or muscular defects opening into the subpulmonary infundibulum) can close because of prolapse of a leaflet of the aortic valve, the prolapsed leaflet forming a plug in the defect (Fig. 8.23d).

COMPLICATIONS

Ventricular septal defects can be associated with many other lesions, and these will be discussed in the appropriate chapters. At this point, we are concerned with mechanisms that can complicate the course of so-called 'isolated' defects. If the defect is large and is not closed surgically, its haemodynamic consequences result in hypertrophy of both the right and left ventricles.[14,15] This hypertrophic response in the right ventricle is almost certainly one cause for the development of muscular subpulmonary obstruction. Perhaps a more significant subarterial obstruction is the variant that accompanies overriding by an arterial valve. We have discussed how, in the normal heart, the outlet septum is an insignificant structure. But, when an arterial valve (be it the pulmonary or aortic valve) overrides the septum, the outlet septum achieves its own identity and becomes crucially important in the production of subarterial obstruction. Deviation of the outlet septum does not automatically produce obstruction to one or other outlet. There is a very characteristic defect, often called the 'Eisenmenger complex',[16] in which the outlet septum is deviated into the right ventricle but the subpulmonary infundibulum remains capacious (Fig. 8.24a). This situation was typically associated with development of pulmonary vascular disease. With more efficient diagnosis and treatment, such

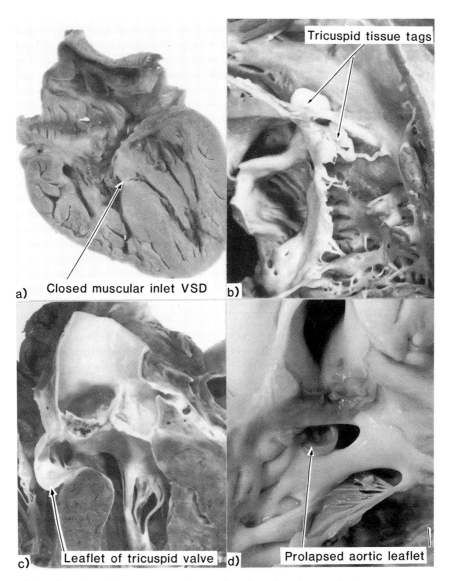

Fig. 8.23 a–d Ventricular septal defects can close through various mechanisms. These illustrations show evidence of closure of (**a**) a muscular defect in the inlet septum; (**b**) a perimembranous defect closing by growth of tissue tags from the tricuspid valve; (**c**) a perimembranous defect closed by fusion with the septal leaflet of the tricuspid valve; and (**d**) a doubly committed muscular outlet defect reduced in size because of prolapse of a leaflet of the aortic valve.

hearts are now rarely seen by the pathologist. Much more frequently, the pathologist will encounter the situation in which the outlet septum, deviated into the right ventricle, produces subpulmonary muscular obstruction (Fig. 8.24b). This is the hallmark of the tetralogy of Fallot, and will be discussed in more detail in

Chapter 12. Malalignment of the septum can also occur in reverse fashion. Then the malaligned septum occupies the left ventricular outflow tract and is associated with the production of subaortic obstruction and overriding of the pulmonary valve. Such subarterial obstruction is distal to the septal defect, and can be converted into a tunnel-

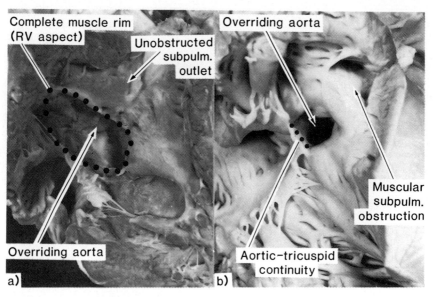

Fig. 8.24 a,b These right ventricular views show the difference between a defect associated with overriding of the aortic valve in the absence of muscular subpulmonary obstruction ((**a**) — the so-called Eisenmenger defect) and (**b**) typical tetralogy of Fallot with muscular subpulmonary obstruction due to deviation of the outlet septum.

type obstruction by development of fibrous circles between the outlet septum and the adjacent mitral valve. This type of obstruction tends to be associated with severe aortic coarctation or interruption of the aortic arch.[17–19] Subaortic obstruction can also be produced distal to the defect, in consequence of formation of a fibrous shelf on the left ventricular aspect of the septum, which may become adherent to the mitral valve with production of an obstructive diaphragm. Often termed a 'membranous' obstruction, this is a misnomer.[20] The shelf is a tough fibrous structure that is almost certainly an acquired lesion. Such fibrous shelves can be found with overriding of the aorta. They can then be a significant cause of postoperative left ventricular obstruction if unrecognized when such a defect is surgically closed. An association of lesions that is well recognized to include such shelves comprises ventricular septal defect, a left ventricular obstructive shelf and anomalous muscle bundles within the right ventricle.[21] The anomalous muscle bundles, almost always hypertrophied septoparietal trabeculations, can complicate ventricular septal defects in their own right without the association of the shelf. Such bundles

may become incorporated, along with hypertrophy of apical trabeculations, into partitions within the right ventricle ('two-chambered right ventricle'). They can be found with ventricular septal defects opening into either ventricular compartment, but usually into the proximal.

Abnormalities of either the atrioventricular or the arterial valves can complicate ventricular septal defects. So-called 'clefts' are seen most frequently in association with atrioventricular septal defects, when the space between the leaflets is part of the overall orifice of the atrioventricular valves. True clefts of the aortic leaflet of the mitral valve can be found along with ventricular septal defects. More significant in the presentation of the defect itself is the finding of deficiency of the septal leaflet of the tricuspid valve. When found in association with a perimembranous defect, such lack of leaflet tissue can produce the anatomical potential for shunting from the left ventricle to the right atrium.[22] This can be produced simply by deficiency of the atrioventricular component of the membranous septum. Such atrioventricular membranous septal defects (Fig. 8.25a) occur in the setting of the normally structured heart, and

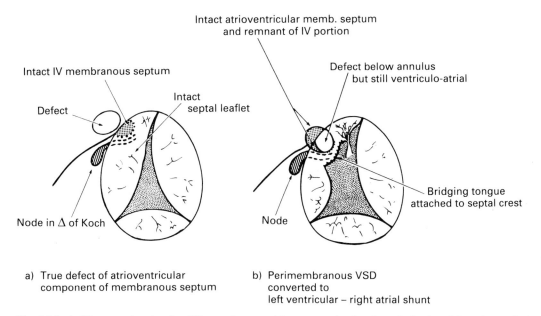

Intact atrioventricular memb. septum
and remnant of IV portion

Intact IV membranous septum

Defect

Intact
septal leaflet

Defect below annulus
but still ventriculo-atrial

Node in Δ of Koch

Node

Bridging tongue
attached to septal crest

a) True defect of atrioventricular
    component of membranous septum

b) Perimembranous VSD
    converted to
    left ventricular – right atrial shunt

Fig. 8.25 a,b Diagrams showing the difference between (**a**) a communication through the site of the atrioventricular component of the membranous septum and (**b**) a perimembranous defect which shunts from left ventricle to right atrium because of a malformation of the septal leaflet of the tricuspid valve.

are not part of the complex described as atrioventricular septal defects. They are rarely seen by the pathologist. Indeed, we are unaware of any convincing autopsy finding of such a defect. Much commoner is the arrangement described above in which a deficiency of the septal leaflet of the tricuspid valve permits a perimembranous septal defect to shunt directly into the right atrium (Fig. 8.25b).

Prolapse is the most significant lesion of an arterial valve, excluding stenosis, to be associated with a ventricular septal defect. This is most frequently seen in the aortic valve and complicates mostly the doubly committed and juxta-arterial defect.[23] Here the prolapse of the valve leaflet can occur along with expansion of the sinus of Valsalva. It is well recognized that aneurysms of the sinus of Valsalva are the extreme end of the spectrum of prolapse of an arterial valve.[24,25] It is presumed that the prolapse in this circumstance reflects the lack of support of the valve leaflet because of absence of the outlet septum. Prolapse of the aortic valve also occurs in perimembranous defects,[25] again where there is a suggestion of lack of septal support for the compromised leaflet. All

of these various complications can predispose to infective endocarditis, as can the insertion of surgical patches. In previous eras, the heart with a ventricular septal defect would often have shown evidence of secondary reactions in terms of ventricular hypertrophy and fibrosis. These changes are rarely seen nowadays. The pathologist is now much more likely to be confronted with post-surgical specimens. In these hearts, patch dehiscence, fibrosis or aneurysm formation at the site of ventriculotomies or damage to the atrioventricular conduction axis are the likely lesions to be seen. Study of the conduction system cannot be performed in every post-surgical case as a matter of routine. Such investigation would be indicated in the presence of electrocardiographic evidence of rhythm problems such as atrioventricular dissociation or so-called 'bifascicular block with left axis deviation', particularly if death was sudden. Of significance to both pathologist and clinician is the state of the pulmonary vasculature in the presence of a ventricular septal defect. It is the normal delayed fall in pulmonary vascular resistance from the high levels of intrauterine life which delays the presentation of most ventricular septal defects until an infant is from 4–6 weeks of age.[26] Sometimes this fall is delayed in patients with large defects and may be limited in its extent. The delay is a consequence of hypertrophy of the muscular coat of the intra-acinar arteries and veins.[27] Once the pulmonary resistance has fallen to its normal levels in the presence of a ventricular septal defect, it will rise

again only if there is pulmonary vascular disease. This occurs in patients with unrestrictive defects and, ideally, should not be seen now that the defects can be corrected surgically during infancy or the lungs be protected by banding of the pulmonary trunk in anticipation of later correction. Rarely, however, patients are still seen with florid changes of pulmonary vascular disease.[27,28]

REFERENCES

1. Anderson RH, Becker AE, Tynan M. Description of ventricular septal defects — or how long is a piece of string? Editorial review. Int J Cardiol 1986; 13: 267–278.
2. Brandt PWT. Axial angled angiocardiography. Cardiovasc Intervent Radiol 1984; 7: 166–169.
3. Hagler DJ, Edwards WD, Seward JB, Tajik AJ. Standardized nomenclature of the ventricular septum and ventricular septal defects, with applications for two-dimensional echocardiography. Mayo Clin Proc 1985; 60: 741–752.
4. Soto B, Becker AE, Moulaert AJ, Lie JT, Anderson RH. Classification of ventricular septal defects. Br Heart J 1980; 43: 332–343.
5. Allwork SP, Anderson RH. Developmental anatomy of the membranous part of the ventricular septum in the human heart. Br Heart J 1979; 41: 275–280.
6. Becu LM, Fontana RS, DuShane JW, Kirklin JW, Burchell HB, Edwards JE. Anatomic and pathologic studies in ventricular septal defect. Circulation 1956; 14: 349–364.
7. Milo S, Ho SY, Macartney FJ et al. Straddling and overriding atrioventricular valves; morphology and classification. Am J Cardiol 1979; 44: 1122–1134.
8. Milo S, Ho SY, Wilkinson JL, Anderson RH. The surgical anatomy and atrioventricular conduction tissues of hearts with isolated ventricular septal defects. J Thorac Cardiovasc Surg 1980; 79: 244–255.
9. Kirklin JW, Kirklin JK, Soto B, Blackstone EA, Bargeron LM Jr. Ventricular septal defects: a surgical viewpoint. In: Anderson RH, Neches WH, Park SC, Zuberbuhler JR, eds. Perspectives in pediatric cardiology, vol. 1. New York: Futura, 1988; pp 91–93.
10. Ruchelli ED, Anderson RH. The significance of discontinuity between the aortic and mitral valves in the presence of 'normally related' arterial trunks. Int J Cardiol (in press).
11. Chesler E, Korns ME, Edwards E. Anomalies of the tricuspid valve, including pouches, resembling aneurysms of the membranous ventricular septum. Am J Cardiol 1968; 21: 661–668.
12. Anderson RH, Lenox CC, Zuberbuhler JR. Mechanisms of closure of perimembranous ventricular septal defects. Am J Cardiol 1983; 52: 341–345.
13. Somerville J. Congenital heart disease — changes in form and function. Br Heart J 1979; 41: 1–22.
14. Jarmakani JMM, Graham TP Jr, Canent RV Jr, Spach MS, Capp MP. Effect of site shunt on left heart-volume characteristics in children with ventricular septal defect and patent ductus arteriosus. Circulation 1969; 40: 411–418.
15. Jarmakani MM, Graham TP Jr, Canent RV Jr, Capp MP. The effect of corrective surgery on left heart volume and mass in children with ventricular septal defect. Am J Cardiol 1971; 27: 254–258.
16. Oppenheimer-Dekker A, Gittenberger-de-Groot AC, Bartelings MM, Wenink ACG, Moene RJ, Van der Harten JJ. Abnormal architecture of the ventricles in hearts with an overriding aortic valve and a perimembranous ventricular septal defect ('Eisenmenger VSD'). Int J Cardiol 1985; 9: 341–355.
17. Moulaert A, Bruins CC, Oppenheimer-Dekker A. Anomalies of the aortic arch and ventricular septal defects. Circulation 1976; 53: 1011–1015.
18. Van Praagh R, Bernhard WF, Rosenthal A, Parisi LF, Fyler DC. Interrupted aortic arch: surgical treatment. Am J Cardiol 1971; 27: 200–211.
19. Freedom RM, Dische MR, Rowe RD. Pathologic anatomy of subaortic stenosis and atresia in the first year of life. Am J Cardiol 1977; 39: 1035–1044.
20. Somerville J. Fixed subaortic stenosis — a frequently misunderstood lesion. Int J Cardiol 1985; 8: 145–148.
21. Baumstark A, Fellows KE, Rosenthal A. Combined double chambered right ventricle and discrete subaortic stenosis. Circulation 1978; 57: 299–303.
22. Warden HE, De Wall RA, Cohen M, Varco RL, Lillehei CW. A surgical pathologic classification for isolated ventricular septal defects and for those in Fallot's tetralogy based on observations made on 120 patients during repair and under direct vision. J Thorac Cardiovasc Surg 1957; 33: 21–44.
23. Ando M, Takao A. Pathological anatomy of ventricular septal defect associated with aortic valve prolapse and regurgitation. Heart Vessels 1986; 2: 117–126.
24. Griffin ML, Sullivan ID, Anderson RH, Macartney FJ. Doubly committed subarterial ventricular septal defect: a morphologic review with echocardiographic and angiocardiographic correlation. Br Heart J 1988; 59: 474–479.
25. Van Praagh R, McNamara JJ. Anatomic types of ventricular septal defect with aortic insufficiency. Am Heart J 1968; 75: 604–619.
26. Hoffman JIE. Ventricular septal defects: overview of management. In: Anderson RH, Neches WH, Park SC, Zuberbuhler JR, eds. Perspectives in pediatric cardiology, vol. 1. New York: Futura, 1988; pp 81–89.

27. Haworth SG, Sauer U, Buhlmeyer K, Reid L. Development of the pulmonary circulation in ventricular septal defect: a quantitative structural study. Am J Cardiol 1977; 40: 781–788.

28. Rabinovitch M, Haworth SG, Castaneda AR, Nadas AS, Reid LM. Lung biopsy in congenital heart disease: a morphometric approach to pulmonary vascular disease. Circulation 1978; 58: 1107–1121.

R.H. Anderson and A.E. Becker

Anomalies of the atrioventricular valves

INTRODUCTION

Congenital malformations can involve the whole or only a part of an atrioventricular valve. When affecting some particular component of the valve, a similar lesion can malform the mitral or tricuspid valve or a common atrioventricular valve. Other lesions have a predilection for one of the valves and affect the others very rarely. An example is Ebstein's malformation, which usually deforms the tricuspid valve but can sometimes affect the right component of a common valve or even a morphologically mitral valve. We will deal with lesions of the individual valves in turn, considering the way in which their different components are involved. These lesions can affect the valve so as to produce either stenosis or incompetence or both. It is often difficult for the pathologist to judge with precision whether a particular valve would have been incompetent, although in the presence of atrial dilatation this can be presumed. Stenosis is somewhat easier to judge. We will not, however, group the lesions according to whether they result in stenosis or incompetence, since each lesion can, in some circumstances, produce varied haemodynamic effects. These should be assessed as far as is possible in each case. In this respect, dysplasia is a protean finding. An entire valve may be dysplastic and, although usually seen in the setting of a hypoplastic left ventricle (see Ch. 10), it may, on occasion, involve all four valves of the heart.[1]

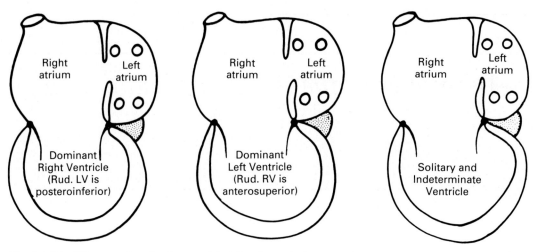

Fig. 9.1 The different settings for absence of the left atrioventricular connexion according to the morphology of the ventricular mass. Only the arrangement with a dominant right ventricle can correctly be termed mitral atresia (rud.= rudimentary).

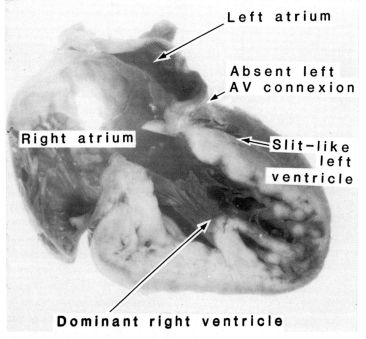

Fig. 9.2 This section in simulated four chamber plane shows the morphology of absent left atrioventricular connexion when the right atrium is connected to a dominant right ventricle in the presence of an incomplete left ventricle (mitral atresia).

LESIONS OF THE MITRAL VALVE

Congenital malformations of the mitral valve can involve the atrioventricular junction, the leaflets, or the tension apparatus, including the papillary muscles. The entire valve can be

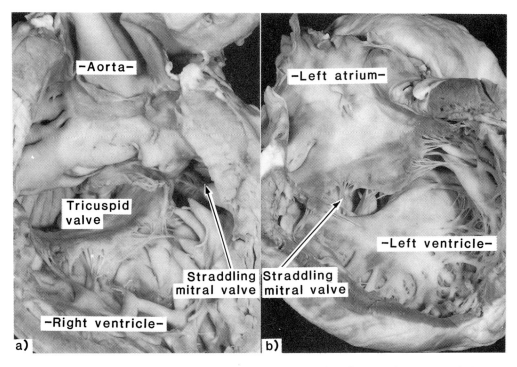

Fig. 9.3 a,b Overriding and straddling of the mitral orifice in the setting of a concordant atrioventricular connexion and double outlet from the right ventricle. The heart is seen (**a**) from the right and (**b**) from the left.

abnormal and miniaturized. The latter feature is almost always associated with ventricular hypoplasia and will be dealt with in the next chapter.

Lesions of the atrioventricular junction

Absent atrioventricular connexion

Absence of one of the two atrioventricular connexions is one form of univentricular atrioventricular connexion. The connexion from the morphologically left atrium can be absent when the right atrium is connected to a dominant right ventricle, a dominant left ventricle or a solitary and indeterminate ventricle (Fig. 9.1). Only the first of these variants can, in strict terms, be considered as mitral atresia (Fig. 9.2). The other two produce similar haemodynamics at atrial level but, had the connexion been formed, the valve would not have been of mitral morphology. This problem in nomenclature will

be considered further in Chapter 19. It must be emphasized that an absent connexion is different from an imperforate valve (see below) although both patterns result in atrioventricular valvar atresia.

Overriding mitral valve

Overriding of the atrioventricular junction is almost always, but not exclusively, associated with straddling of the tension apparatus. This lesion affects the morphologically mitral valve irrespective of its position. In most cases the affected heart has usual atrial arrangement and right-hand ventricular topology (Fig. 9.3). According to the degree of override of the junction, the malformation ranges from the extreme of a concordant atrioventricular connexion to that of a double inlet to the right ventricle. The atrioventricular junction supporting the mitral valve can also override in hearts with usual atrial arrangement and left-hand ventricular topology. This

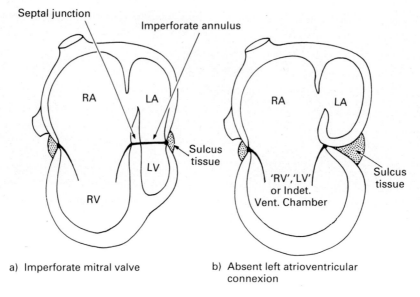

a) Imperforate mitral valve   b) Absent left atrioventricular connexion

Fig. 9.4 a,b There is a fundamental difference morphologically between absence of the left atrioventricular connexion (**b**) and an imperforate mitral valve (**a**) although both produce the same haemodynamic effect.

produces a spectrum of lesions between the extremes of discordant atrioventricular connexion and of double inlet right ventricle with rudimentary and incomplete right-sided left ventricle. This spectrum is described further in Chapter 17.

Lesions of the valvar leaflets

Imperforate mitral valve

For the valve to be imperforate, there must have been formation of the atrioventricular junction. It is this feature which distinguishes this variant of valvar atresia from absence of the atrioventricular connexion (Fig. 9.4). The mitral valve can be imperforate along with aortic atresia as part of the hypoplastic left heart syndrome (see Ch. 10). An imperforate mitral valve can also be seen with a patent aortic root, when the aorta is connected either to the left (Fig. 9.5) or to the right ventricle. Usually, when the mitral valve is imperforate, the tension apparatus is poorly formed, being represented as columns in the wall of the hypoplastic left ventricle.

Prolapse of the leaflets

Prolapse is said to occur when, during ventricular systole, the leaflets balloon back across the atrioventricular junction into the cavity of the atrium. In florid cases there is no problem in recognizing such prolapse, which can affect a solitary scallop of the mural leaflet (Fig. 9.6), rarely only the aortic leaflet or, more commonly, the whole valve. When the whole valve is involved, the leaflets are almost always thickened and dysplastic, producing the lesion known as the 'floppy valve'.[2] In some hearts the picture may not be as clear cut as, for instance, when individual scallops of the valve may show so-called hooding. It seems probable that, with increasing age, hooded valves can become prolapsed. The pathologist cannot observe this progression in any one heart, since he only sees the specimen at one phase in its evolution. It seems likely, nonetheless, that prolapse is an acquired condition promoted by congenital precursors. The most florid cases seen in children are in those with collagen diseases such as Marfan's syndrome. Biochemical disorders, probably congenital, can be identified in many

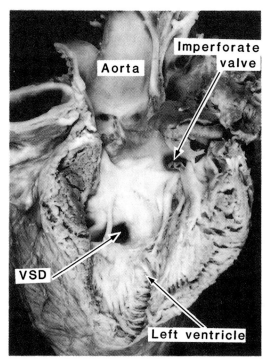

Fig. 9.5 An imperforate mitral valve is shown in the setting of concordant ventriculo–arterial connexions. Note the rudimentary nature of the tension apparatus.

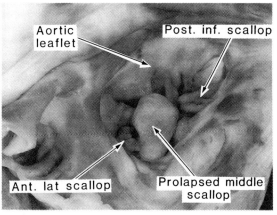

Fig. 9.6 Either leaflet of the mitral valve may show prolapse, or the whole valve may be involved. This illustration shows florid prolapse of the middle scallop of the mural leaflet in a patient with Marfan's syndrome.

adults with prolapse.[3] There is also strong evidence which points to the prolapsed valves

having had insufficient support by the tendinous cords during early life.[4] The overall picture, therefore, points strongly towards a congenital basis for the prolapsed valve.

Straddling mitral valve

'Straddling' describes the condition in which the tension apparatus is contained within both the right and left ventricles, crossing the crest of a ventricular septal defect. The mitral valve always straddles a defect which communicates with the outlet component of the right ventricle[5] and is almost always found with either discordant or double outlet ventriculo–arterial connexions.[6] Straddling almost always accompanies override of the junction (see Fig. 9.3) but, rarely, can be found in isolation.

Mitral arcade

The normal arrangement of the tension apparatus is for the papillary muscles to give rise to tendinous cords which are inserted into the leaflets. When muscle of the papillary muscles continues on to the leading edge of the leaflet, so that a bar of muscle extends across the leaflet (Fig. 9.7), the condition is described as the 'arcade' lesion.[7] Surgeons sometimes call this arrangement a 'hammock' malformation.[8]

Ebstein's malformation of the mitral valve

When the left-sided atrioventricular valve is affected by Ebstein's malformation in a heart with usual atrial arrangement, almost always it is in the setting of discordant atrioventricular connexions and the valve is of tricuspid morphology. This is discussed in Chapter 17. Very rarely, the left-sided mitral valve in hearts with concordant atrioventricular connexions can be malformed in the way that characterizes Ebstein's malformation of the tricuspid valve.[9] The leaflet is adherent to the wall of the ventricle so that it seems to arise within the cavity of the ventricle, although the atrioventricular junction is formed at the appropriate level. In the tricuspid valve, as will be described below, it is the septal and mural leaflets

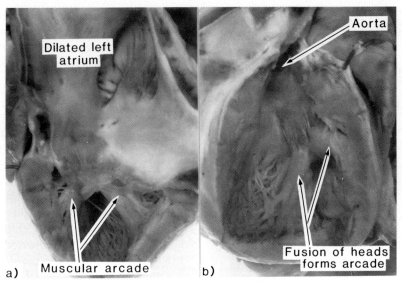

Fig. 9.7 a,b This lesion, seen from the atrial (**a**) and ventricular (**b**) aspects, in which the papillary muscles join on the undersurface of the leading edge of the valve leaflet, is called an arcade.

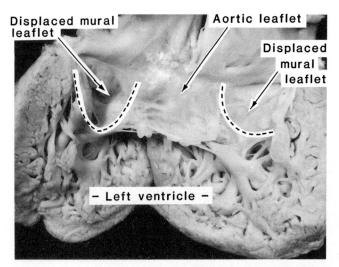

Fig. 9.8 The mural leaflet of this valve is adherent to the ventricular surface, producing downward displacement and fulfilling the criteria for diagnosis of Ebstein's malformation in a morphologically mitral valve.

which are predominantly involved. When Ebstein's malformation affects the mitral valve, however, it is the mural leaflet which is deformed and adherent to the ventricular wall (Fig. 9.8). The aortic leaflet is attached in its normal fashion.[10]

Dual orifice

Hearts with a dual orifice in the left atrioventricular valve most usually have deficient atrioventricular septation and the deformed valve is the left component of a common valve (see Ch. 7). The

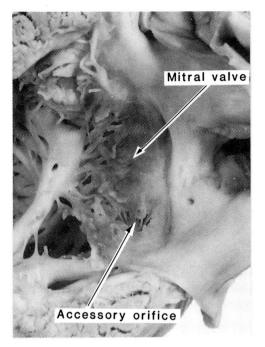

Fig. 9.9 This mitral valve possesses a dual orifice due to interconnexion of its leaflets.

mitral valve can also exhibit dual orifices, usually with each orifice supported by a solitary papillary muscle (Fig. 9.9).

Anomalous attachment of tendinous cords

The extreme form of anomalous attachment is found in one variant of the 'parachute' valve, where all the tendinous cords focus on one papillary muscle (see below). Lesser forms of the anomaly are found where the cords are attached across the subaortic outflow tract, often producing obstruction. This is seen most frequently in atrioventricular septal defect or in hearts with discordant ventriculo–arterial connexions (when the anomaly produces subpulmonary obstruction).

Cleft mitral valve

An isolated cleft of the mitral valve in a heart with normal atrioventricular septation (Fig. 9.10a) differs markedly from the functional commissure

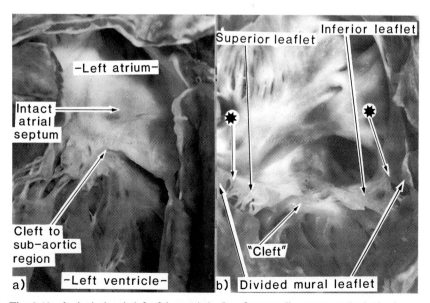

Fig. 9.10 a,b An isolated cleft of the aortic leaflet of a normally constructed mitral valve (**a**), which 'points' to the subaortic outflow tract, is totally dissimilar morphologically to the space (asterisks) between the left ventricular components of the bridging leaflets in an atrioventricular septal defect (**b**).

between the left ventricular components of the bridging leaflets in an atrioventricular septal defect (Fig. 9.10b). The latter malformation has been discussed at length in Chapter 7. The true mitral cleft produces incompetence of the valve and can be remedied simply by surgical suturing of the edges of the cleft. The condition can be found in an otherwise normal heart, or it may be associated with other lesions such as double outlet right ventricle or discordant atrioventricular connexions. Straddling mitral valves often have clefts in the leaflet which extend into the right ventricle.

Lesions of the tension apparatus

It could be argued that some malformations described above as lesions of the leaflets, notably the arcade lesion and dual orifices, would better be considered as anomalies of the tension apparatus. While accepting such an approach, we preferred to include them in the section concerned with the leaflets. In this section on the tension apparatus, therefore, we are left with only the so-called 'parachute' lesion.

'Parachute' mitral valve

First described in the setting of a heart with discordant atrioventricular connexions,[11] the significance of the malformations which produced a parachute-like deformity of the valve was emphasized subsequently by Shone and his colleagues.[12] They described the association with supravalvar ring of the left atrium, subaortic fibrous shelf and aortic coarctation, a complex which has since become known as the Shone syndrome. The 'parachute' lesion is most commonly found in association with aortic coarctation or in hearts with atrioventricular septal defects. It can be produced by two distinct anatomical mechanisms, both of which produce an unequivocal parachute-like arrangement, with the tension apparatus originating from a solitary papillary muscle mass. In the more common format, the solitary muscle mass is produced by fusion of the paired papillary muscles usually found supporting the mitral valve. To an extent, this arrangement is seen in the normal valve, since

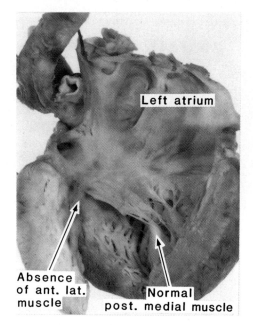

Fig. 9.11 In this heart with tricuspid atresia, all the tension apparatus is inserted into a solitary papillary muscle, giving the appearance of a parachute. The other papillary muscle is congenitally absent.

the muscles are adjacent when examined in their 'in situ' position. The parachute arrangement is an exaggeration of this, usually seen in somewhat hypoplastic ventricles. A much more striking anomaly is seen when one papillary muscle is grossly hypoplastic or absent. The most florid example of this in our collections is in a heart with tricuspid atresia (Fig. 9.11), but it is also described as an isolated lesion or in hearts with a hypoplastic left ventricle.[13]

LESIONS OF THE MORPHOLOGICALLY TRICUSPID VALVE

As with the mitral valve, congenital malformations of the tricuspid valve can be considered in terms of the junction, the leaflets and the tension apparatus.

Ebstein's malformation

The essence of Ebstein's malformation[14] is downward displacement of the 'annular' attach-

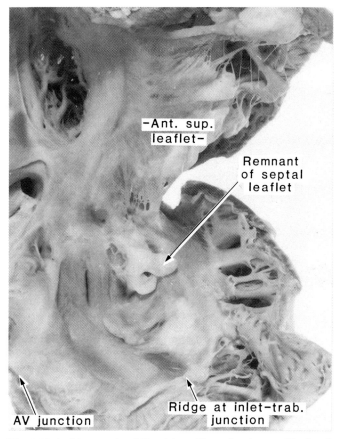

Fig. 9.12 In this example of Ebstein's malformation the septal leaflet of the tricuspid valve is represented only by dysplastic excrescences pointing towards the ventricular apex. The valve is seen from its atrial aspect.

ment of the leaflets so that they arise from the ventricular myocardium rather than the atrioventricular junction, the latter remaining at its appropriate site. In the area of displacement, the leaflets are apparently absent. Indeed, in some hearts, the septal leaflet may be totally lacking or represented by cauliflower-like excrescences of valve tissue found towards the ventricular apex (Fig. 9.12). The leaflets affected in this fashion are primarily the septal and mural ones, although in some hearts there may be minimal displacement of the anterosuperior leaflet along the ventriculo-infundibular fold. The extent of displacement can vary markedly and the severity of the lesion reflects this. The leaflets, however, are never displaced beyond the junction of the inlet and apical trabecular components of the

right ventricle. In addition to this displacement, which affects the proximal part of the valves, there is variability in the distal attachments. This largely concerns the anterosuperior leaflet, which may be attached in the usual focal fashion to the right ventricular papillary muscles (Fig. 9.13a), or else have a grossly abnormal linear attachment to the junction between the inlet and apical components (Fig. 9.13b). Intermediate patterns can be found which show a series of interrupted attachments along a linear attachment.[15] The most severe form of linear attachment produces an imperforate variant of Ebstein's malformation causing tricuspid atresia (Fig. 9.14). In addition to these malformations of attachment, almost always the leaflets are also dysplastic.[16] Furthermore, the more severe the lesion, the more obvious is

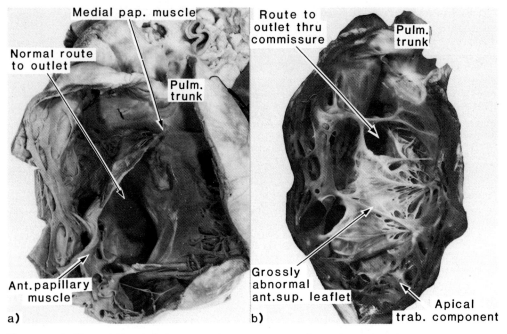

Fig. 9.13 a,b Views of the ventricular aspect of the two extremes of the attachments of the anterosuperior leaflet of the tricuspid valve seen in Ebstein's malformation: (**a**) shows focal attachment, which provides unobstructed flow to the ventricular outlets; in the presence of linear attachment (**b**), the blood reaches the outlet component through what normally would be the commissures.

the thinning and dilatation of the inlet part of the right ventricle, which becomes part of the right atrium as a consequence of the annular displacement ('physiological atrialization'). When the thinning of this part is particularly severe the arrangement is called 'anatomical atrialization'. The outlet part of the ventricle can also be thinned. This is of functional significance since it is the apical trabecular and outlet components which represent the working right ventricle. Ebstein's malformation can exist in isolation but usually is found with other associated lesions. Almost always there is an atrial septal defect in the oval fossa. Ventricular septal defects may also be present. The malformation often affects the tricuspid valve in association with pulmonary atresia with intact ventricular septum.

Other lesions of the tricuspid valve

Absent atrioventricular connexion

Absence of the right atrioventricular connexion can be found with the left atrium connected to a left, right or solitary and indeterminate ventricle. The variant with a dominant left ventricle provides the pattern known as classic tricuspid atresia, and is considered in Chapter 19. We emphasize that absent atrioventricular connexion is an entity in its own right (Fig. 9.15). It is by far the commonest cause of tricuspid atresia and is distinct from an imperforate tricuspid valve (see below).

Overriding tricuspid annulus

This lesion almost always co-exists with straddling of the tension apparatus of the valve (Fig. 9.16) (see below). When found in hearts with usual atrial arrangement and right-hand ventricular topology, the degree of override determines the categorization of the anomaly between the extremes of concordant atrioventricular connexions and double inlet left ventricle with right-sided rudimentary and incomplete right ventricle. This arrangement is associated with an

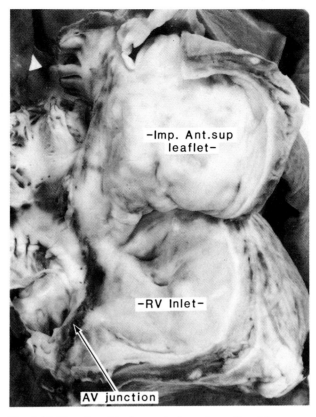

Fig. 9.14 The tricuspid valve can be imperforate (Imp.) in cases of Ebstein's malformation, giving tricuspid atresia.

anomalous disposition of the atrioventricular conduction axis (see Ch. 8). Overriding of the morphologically tricuspid valve can also be found in hearts with usual atrial arrangement and left-hand ventricular topology. A spectrum of malformations then exists between hearts having discordant atrioventricular connexions and those with double inlet left ventricle and left-sided rudimentary and incomplete right ventricle. These hearts also have an abnormal disposition of their conduction tissues (see Chs 14 and 15).

Imperforate tricuspid valve

As with imperforate mitral valve, an imperforate membrane in tricuspid position requires the formation of the atrioventricular junction. The arrangement must, therefore, be distinguished from absence of the atrioventricular connexion (see above). Imperforate tricuspid valves are probably found most frequently in the setting of Ebstein's malformation (Fig. 9.14). They can be found blocking a normally positioned junction in hearts with concordant atrioventricular connexions but are commoner in those with double inlet left ventricle (see Ch. 18).

Straddling tricuspid valve

This malformation, defined as attachment of the tendinous cords of the valve within both right and left ventricles, is found almost always with overriding of the junction (see above). The valve almost always straddles in the setting of a malalignment defect between the atrial and muscular ventricular septal structures. As such, the valve straddles the inlet part of the septum.

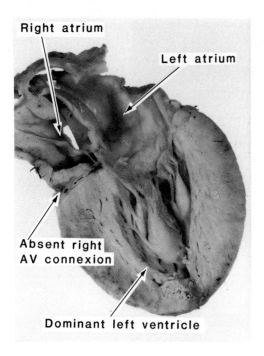

Right atrium

Left atrium

Absent right
AV connexion

Dominant left ventricle

Fig. 9.15 Classic tricuspid atresia is produced by complete absence of the right atrioventricular connexion. This is best illustrated, as shown, in simulated four chamber section.

Rarely, tendinous cords may be found straddling a muscular inlet defect.

'Parachute' tricuspid valve

This rare lesion is found when all the tendinous cords from the three leaflets of the valve are inserted to a solitary papillary muscle.[17]

Congenitally unguarded orifice

This lesion is due to failure of formation of the leaflets of the tricuspid valve. Most frequently it is part of the syndrome of pulmonary atresia with intact ventricular septum.[18] Although sometimes found when the tricuspid orifice and right ventricular cavity are hypoplastic, usually it is seen when the right side of the heart is thinned and dilated (see Ch. 10). Absence of the leaflets of the tricuspid valve is also seen when there is isolation of the inlet component of the right ventricle, a

muscular partition interposing between the inlet and the rest of the ventricle.[19] This lesion has much in common with imperforate Ebstein's malformation (compare Figs 9.14 and 9.17) and, like this lesion, results in tricuspid atresia.

Dysplastic tricuspid valve

Dysplasia of the leaflets of the tricuspid valve is seen most frequently as part of Ebstein's malformation. Less commonly it can be found in the setting of a valve attached normally to the atrioventricular junction (Fig. 9.18) when it can produce stenosis, incompetence or both.

LESIONS OF A COMMON ATRIOVENTRICULAR VALVE

These abnormalities are found predominantly with an atrioventricular septal defect and have been described in Chapter 7. It is important in this context to realize that the common valve seen with deficient atrioventricular septation is morphologically different from the normal valves, particularly its left component, which has scant resemblance to a mitral valve. This has been emphasized in the difference between an isolated cleft of the mitral valve and the so-called 'cleft' in atrioventricular septal defects, the 'cleft' in the latter case being the space between the left ventricular components of the bridging leaflets. Despite these differences the various lesions described above as affecting the mitral and tricuspid valves can also affect the common valve, with the obvious exception of the isolated cleft. It should be noted that usually, but not always, the common valve straddles and overrides. It does not exhibit these features when committed exclusively to one ventricle in the setting of double inlet ventricle (see Ch. 18). The degree of override does, nonetheless, vary and produces another spectrum of anomalies between the extremes of double inlet ventricle and hearts having an atrioventricular septal defect with concordant, discordant or ambiguous atrioventricular connexions, depending on the chamber combinations present. It is often difficult to eluci-

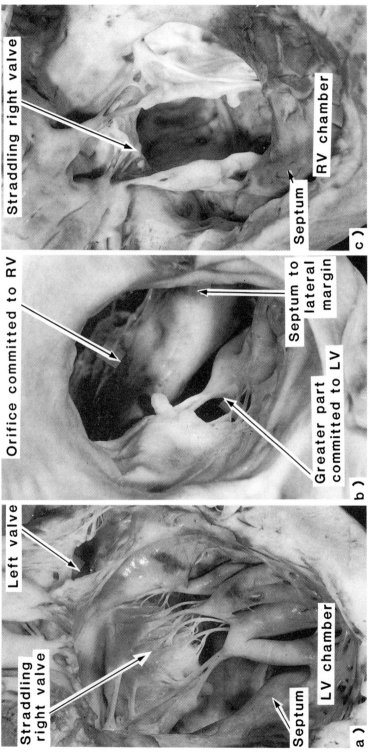

Fig. 9.16 a–c This heart shows overriding of the orifice of the morphologically tricuspid valve and straddling of its tension apparatus viewed (**a**) from the left ventricle, (**b**) from the right atrium, and (**c**) from the right ventricle. This specimen is intermediate between the extremes of a concordant atrioventricular connexion and double inlet to the morphologically left ventricle.

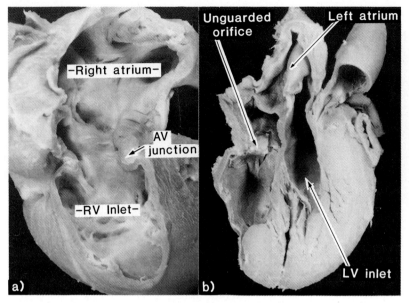

Fig. 9.17 a,b This heart has a congenitally unguarded tricuspid orifice with the inlet component of the right ventricle isolated by a complete muscular shelf from the rest of the right ventricle (**a**). The four chamber section (**b**) shows the unguarded junction.

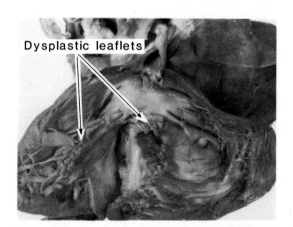

Fig. 9.18 This illustration shows dysplasia of the leaflets of a normally located tricuspid valve.

date the nature of the connexion and therefore to decide whether the lesion is an atrioventricular septal defect or a double inlet ventricle. In these circumstances it is probably better simply to describe the anatomical findings.

In lesions affecting the common valve, the right or left components may be imperforate, usually when associated with an atrioventricular septal defect. 'Parachute' lesions are also most frequently seen in this setting. The right component may exhibit Ebstein's malformation, either with an atrioventricular septal defect or when there is double inlet ventricle. Any of the other lesions described above may also be seen when there is a common valve.

REFERENCES

1. Bharati S, Lev M. Congenital polyvalvular disease. Circulation 1973; 47: 575–586.
2. Angelini A, Becker AE, Anderson RH, Davies MJ. Mitral valve morphology: normal and mitral valve prolapse. In: Boudoulas H, Wooley CF, eds. Mitral valve prolapse and the mitral valve prolapse syndrome. New York: Futura, 1988; 13–54.
3. Liss Y, Burleigh MC, Parker DJ, Child AH, Hobb J, Davies MJ. Biochemical characterization of individual normal, floppy and rheumatic forms of mitral valves. Biochem J 1987; 244: 597–603.
4. Van der Bel-Kahn J, Duren DR, Becker AE. Isolated mitral valve prolapse: chordal architecture as an anatomic basis in older patients. J Am Coll Cardiol 1985; 5: 1335–1340.
5. Wenink ACG, Gittenberger-de-Groot AC. Straddling mitral and tricuspid valves: morphologic differences and

developmental backgrounds. Am J Cardiol 1982; 49: 1959–1971.

6. Kitamura N, Takao A, Ando M, Imai Y, Konno S. Taussig-Bing heart with mitral valve straddling: case reports and post-mortem study. Circulation 1974; 49: 761–767.

7. Layman TE, Edwards JE. Anomalous mitral arcade: a type of congenital mitral insufficiency. Circulation 1967; 35: 389–395.

8. Carpentier A, Branchini B, Cour JC et al. Congenital malformations of the mitral valve in children. Pathology and surgical treatment. J Thorac Cardiovasc Surg 1976; 72: 854–866.

9. Ruschhaupt DG, Bharati S, Lev M. Mitral valve malformation of Ebstein type in absence of corrected transposition. Am J Cardiol 1976; 38: 109–112.

10. Leung M, Rigby ML, Anderson RH, Wyse RKH, Macartney FJ. Reversed off-setting of the septal attachments of the atrioventricular valves and Ebstein's malformation of the morphologically mitral valve. Br Heart J 1987; 57: 184–187.

11. Swan H, Trapnell JM, Denst J. Congenital mitral stenosis and systemic right ventricle with associated pulmonary vascular changes frustrating surgical repair of patent ductus arteriosus and coarctation of the aorta. Am Heart J 1949; 38: 914–923.

12. Shone JD, Sellers RD, Anderson RC, Adams PJ, Lillehei CW, Edwards JE. The developmental complex of "parachute mitral valve", supravalvular ring of left atrium, subaortic stenosis, and coarctation of the aorta. Am J Cardiol 1963; 11: 714–725.

13. Ruckman RN, Van Praagh R. Anatomic types of congenital mitral stenosis: report of 49 cases with consideration of diagnosis and surgical implications. Am J Cardiol 1978; 42: 592–601.

14. Mann RJ, Lie JT. The life story of Wilhelm Ebstein (1836–1912) and his almost overlooked description of a congenital heart disease. Mayo Clin Proc 1979; 54: 197–204.

15. Leung MP, Baker EJ, Anderson RH, Zuberbuhler JR. Cineangiographic spectrum of Ebstein's malformation: its relevance to clinical presentation and outcome. J Am Coll Cardiol 1988; 11: 154–161.

16. Becker AE, Becker MJ, Edwards JE. Pathologic spectrum of dysplasia of the tricuspid valve. Features in common with Ebstein's malformation. Arch Pathol 1971; 91: 167–178.

17. Milo S, Stark J, Macartney FJ, Anderson RH. Parachute deformity of the tricuspid valve (case report). Thorax 1979; 34: 543–546.

18. Kanjuh VI, Stevenson JE, Amplatz K, Edwards JE. Congenitally unguarded tricuspid orifice with co-existent pulmonary atresia. Circulation 1964; 30: 911–917.

19. Zuberbuhler JR, Allwork SP, Anderson RH. The spectrum of Ebstein's anomaly of the tricuspid valve. J Thorac Cardiovasc Surg 1979; 77: 202–211.

Ventricular hypoplasia

INTRODUCTION

A malformed ventricle can be small in many circumstances. The ventricular cavity may be smaller than usual while the ventricular walls are obviously and grossly hypertrophic. Not all hearts exhibiting such features will be discussed in this chapter. For example, those ventricles which are small because they lack one or more of their component parts (as with the incomplete and rudimentary ventricles to be found in hearts with a univentricular atrioventricular connexion to a dominant ventricle) are considered in Chapters 18 and 19. The small right or left ventricles found in hearts with deficient atrioventricular septation and unbalanced commitment of the atrioventricular junction are described in Chapter 7. In this chapter we are specifically concerned with those hearts which have ventricular cavities of reduced volume, usually with mural hypertrophy, when the ventricular septum is intact. This pattern may be encountered in either the right or the morphologically left ventricle. When the right ventricle is involved, almost always there is co-existing pulmonary atresia and the combination is called 'pulmonary atresia with intact ventricular septum'. Some hearts in this group have dilated rather than hypertrophic ventricles but they will be included here even though they do not strictly have ventricular hypoplasia. Hearts with small left ventricular cavities and hypertrophy of the left ventricular wall are usually grouped together as the hypoplastic left heart syndrome.

PULMONARY ATRESIA WITH INTACT VENTRICULAR SEPTUM

The dominant lesion in this condition is complete blockage of the pulmonary arterial pathways at the ventriculo–arterial junction. Almost always the combination of pulmonary atresia and an intact ventricular septum is found in association with concordant atrioventricular and ventriculo–arterial connexions. Rarely it may be found when there is either complete[1] or corrected[2] transposition where the left ventricle is hypoplastic. In this section we are concerned with pulmonary atresia associated with a malformed right ventricle. Because of the atretic ventricular outlet, the circulatory pathways depend upon the presence of an interatrial communication and patency of the arterial duct (ductus arteriosus) (Fig. 10.1). Sometimes the pulmonary blood supply can be derived from systemic–pulmonary collateral arteries, but these are rare. This is in contrast to pulmonary atresia with a ventricular septal defect where collateral arteries from the aorta supply the lungs in up to half the cases (see Ch. 12). When the ventricular septum is intact, the obligatory interatrial communication is most often due to exaggerated patency of the oval foramen, since the circulation is an exaggeration of the fetal arrangement. Sometimes there may be a true deficiency of the atrial septum within the oval fossa. All the other types of interatrial defects (see Ch. 6) may also occur although we have not seen them in this setting. The most significant variability in morphology is found within the right ventricle and at the ventriculo–arterial junction.

Variability in the ventricular mass

Hearts with pulmonary atresia and an intact ventricular septum are often categorized as having either a small right ventricle (so-called 'type 1') or

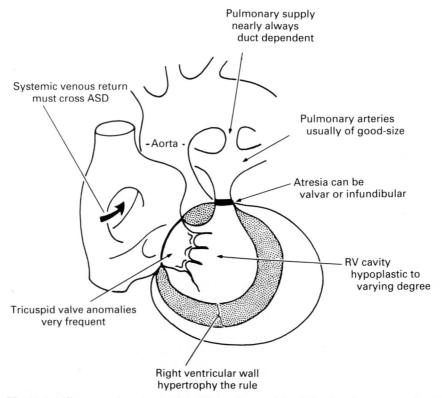

Pulmonary supply
nearly always
duct dependent

Systemic venous return
must cross ASD

Pulmonary arteries
usually of good-size

-Aorta-

Atresia can be
valvar or infundibular

RV cavity
hypoplastic to
varying degree

Tricuspid valve anomalies
very frequent

Right ventricular wall
hypertrophy the rule

Fig. 10.1 A diagrammatic representation of the pathways of circulation in pulmonary atresia with intact ventricular septum.

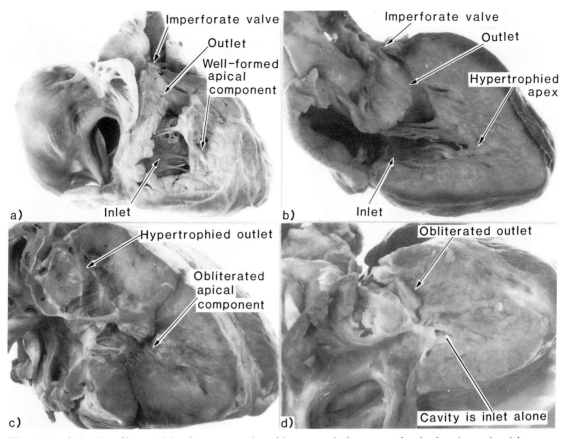

Fig. 10.2 a–d A series of hearts with pulmonary atresia and intact ventricular septum showing how increasing right ventricular cavitary hypoplasia (**a–d**) is dependent upon hypertrophy and overgrowth of the wall of first the apical trabecular (**a–c**) and then the outlet (**d**) components of the ventricle.

a normally sized or dilated ventricle ('type 2').[3] This categorization is too restrictive. The hypoplasia of the ventricular cavity presents as a spectrum of malformations from tiny to dilated, with very few hearts having chambers of normal volume.[4] The spectrum can be extended to include cases with critical pulmonary stenosis (see Ch. 11). This is because the right ventricle is often proportionately hypoplastic in terms of cavity size and hypertrophied in terms of wall thickness when the pulmonary valve is minimally patent. It is much more helpful, therefore, to analyse the hypoplasia of the cavity in terms of overgrowth of its inlet, outlet or apical trabecular components by the mural hypertrophy. This analysis — called the tripartite approach to cavity hypoplasia,[5] — has considerable implications for surgical management.[6] The concept originates

from the observation that those hearts with the best-formed ventricles have reasonable formation of all components, although all may be somewhat small in terms of volume (Fig. 10.2a). With increasing hypertrophy of the right ventricular myocardium, presumably in response to the atretic outflow, the cavity becomes 'squeezed in' by the thickened walls. This starts within the apical trabecular component. Thus, hearts with reasonably sized ventricles have overgrowth of the apical zone (Fig. 10.2b). Increasing degrees of hypertrophy then produce tubular narrowing of the subpulmonary outflow (Fig. 10.2c). In those cases with the smallest cavities, the infundibulum is obliterated and the ventricular cavity is effectively represented only by the inlet (Fig. 10.2d). The size of the cavity is directly related to the diameter of the tricuspid valve orifice.[4,5] This is a

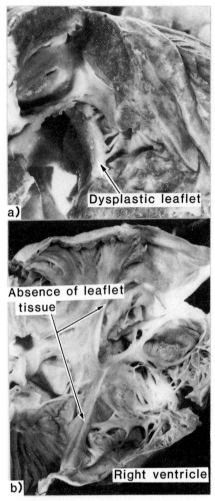

a)

Dysplastic leaflet

Absence of leaflet tissue

Right ventricle

b)

Fig. 10.3 a,b Changes in the tricuspid valve are frequent in the setting of pulmonary atresia with intact ventricular septum. These examples show (**a**) dysplastic leaflets and (**b**) a congenitally unguarded orifice (absent leaflets).

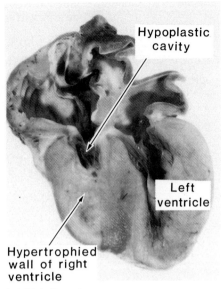

Hypoplastic cavity

Left ventricle

Hypertrophied wall of right ventricle

Fig. 10.4 This 'four chamber' section shows severe hypertrophy of the right ventricular wall in a case where the cavity was, effectively, represented by only the inlet.

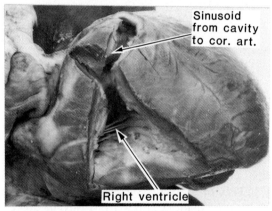

Sinusoid from cavity to cor. art.

Right ventricle

Fig. 10.5 This dissection shows a large sinusoid connecting the hypoplastic right ventricular cavity to the anterior interventricular coronary artery.

useful measurement which can be made during life, either echocardiographically or by angiocardiography.

The tricuspid valve is malformed in most cases, with thickened and dysplastic leaflets and cords (Fig. 10.3a). Some show evidence of downward displacement of the leaflets (Ebstein's malformation). The grossest examples of this lesion are seen in hearts with dilatation of the right ventricle and pulmonary atresia (see below). Dilated ventricles can also be seen when the tricuspid orifice is unguarded (absence of leaflets). Rarely,

the leaflets may be absent when the cavity is hypoplastic (Fig. 10.3b). The myocardium is usually grossly thickened, the greater degrees of hypertrophy being associated with the smaller cavities. The hypertrophied septum bulges markedly into the left ventricle and, in the most severe cases, the right ventricle resembles a fruit, the cavity being the stone with the myocardium being the pulp (Fig. 10.4).

The endocardial layer of the right ventricle often shows minimal fibro-elastic changes. The most severe myocardial lesions are the so-called 'sinusoids'.[7] These are found in the cases with the thickest walls and the smallest cavities, in which the apical trabecular component is virtually obliterated. Within the wall, however, there are multiple intercommunicating channels lined with endothelium. These are the sinusoids, often considered to represent embryonic myocardium.[8] They have much more sinister clinical and prognostic significance when they also communicate with the epicardial branches of the coronary arteries (Fig. 10.5). Cases with large communications between sinusoids and the coronary arteries

also show multiple malformations of the coronary arteries themselves.[7,9] In the most extreme examples, neither coronary artery is patent at its aortic origin.[10] Lesser malformations involve atresia of one coronary arterial orifice and interruption of segments of the major epicardial branches. The left coronary artery has also been identified arising anomalously from the pulmonary trunk.

The ventriculo–arterial junction

The precise morphology at the ventriculo–arterial junction is closely related to the degree of cavity hypoplasia. There are two possible arrangements. In one, the leaflets of the pulmonary valve are present but imperforate (Fig. 10.6a). They form a domed membrane, set at the base of the sinuses of Valsalva, which separates the cavities of the ventricle and the pulmonary trunk. Of necessity, the infundibular cavity must be patent to the underside of the imperforate valve. In the other pattern, there is no evidence of formation of the valve leaflets (Fig. 10.6b). Instead, the subpulmonary infundibulum is obliterated at the ventriculo–arterial junction (muscular atresia, often with obliteration of virtually the entire outlet component). The pulmonary trunk then originates as a blind structure above the radiating sinuses of Valsalva. Irrespective of the type of atresia and the size of the ventricular cavity, the pulmonary trunk and its branches are almost always of good size.[4] The arterial duct is usually the source of pulmonary supply and, unless the supply is supplemented by other means, closure of the duct will cause death. The course of the duct is different from the usual arrangement in some cases. The angle of inclination of the duct may reflect the stage of fetal life at which the atresia developed,[11] although this has yet to be proved. Nonetheless, echocardiographic studies have now documented the progression of pulmonary stenosis to atresia during fetal life.[12,13]

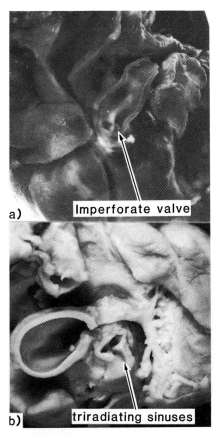

a)

Imperforate valve

b)

triradiating sinuses

Fig. 10.6 a,b The nature of the pulmonary atresia depends upon whether there is a potential connexion between the cavities of right ventricle and pulmonary trunk, in which case there is an imperforate valve membrane (**a**), or whether there is muscular outlet atresia, in which case there is no evidence of formation of a pulmonary valve (**b**).

Pulmonary atresia with dilated right ventricle

Although not strictly an example of right ventric-

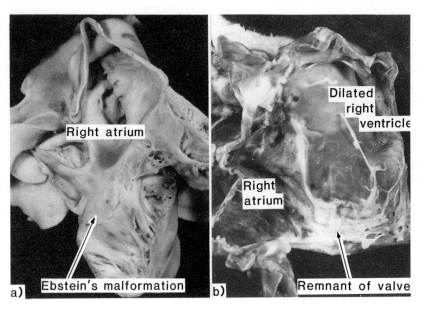

Fig. 10.7 a,b These hearts show the changes to be found at the atrioventricular junction when pulmonary atresia is associated with a dilated right ventricle. There is either Ebstein's malformation (**a**) or a congenitally unguarded junction (**b**).

ular hypoplasia, the variant of pulmonary atresia with intact ventricular septum in which the ventricular cavity is grossly dilated is described here. Such cases form a special group. The condition presents clinically in the neonatal period if it does not lead to death of the fetus prior to birth.[14] The dilated right atrium and ventricle fill the chest, giving the so-called 'wall-to-wall' appearance of the heart in the chest radiograph. The enlarged heart also compresses the lungs, and it is the accompanying hypoplasia of the lungs themselves which probably contributes most to the bad prognosis. The tricuspid valve either shows evidence of gross Ebstein's malformation (Fig. 10.7a) or else there are various degrees of absence of the leaflets (Fig. 10.7b). Usually it is the septal and mural leaflets which are lacking, the anterosuperior leaflet being found in rudimentary form. In other cases, all the leaflets are missing. The atresia at the ventriculo–arterial junction is almost always of the muscular type. The pulmonary trunk is well formed but the pulmonary arteries are often hypoplastic, reflecting the hypoplasia of the lungs. The thin

walls of the ventricle are, almost certainly, the consequence of acquired change during fetal life. These hearts should be distinguished from Uhl's anomaly (see Ch. 23) in which there is congenital absence of the myocardium of the parietal ventricular wall.

'SAUSAGE' RIGHT VENTRICLE

There is a small group of patients, well-recognized clinically,[15] who have right ventricular hypoplasia in association with normally structured tricuspid and pulmonary valves. When seen angiographically, the residual cavity of the right ventricle bears a striking resemblance to a sausage. We have seen one heart with this arrangement.[16] The hypoplasia was due to absence of formation of the ventricular apical trabecular component — the cavity, as a result, being a smooth tube connecting the tricuspid and pulmonary valves (Fig. 10.8). The apical trabecular component of the left ventricle was also grossly malformed.

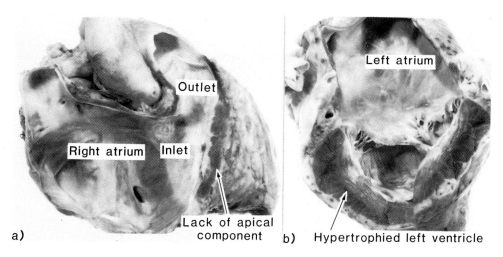

a) b)

Outlet

Right atrium Inlet

Lack of apical component

Left atrium

Hypertrophied left ventricle

Fig. 10.8 a,b These illustrations show the right (**a**) and left (**b**) ventricles in a case with congenital absence of the apical trabecular component of the right ventricle — the so-called 'sausage' ventricle.

THE HYPOPLASTIC LEFT HEART SYNDROME

There is a group of anomalies which have in common the presence of a small left ventricle, usually with an intact ventricular septum, and with various degrees of hypoplasia of the aortic pathways. First grouped together by Lev under the title of 'hypoplasia of the aortic tract complexes',[17] they were subsequently described as the 'hypoplastic left heart syndrome' by Noonan and Nadas.[18] Patients with aortic coarctation often have some degree of left ventricular hypoplasia. Indeed, the majority of the cases described by Noonan and Nadas[18] were characterized by coarctation. It is difficult in these cases to determine when the left ventricle is truly hypoplastic. Nowadays, the hearts considered to represent hypoplastic left heart syndrome tend to have aortic atresia or critical aortic stenosis. These are the lesions we will describe. This is not to deny that some patients with coarctation have left ventricular hypoplasia. In those who show this association, the hypoplastic ventricle is often the cause for a fatal outcome at surgery. We will, nonetheless, defer consideration of these hearts to Chapter 13. Neither will we discuss here those hearts having aortic atresia in association with a well-formed left ventricle.

Aortic atresia is not synonymous with the hypoplastic left heart syndrome. The characteristic feature of the latter entity is cavity hypoplasia of the left ventricle, usually with mural hypertrophy and an intact ventricular septum. The flow pathways are dependent upon patency or otherwise of the atrial septum and the arterial duct (Fig. 10.9). As with hypoplastic right ventricle, anatomical variability can be found at various levels within the heart. Until recently, these variables were largely of pathological interest but, in the past decade, it has been shown that such hearts are amenable to surgical 'correction'. This surgical experience has emphasized the practical importance of these various anatomical patterns.

The atrial chambers

Irrespective of the nature of the obstruction within the left heart, the major flow pathway for pulmonary venous return is to the right atrium. Almost always, therefore, there is an interatrial communication through the oval fossa which, by virtue of the design of the fossa, usually obstructs the flow of blood from left to right. In a minority of cases, the atrial septum is intact. This arrangement is of little significance during fetal life although it is certainly possible that premature closure of the oval foramen could promote development of left ventricular hypoplasia. It might

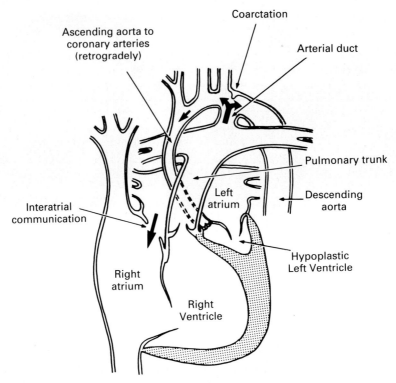

Fig. 10.9 This diagrammatic representation shows the circulatory pathways in so-called hypoplastic left heart syndrome.

be thought that an intact atrial septum would be incompatible with life after birth. When there is an intact septum, therefore, alternative routes are developed whereby the pulmonary venous return can reach the systemic circulation. Possibilities are a laevo-atrial cardinal vein (see Ch. 5), anomalous pulmonary venous connexion, and unroofing or fenestrations of the coronary sinus. There are exceptional cases, nonetheless, in which there is no apparent route for pulmonary venous return, yet the baby may have survived for several months. Presumably there are collateral channels which are not obvious on gross examination.

The atrioventricular junction

The major variable is whether the mitral valve is patent and stenotic or imperforate. Cases with a patent valve are those which show left ventricular mural hypertrophy and fibro-elastosis (see below). When the mitral valve is atretic, the left ventricle

is thin-walled but grossly hypoplastic, often represented by a mere slit within the postero-inferior wall of the ventricular mass. The mitral valve may be imperforate (Figs. 10.10a, b) but more usually the entire left atrioventricular connexion is absent (Fig. 10.10c). The heart then exhibits univentricular atrioventricular connexion to a dominant right ventricle. The left ventricle is not only hypoplastic but also incomplete, lacking its inlet component and often its outlet component. It has been suggested[19] that these hearts with mitral atresia have much better ventricular myocardium than those with patent valves and fibro-elastosis, which might suggest that they are more amenable to surgical 'correction': so far, there is no substantiating evidence to support this concept.

The ventricular mass

The major feature is that the right ventricle forms

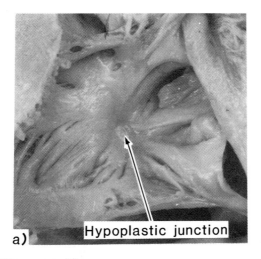

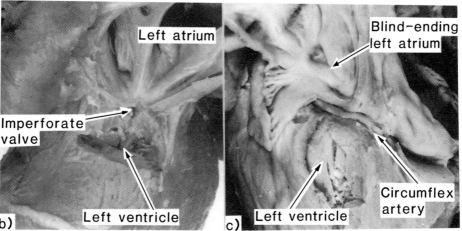

Fig. 10.10 a–c These photographs of the left atrioventricular junction show the difference between an imperforate valve which blocks a formed but hypoplastic orifice (**a & b**) and complete absence of the atrioventricular connexion (**c**).

the apex of the ventricular mass. This feature becomes increasingly obvious with diminishing size of the left ventricle although, when the mitral valve is atretic, the left ventricle may not be immediately evident on gross examination. The ventricular mass is then effectively formed in total by the right ventricle (Fig. 10.11). In extreme examples, it may be necessary to examine the myocardial mass histologically to identify the left ventricle. Under all these conditions, the extent of the left ventricle will still be delineated by the descending branches of the major coronary arteries.

The effect of atresia of the mitral valve on the left ventricle differs from that of mitral stenosis. The latter lesion leads to mural hypertrophy and subendocardial fibroelastosis (Fig. 10.12). This process, as with right ventricular hypoplasia (see earlier in this Chapter), is associated with the development of myocardial sinusoids and coronary arterial lesion.[20] Changes can also be seen within the right ventricle. Often the septomarginal trabeculation is particularly obvious as a discrete muscle bar. This bar can rarely divide the right ventricle into a two-chambered structure. The tricuspid valve may also be dysplastic.

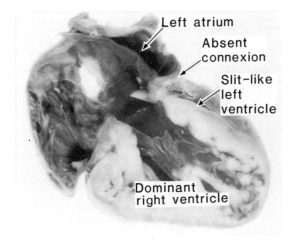

Fig. 10.11 This 'four chamber' section shows the typical morphology when the left atrioventricular connexion is absent and the left ventricle is a mere slit in the posterior wall of the ventricular mass.

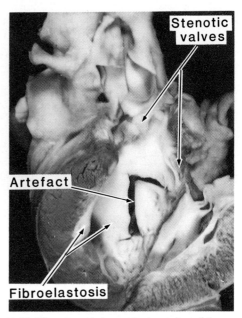

Fig. 10.12 Fibroelastosis is seen in the setting of the hypoplastic left heart syndrome only when the mitral valve is patent, as in this case with mitral and aortic stenosis.

The ventriculo–arterial junction

Changes here reflect the presence of stenosis (Fig. 10.13a) or atresia of the aortic valve. Atresia of the valve may take the form simply of an imperforate membrane (Fig. 10.13b). More usually, it is due to muscular or fibromuscular obliteration of the orifice (Fig. 10.13c). The aorta then commences above the sinuses of Valsalva as a blind sack from which arise the coronary arteries.

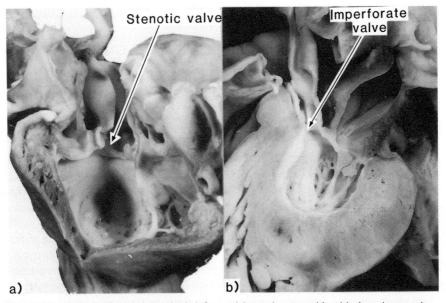

Fig. 10.13 a–c A significantly hypoplastic left ventricle can be seen with critical aortic stenosis (**a**) or with aortic atresia due to an imperforate valve (**b**) or a fibromuscular segment (**c**).

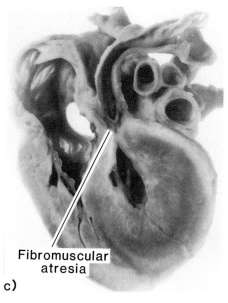

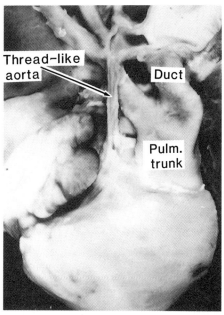

Fibromuscular
atresia

c)

Fig. 10.13 c

Fig. 10.14 The major flow pathway in aortic atresia is from the pulmonary trunk through the duct to the aorta. The head and neck arteries are supplied retrogradely through the isthmus, and the ascending aorta, often thread-like as in this example, supplies the coronary arteries in retrograde fashion.

The arterial pathways

The major flow pathway from the heart is through the pulmonary trunk and the arterial duct. The ascending aorta is hypoplastic to a degree that depends on whether the aortic valve is stenotic or atretic. In extreme situations, the calibre of the aorta can be no greater than that of the coronary

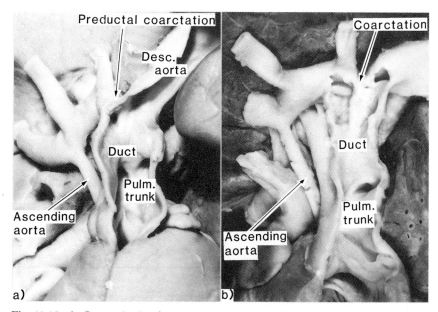

Fig. 10.15 a,b Coarctation is a frequent accompaniment of the hypoplastic left heart syndrome and can be seen in either preductal (**a**) or paraductal (**b**) location.

arteries (Fig. 10.14). It should not be mistaken for anomalous origin of the coronary arteries from the brachiocephalic artery in the presence of a common arterial trunk. The entire blood supply to the head and neck, to the arms and to the upper part of the trunk, together with the coronary arterial supply, is through the arterial duct and then in retrograde fashion through the aortic isthmus. Co-existing coarctation is of utmost significance in this setting. Examination of the heart in such cases reveals discrete lesions at the isthmus in up to three-quarters.[21] The coarctation shelves can be found in either preductal or paraductal position (Fig. 10.15). Most of the lesions that we have seen were preductal, the shelf being composed of ductal tissue. The Leiden group, in contrast, found that the majority of the lesions were paraductal.[22]

REFERENCES

1. Ho SY, Angelini A, Russell G. Pulmonary atresia with hypoplastic left ventricle. Int J Cardiol 1987; 15: 349–352.
2. Steeg CN, Ellis K, Bransilver B, Gersony WM. Pulmonary atresia and intact septum complicating corrected transposition of the great vessels. Am Heart J 1971; 82: 382–386.
3. Davignon AL, Greenwold WE, Dushane JW, Edwards JE. Congenital pulmonary atresia with intact ventricular septum: clinicopathologic correlation of two anatomic types. Am Heart J 1961; 62: 591–602.
4. Zuberbuhler JR, Anderson RH. Morphological variations in pulmonary atresia with intact ventricular septum. Br Heart J 1979; 41: 281–288.
5. Bull C, de Leval MR, Mercanti C, Macartney FJ, Anderson RH. Pulmonary atresia with intact ventricular septum: a revised classification. Circulation 1982; 66: 266–271.
6. de Leval M, Bull C, Stark J, Anderson RH, Taylor JFN, Macartney FJ. Pulmonary atresia and intact ventricular septum: surgical management based on a revised classification. Circulation 1982; 66: 272–280.
7. Gittenberger-de-Groot AC, Sauer U, Bindl L, Babic R, Essed CE, Buhlmeyer K. Competition of coronary arteries and ventriculo-coronary arterial communications in pulmonary atresia with intact septum. Int J Cardiol 1988; 18: 243–258.
8. Dusek J, Ostadal B, Duskova M. Postnatal persistence of spongy myocardium with embryonic blood supply. Arch Pathol 1975; 99: 312–317.
9. Calder AL, Sage MD. Coronary arterial abnormalities in pulmonary atresia with intact ventricular septum. Am J Cardiol 1987; 59: 436–442.
10. Lenox CC, Briner J. Absent proximal coronary arteries associated with pulmonary atresia. Am J Cardiol 1972; 30: 666–669.
11. Santos MA, Moll JN, Drumond C, Araujo WB, Romao N, Reis NB. Development of the ductus arteriosus in

right ventricular outflow tract obstruction. Circulation 1980; 62: 818–822.
12. Todros T, Presbitero P, Gaglioti P, Demarie D. Pulmonary stenosis with intact ventricular septum: documentation of development echocardiographically during fetal life. Int J Cardiol 1988; 19: 355–360.
13. Allan LD, Crawford DC, Tynan MJ. Pulmonary atresia in prenatal life. J Amer Coll Cardiol 1986; 8: 1131–1136.
14. Allan LD. Development of congenital lesions in mid or late gestation. Editorial Note. Int J Cardiol 1988; 19: 361–362.
15. Van der Hauwaert LG, Michaelson M. Isolated right ventricular hypoplasia. Circulation 1971; 44: 466–474.
16. Oldershaw P, Ward D, Anderson RH. Hypoplasia of the apical trabecular component of the morphologically right ventricle. Am J Cardiol 1985; 55: 862–863.
17. Lev M. Pathologic anatomy and interrelationship of hypoplasia of the aortic tract complexes. Lab Invest 1952; 1: 61–70.
18. Noonan JA, Nadas AS. The hypoplastic left heart syndrome. Pediatr Clin North Am 1958; 5: 1029–1056.
19. Freedom RM, Benson L, Wilson GJ. The coronary circulation and myocardium in pulmonary and aortic atresia with an intact ventricular septum. In: Marcelletti C, Anderson RH, Becker AE, Corno A, Di Carlo D, Mazzera E, eds. Paediatric cardiology, vol. 6. Edinburgh: Churchill Livingstone, 1986; 78–96.
20. O'Connor WN, Cash JB, Cottrill CM, Johnson GL, Noonan JA. Ventriculocoronary connections in hypoplastic left hearts: an autopsy microscopic study. Circulation 1982; 66: 1078–1086.
21. Von Rueden TJ, Knight L, Moller JH, Edwards JE. Coarctation of aorta associated with aortic valve atresia. Circulation 1975; 52: 951–954.
22. Elzenga NJ, Gittenberger-de-Groot AC. Coarctation and related aortic arch anomalies in hypoplastic left heart syndrome. Int J Cardiol 1985; 8: 379–389.

Abnormalities of the ventricular outlets and arterial valves

INTRODUCTION

When assessing malformations of the outflow tracts, it is necessary to consider lesions of the ventricular outlets themselves and also anomalies of the arterial valves. Since lesions of the ascending portions of the great arteries produce comparable symptoms, they too will be discussed in this chapter. When describing pathology of the outflow tracts, we will deal with lesions of the outlets of the morphologically left and right ventricles as separate entities irrespective of the arterial trunk they supply. This is because the nature of the obstructive lesions is basically the same irrespective of the presence of concordant or discordant ventriculo–arterial connexions. We will not, however, discuss here obstruction in the presence of double outlet ventricle or common arterial trunk: they are considered in Chapters 21 and 22 respectively.

THE OUTLET FROM THE MORPHOLOGICALLY LEFT VENTRICLE

The left ventricular outflow tract (Fig. 11.1) is in part a muscular structure (the origin of the leaflets of the arterial valve being from the septal musculature and the muscular ventriculo-infundibular fold) and in part a fibrous structure (the central fibrous body, the area of fibrous continuity between the arterial and atrioventricular valves and the left fibrous trigone). On rare occasions, the left ventricular outlet may be a completely muscular structure, very rarely with concordant

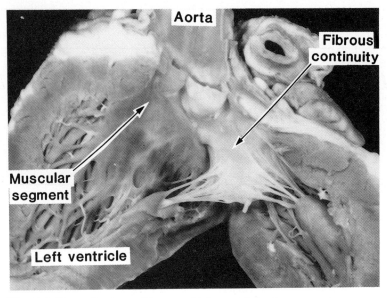

Fig. 11.1 The outflow tract of the normal left ventricle has been opened through its anterolateral quadrant to show its partly fibrous and partly muscular nature.

ventriculo–arterial connexions[1] but more usually, in this context, with discordant connexions (see Ch. 20). In most instances, nonetheless, it is the partly fibrous and partly muscular arrangement which dictates the nature of outflow obstruction.

Fibrous shelf

A fibrous shelf which extends from the ventricular septum beneath the arterial valve on to the facing surface of the mitral valve is a common cause of either aortic obstruction with concordant ventriculo–arterial connexions (Fig. 11.2) or pulmonary obstruction with discordant ventriculo–arterial connexions (see Ch. 20). Only rarely is the lesion a completely circular obstruction; more usually it is like a horseshoe which attaches to the base of the non-facing leaflet of the arterial valve. The septal component of the shelf is adherent to the endocardium directly covering the origin of the left bundle branch from the conduction axis. Because of this, its surgical removal without production of heart block may be difficult.

Fibromuscular tunnel

A fibromuscular tunnel produces a longer segment of outflow tract stenosis (Fig. 11.3). It also can be found with either concordant or discordant ventriculo–arterial connexions.

Aneurysmal tissue tags

These grape-like structures may arise from the membranous septum, be it intact or partially formed, or from the mitral valve or the tricuspid valve when they herniate through a co-existing ventricular septal defect into the left ventricle. When there are concordant ventriculo–arterial connexions, the tissue tags are not as frequent a cause of obstruction since they are directed to the right ventricle by the higher left ventricular pressure. They are more significant in the setting of atrioventricular septal defects (see Ch. 7), when they further obstruct an already narrowed outflow tract. They are particularly significant when there are discordant ventriculo–arterial connexions, because the pressure differential between the ventricles favours their protrusion

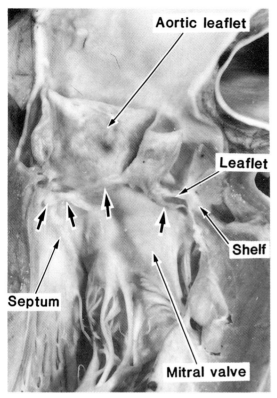

Fig. 11.2 This specimen shows a fibrous shelf of relatively minor size positioned very close to the base of the leaflets of the aortic valve. Note that the shelf extends on to the leaflet of the valve but is largely fixed to the septum (left-hand arrows).

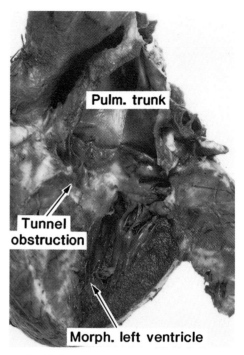

Fig. 11.3 In this heart, an entire segment of the outflow tract is narrowed to produce tunnel-like obstruction.

into the subpulmonary left ventricular outflow tract.

Anomalous insertion of atrioventricular valvar tension apparatus

This lesion is also seen most frequently in hearts with deficient atrioventricular septation (see Ch. 7) but can be an important cause of obstruction in the setting of discordant ventriculo–arterial connexions.

Deviation of the ventricular septum

Malalignment of the outlet component of the ventricular septum with deviation into the left ventricle is an important cause of subaortic obstruction when there is a ventricular septal defect and concordant ventriculo–arterial connexions. It is now well-recognized that with this type of ventricular septal defect there is a high frequency of association with coarctation or interruption of the aortic arch.[2,3] Indeed, all forms of left ventricular outflow tract obstruction in the presence of concordant ventriculo–arterial connexions are frequently accompanied by obstructive lesions of the aortic arch (see Ch. 13). When the outlet septum is deviated into the left ventricle with discordant ventriculo–arterial connexions it results in subpulmonary obstruction.

Hypertrophy of the anterolateral muscle bundle

The anterolateral muscle bundle is normally an inconspicuous trabeculation which descends the anterior parietal wall of the outflow tract from its junction with the ventricular septum (Fig. 11.1). If hypertrophied,[4] it can cause or exacerbate left ventricular outflow tract obstruction with either

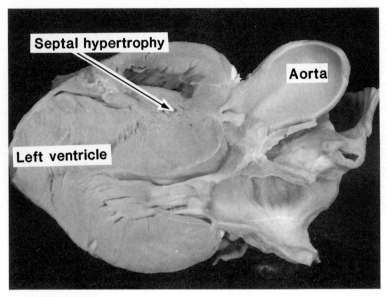

Fig. 11.4 This specimen shows gross hypertrophy of the ventricular septum as part of the process known as hypertrophic cardiomyopathy. The heart is sectioned to replicate the parasternal long axis echocardiographic plane.

concordant or discordant ventriculo–arterial connexions.

Dynamic obstructive lesions

Dynamic obstruction of the left ventricular outflow tract is characterized by bulging or muscular thickening of the septal surface. The thickening can be minimal and not necessarily recognized as pathological. When extreme, its obstructive nature cannot be in doubt (Fig. 11.4) and it is identical with the process described as hypertrophic obstructive cardiomyopathy. As with the lesions described above, dynamic obstruction may be found with both concordant and discordant ventriculo–arterial connexions.

ABNORMALITIES OF THE MORPHOLOGICALLY RIGHT VENTRICULAR OUTLET

The right ventricular outflow tract, in contrast to the left ventricular outflow tract, is a completely muscular structure (Fig. 11.5). In hearts with normal outflow tracts, the ventriculo-infundibular fold and parietal wall form most of the infundibulum, the outlet septum being an insignificant structure. In keeping with the architecture, obstruction of the right ventricular outflow tract is almost invariably muscular. Obstruction may rarely be produced by extreme herniation of a fibrous tissue tag from the area of the central fibrous body,[5] or even by prolapse of the Eustachian valve into the right ventricular outlet.

Muscular obstruction can exist either within the trabecular zone of the right ventricle, at the junction of the trabecular and outlet portions, or as a concentric thickening of the outlet itself (Fig. 11.6). Obstruction in the trabecular zone is not strictly outflow tract obstruction, but can be conveniently considered here. In the normal heart, the supraventricular crest inserts between the limbs of the septomarginal trabeculation. The body of the trabeculation, together with the moderator band, then completes a muscular loop around the trabecular part of the ventricle. It is hypertrophy of one or more of these muscular structures which produces obstruction, a condition usually known as 'two-chambered right ventricle'. There are two distinct forms. In the

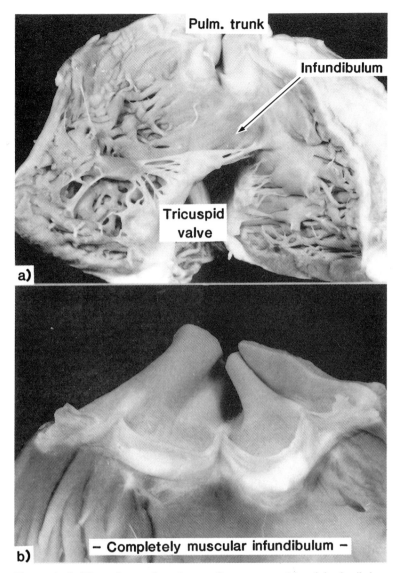

Fig. 11.5 a,b These pictures show the overall arrangement (**a**) and the detailed morphology (**b**) of the completely muscular outflow tract of the morphologically right ventricle.

milder type, the moderator band (or, more likely, an anomalous septoparietal trabeculation) takes off from the septomarginal trabeculation much higher than usual and crosses the cavity of the ventricle. This arrangement is frequently a chance finding in an otherwise normal heart (Fig. 11.7). In the more severe form, the apical extent of the septomarginal trabeculation is enlarged and forms a shelf dividing the apical trabecular component of the ventricle into two cavities (Fig. 11.8). The inlet and outlet portion each then possesses part of the trabecular component as an apical extension. Such two-chambered right ventricles can exist with and without ventricular septal defects and with co-existing tetralogy of Fallot. In extreme cases, the inlet and outlet chambers may be totally divorced by a complete muscular septum. These anomalies have an unguarded

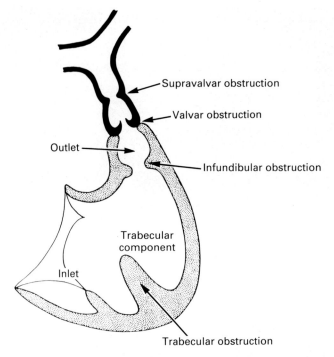

Fig. 11.6 This diagram shows the potential sites for obstruction in the outflow pathways from the right side of the heart.

tricuspid orifice and present as 'tricuspid atresia' (see Ch. 19).

Stenosis at the junction of the trabecular and outlet parts of the right ventricle is the most common form of muscular pulmonary stenosis. This can exist either as a localized narrowing, when the outlet part of the right ventricle forms an expanded chamber above the stenotic ring, or else the entire infundibular region of the right ventricle is concentrically narrowed. The finding of a discrete infundibular chamber is most frequent in the tetralogy of Fallot when the infundibular narrowing is superimposed on the malalignment of the outlet septum (see Ch. 12). In contrast, isolated tubular muscular stenosis occurs most frequently with an intact ventricular septum.

ABNORMALITIES OF THE ARTERIAL VALVES

Stenosis of the aortic or pulmonary valves can

be considered irrespective of their relation to either the left or the right ventricle. Aortic valvar stenosis, while common in the setting of concordant ventriculo–arterial connexions, is exceedingly rare with discordant ones. Pulmonary valvar stenosis, in relative rather than absolute terms, is more common with discordant than concordant ventriculo–arterial connexions. It is important to restate that the arterial valves possess no ring (or 'annulus') in the sense of a fibrous circular structure which supports the valvar leaflets. The morphology of all arterial valves is dictated by the semilunar attachments of the leaflets (Figs 11.1 and 11.5).

Arterial valvar dysplasia

Dysplastic arterial valves are characterized by uniform thickening in which the trifoliate structure of the valve can still be recognized. The valve leaflets are composed of mucoid connective tissue. The lesion may affect either aortic or

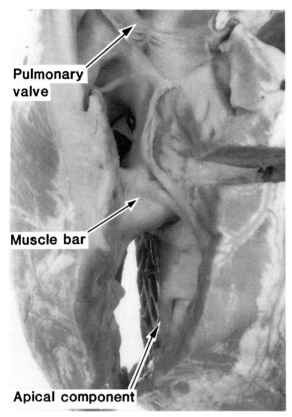

Fig. 11.7 This heart had, as an incidental finding, a discrete septoparietal trabeculation crossing the cavity of the junction of the apical trabecular and outlet components of the right ventricle.

pulmonary valves, and is the major obstructive lesion in Noonan's syndrome ('pseudo-Turner's syndrome') — the male phenotype of Turner's syndrome, with various external malformations and usually malformations of the heart, particularly right-sided lesions.[6]

Dome-shaped valvar stenosis

This condition is characterized by a dome-shaped diaphragm with a central perforation. Three shallow raphes are usually recognizable (Fig. 11.9). It tends to occur in the pulmonary rather than in the aortic valve.

Unicuspid and unicommissural valvar stenosis

This stenosis is characterized by a keyhole-shaped eccentric orifice in which a single leaflet takes origin from the arterial wall and swings around to insert close to its point of departure (Fig. 11.10). The plane of the orifice is oblique, being more shallow at the site of the commissure than on the opposite aspects. Two raphes can often be recognized, suggesting that the lesion results from failure of formation of two of the commissures of

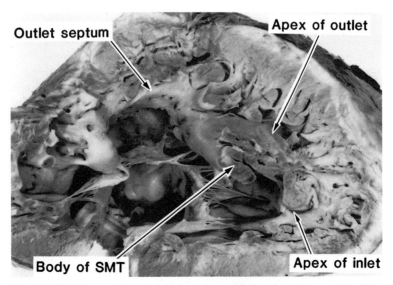

Fig. 11.8 This heart, with co-existing tetralogy of Fallot, shows hypertrophy of the apical extent of the septomarginal trabeculation (SMT) producing discrete apical components of both the inlet and outlet parts of the right ventricle.

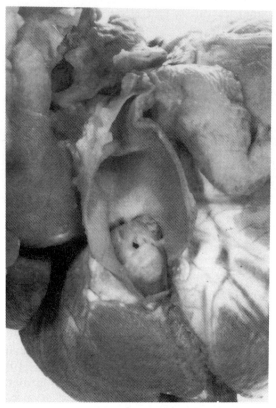

Fig. 11.9 This illustration shows domed stenosis of a pulmonary valve which, initially, had three leaflets.

a tricommissural valve. It is seen most frequently in the aortic position.

The arterial valve with two leaflets

Valves with only two leaflets are not intrinsically stenotic unless there is also dysplasia of the leaflets or other superimposed pathological change.[7] Pathological changes are acquired with increasing age and may take various forms. The valve may become stenotic due to sclerosis and calcification (Fig. 11.11a) or one of the leaflets may prolapse into the ventricle with subsequent valvar insufficiency (Fig. 11.11b). Such valves are highly susceptible to infective endocarditis. The form of the leaflets also varies, in one variant the leaflets being of equal size, in the other the size being unequal. The larger leaflet, termed the conjoined cusp, almost always has a shallow raphe in its middle part. The valve with two leaflets of unequal size, one representing a conjoined leaflet, occurs more commonly in the aorta. The conjoined leaflet is then usually anterior and both coronary arteries arise from the sinus above it. The processes of acquired disease have a predilection for this type of valve rather than for the one with leaflets of equal size. The inference can be

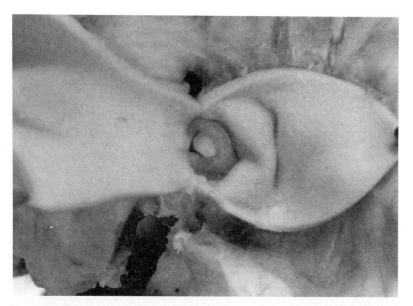

Fig. 11.10 This stenotic aortic valve shows the arrangement said to be unicuspid and unicommissural.

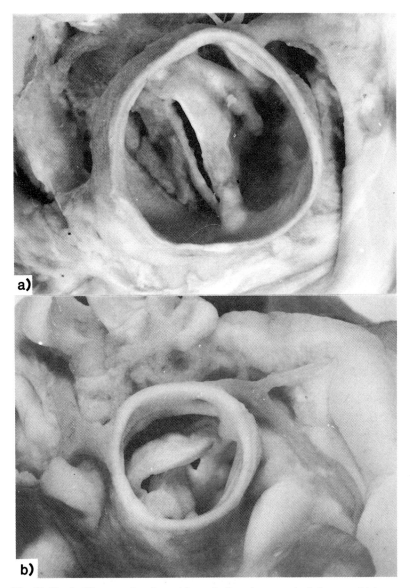

Fig. 11.11 a,b These aortic valves with two leaflets show acquired changes of (**a**) calcification and stenosis and (**b**) prolapse and regurgitation.

made that this type of valve is the result of fusion of two leaflets during development. This is supported by the finding that most have three aortic sinuses (Fig. 11.12a). Some valves, however, not only have two leaflets but also have two sinuses (Fig. 11.12b), evidence that there is a truly bicuspid valve.[8] A valve with two leaflets is found in approximately half the cases of aortic coarctation: in these, the leaflets are usually of equal size.

Arterial valves with three leaflets

The normal arterial valve has three leaflets but these are rarely of equal size, irrespective of whether the valve guards the pulmonary or aortic orifice. The occurrence of leaflets of unequal area in the high pressure systemic circuit may be significant for the development of the type of isolated aortic valve stenosis which occurs most frequently in elderly patients.[9]

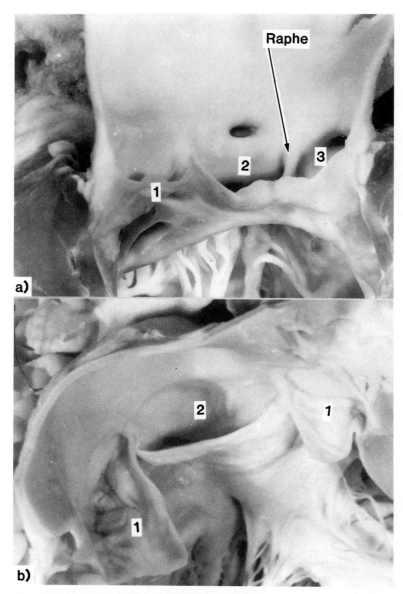

Fig. 11.12 a,b These illustrations show aortic valves having two leaflets but with either (**a**) three or (**b**) two sinuses. The heart shown in (**a**) has discordant ventriculo–arterial connexions (complete transposition).

Arterial valves with four leaflets

An arterial valve with four leaflets is of no functional significance. The leaflets may be of equal size, or three leaflets may be of similar size with one miniature leaflet. Such valves are extremely rare in the aortic position but not infrequent in the pulmonary position. A valve with four leaflets is commonly found at the orifice of a common arterial trunk (see Ch. 22).

Incompetent arterial valves

There is no specific congenital pathology producing valvar incompetence. Prolapse of a

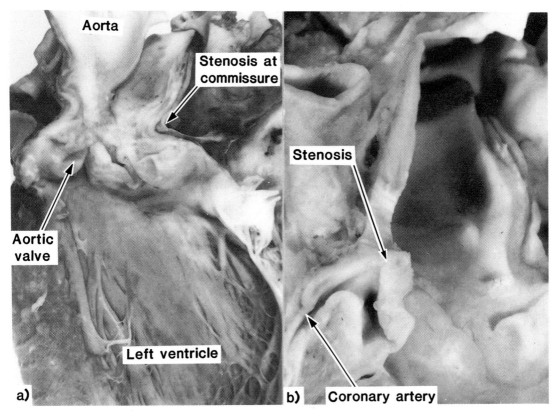

Fig. 11.13 a,b This heart shows an example of the so-called 'hour-glass' variant of supravalvar stenosis, in this case (**a**) at the level of the commissures of the aortic valve. The coronary arteries arise proximal to the stenotic lesion (**b**) and are dilated.

valve with two leaflets has been discussed above. 'Floppy' valves, those which are the seat of mucoid change, are found in children with Marfan's syndrome.

SUPRAVALVAR ARTERIAL STENOSIS

Obstructive lesions of the ascending arterial trunks are justifiably considered along with valvar and subvalvar obstructions, since in most cases they occur at the level of the commissures or involve the latter. They occur most frequently in the aorta[10,11] and they may take one of three forms. The lesion may be present as a discrete shelf, as a so-called hour-glass deformity or as a tubular variety in which most of the aortic arch and its branches are also involved. The tubular type is probably the rarest. The other varieties show an underlying disordered mosaic architecture of the aortic wall which may also occur in the pulmonary vascular tree, where it produces narrowing of the pulmonary trunk and so-called peripheral coarctation of pulmonary arterial branches. When a supravalvar lesion obstructs the outlet from the left ventricle, the ascending aorta becomes divided into segments at high and lower pressures (Fig. 11.13a). The coronary arteries arise from the segment under high pressure (Fig. 11.13b), this feature accounting for their dilated and tortuous course and probably explaining the development of premature atherosclerosis. This, in combination with ventricular hypertrophy, underlies the common occurrence of sudden death in this condition. As indicated above, whatever the nature of the supravalvar stenosis, the abnormality of the wall involves the commissural attachments of the leaflets. The abnormal commissural attach- ments predispose to early degeneration of the leaflets.

REFERENCES

1. Rosenquist GC, Clark EB, Sweeney LJ, McAllister HA. The normal spectrum of mitral and aortic valve discontinuity. Circulation 1976; 54: 298–301.
2. Becu LM, Tauxe WN, DuShane JW, Edwards JE. A complex of congenital cardiac anomalies: ventricular septal defect, biventricular origin of the pulmonary trunk and subaortic stenosis. Am Heart J 1955; 50: 901–911.
3. Moulaert A, Bruins CC, Oppenheimer-Dekker A. Anomalies of the aortic arch and ventricular septal defects. Circulation 1976; 53: 1011–1015.
4. Moulaert AJ, Oppenheimer-Dekker A. Anterolateral muscle bundle of the left ventricle, bulboventricular flange and subaortic stenosis. Am J Cardiol 1976; 37: 78–81.
5. Bonvicini M, Piovaccari G, Picchio F. Severe subpulmonary obstruction caused by an aneurysmal tissue tag complicating an infundibular perimembranous ventricular septal defect. Br Heart J 1982; 48: 189–191.
6. Noonan JA. Hypertelorism with Turner phenotype. A new syndrome with associated congenital heart disease. Am J Dis Child 1968; 116: 373–380.
7. Edwards JE. The congenital bicuspid aortic valve. Circulation 1961; 23: 485–488.
8. Angelini A, Ho SY, Anderson RH, Devine WE, Zuberbuhler JR, Becker AE, Davies MJ. The morphology of the normal as compared to the bifoliate aortic valve. J Thorac Cardiovasc Surg 1989; 98: 363–367.
9. Vollebergh FEMG, Becker AE. Minor congenital variations of cusp size in tricuspid aortic valves. Possible link with isolated aortic stenosis. Br Heart J 1977; 39: 1006–1011.
10. Edwards JE. Pathology of left ventricular outflow tract obstruction. Circulation 1965; 31: 586–599.
11. Peterson TA, Todd DB, Edwards JE. Supravalvular aortic stenosis. J Thorac Cardiovasc Surg 1965; 50: 734–741.

Tetralogy of Fallot with pulmonary stenosis or atresia

INTRODUCTION

In 1888, Etienne-Louis Arthur Fallot published the morphological findings in the hearts of patients presenting with 'la maladie bleue'. He identified, in three-quarters of the cases studied, a relatively constant association of four features, namely an interventricular communication, subpulmonary muscular obstruction, a biventricular connexion of the leaflets of the aortic valve and concentric hypertrophy of the right ventricle.[1] We now recognize this entity as the tetralogy of Fallot although, in retrospect, it is clear that similar cases had been observed and described well before Fallot made his clinicopathological correlations.[2] In this chapter we will describe the distinctive features of the lesion and the subtle differences to be found in individual cases, such that, despite their obvious similarities, no two cases are exactly alike.[3] We will also include a description of the lesion when complicated by subpulmonary atresia rather than stenosis, emphasizing how, when the outflow tract is atretic, it is the morphology of the pulmonary arterial supply which is the crucial feature.

TETRALOGY OF FALLOT WITH PULMONARY STENOSIS

The essential feature that determines the effect of the lesions of the tetralogy of Fallot is anterocephalad deviation of the insertion of the outlet septum. In the normal heart (see Ch. 1), the

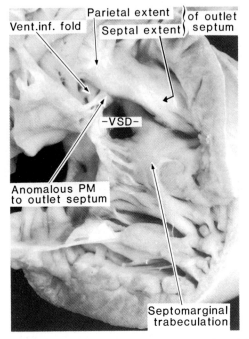

Parietal extent ⎫ of outlet
Vent.inf. fold   Septal extent ⎭ septum

–VSD–

Anomalous PM
to outlet septum

Septomarginal
trabeculation

Fig. 12.1 The essence of the tetralogy is separation of the hypertrophic outlet septum from the rest of the muscular interventricular septum. This specimen shows how the outlet septum, which is not recognizable in the normal heart, has septal and parietal extensions. The septal extension joins the rest of the septum anterocephalad to the septomarginal trabeculation, thus narrowing the subpulmonary infundibulum. Because of the overriding of the aortic valve, the ventriculo-infundibular (vent. inf.) fold now separates the aortic and tricuspid valves. In this particular heart the medial papillary muscle (PM) is anomalously attached to the outlet septum.

outlet septum is an insignificant structure inserted and buried between the limbs of the septomarginal trabeculation. Indeed, it is so fully incorporated into the septum that it is not possible to distinguish it from the dominant component of the supraventricular crest, namely the ventriculo-infundibular fold. In the tetralogy, however, the outlet septum and the ventriculo-infundibular fold are divorced relative to the septomarginal trabeculation, the ventricular septal defect and overriding aortic valve being situated between and bordered by them (Fig. 12.1). The very fact that these muscular structures are separated and distinct in the tetralogy is at the root of much of the confusion and controversy which surrounds its description.

This is because each of these three structures has at various times and in various places been called the 'crista'. Consequently, when the term 'crista' is encountered in accounts of the tetralogy, it is difficult to be sure to which of the different structures it refers. Kjellberg and his colleagues[4] designated the outlet septum as the 'body of the crista' and then recognized its septal and parietal extensions. These are designated as the 'septal bands' and 'parietal bands' respectively (Fig. 12.2a). But others[5,6] had designated the outlet septum itself as the 'parietal band' while the structure we now describe as the septomarginal trabeculation was described as the 'septal band' (Fig. 12.2b). The structure thus nominated as the 'septal band' (our 'septomarginal trabeculation' — see below) had not been named at all by Kjellberg and his colleagues.[4] Instead, confusingly, their 'septal band' is the septal insertion of the outlet septum. It was against this background that we suggested[7] that the term 'crista' (or 'supraventricular crest') be reserved for description of the muscular crest separating the tricuspid and pulmonary valves in a normal right ventricular outflow tract. In situations where the muscular constituents of the outflow tracts are separated one from the other, as is the case in the tetralogy, we suggest that each be accounted for separately, using descriptive and mutually exclusive terms. This is the basic convention to be followed here. As described in Chapter 4, any muscular structure interposing between the ventricular outflow tracts is called the outlet (infundibular) septum and has septal and parietal insertions. Any muscular structure separating an arterial valve from an atrioventricular valve is called the ventriculo-infundibular fold. The extensive septal trabeculation of the morphologically right ventricle is called the septomarginal trabeculation. It has a body and anterior and posterior limbs, these limbs usually cradling the ventricular septal defect. The moderator band arises apically from the body of the septomarginal trabeculation and crosses to the anterior papillary muscle supporting the tricuspid valve, often then continuing to the free ventricular wall. The moderator band, however, is only one of a series of muscle bars which extend to the parietal wall. The others are the septoparietal trabeculations[8] (Fig. 12.2c). Using

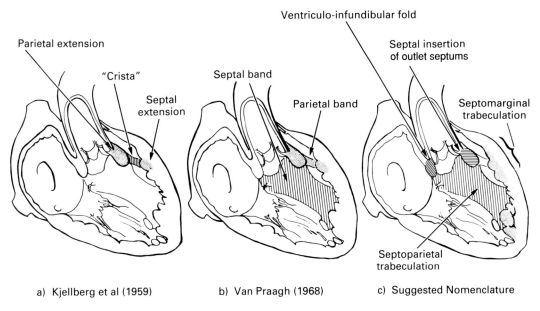

Fig. 12.2 a–c Potential problems exist in the use of the terms 'crista', 'parietal band' and 'septal band' because of the various ways they have been used by different authors. This diagram illustrates the conventions used by Kjellberg and his colleagues (**a**) and Van Praagh (**b**) and compares them with our preferred nomenclature (**c**).

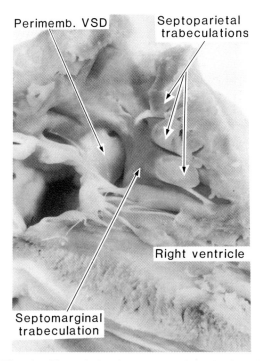

Fig. 12.3 The typical perimembranous defect (perimemb. VSD) is roofed by extensive fibrous continuity between the aortic, mitral and tricuspid valves. Note the hypertrophied septoparietal trabeculations.

these various terms, the different structures surrounding the ventricular septal defect can be described simply and with less likelihood of confusion.

Variability in the ventricular septal defect

When viewed from the right ventricle, the typical defect is related to the outflow portion of the ventricles. It is essentially juxta-aortic and, at the same time, a malalignment defect because of the right ventricular location of the outlet septum. Because of this septal malalignment, the roof of the defect is formed partly by the leaflets of the overriding aortic valve and partly by their attachment to the ventriculo-infundibular fold (Fig. 12.3). The floor of the defect is the crest of the ventricular septum, reinforced on its right ventricular aspect by the limbs of the septomarginal trabeculation. The area of the defect most liable to variation is its postero-inferior quadrant. In about four-fifths of cases, the margin in this area is formed by fibrous continuity between the leaflets of the aortic, mitral

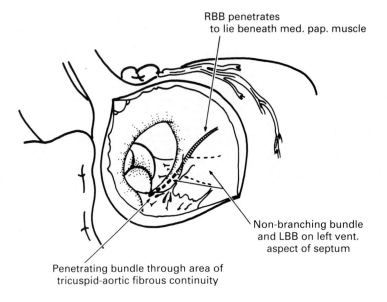

RBB penetrates
to lie beneath med. pap. muscle

Non-branching bundle
and LBB on left vent.
aspect of septum

Penetrating bundle through area of
tricuspid-aortic fibrous continuity

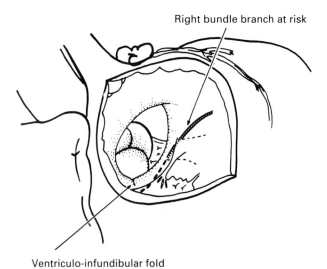

Right bundle branch at risk

Ventriculo-infundibular fold
fuses with septomarginal trabeculation
— safe conduction axis

Fig. 12.4 Drawings showing the surgeon's view through a right
infundibulotomy of a perimembranous defect (upper) and a defect with a
muscular postero-inferior rim (lower). It shows how the presence of this rim
modifies the portion of the ventricular conduction axis which is potentially at
risk from surgical trauma. The usual arrangement is shown for a
perimembranous defect in which the axis and left bundle branch (LBB) are
carried on the left aspect of the septum well below its crest.

and tricuspid valves (Fig. 12.3). Because of this
feature, the defect that characterizes the tetralogy

is very similar to a perimembranous defect
opening to the outlet of the right ventricle without

aortic overriding. These anatomical features are reflected in the distribution of the atrioventricular conduction tissues. As in other hearts with concordant atrioventricular connexions, the guides to the atrioventricular node are the landmarks of the triangle of Koch (see Ch. 1). The penetrating bundle perforates the central fibrous body through the area of aortic–mitral–tricuspid valvar continuity (Fig. 12.4). Here the bundle is frequently overlaid by a remnant of the interventricular membranous septum. In cardiac surgery the septal remnant itself is relatively safe tissue for suture anchorage, but it lies directly superficial to the penetrating bundle. Deeply placed sutures in this area, therefore, are liable to produce complete heart block. Having perforated, the non-branching atrioventricular bundle enters the left ventricular part of the aortic outflow tract and then almost always veers away from the septal crest. In the majority of cases, the branching atrioventricular bundle is carried on the left ventricular aspect of the septum and is remote from the septal crest. In a minority, however, the bundle may branch directly astride the septum, being at risk when sutures are placed into the septal crest.[9, 10]

The second type of ventricular septal defect, occurring in about one-fifth of cases, is characterized by interruption of the area of aortic–tricuspid–mitral valvar continuity by a muscle fold which separates the attachments of the leaflets of the aortic and tricuspid valves (Fig. 12.5). When viewed from the right ventricular aspect, the defect has a complete muscular rim. It is fusion of the posterior limb of the septomarginal trabeculation with the ventriculo-infundibular fold which produces the muscle between the aortic and tricuspid valves and which separates the ventricular conduction tissues from the edge of the defect.

A third variety of septal defect is described in association with the tetralogy. This is the doubly committed and juxta-arterial defect, existing as a consequence of absence or extreme hypoplasia of the outlet septum (Fig. 12.6). Because the outlet septum is absent, however, we now prefer not to consider the hearts as examples of Fallot's tetralogy, since, to us, the hallmark

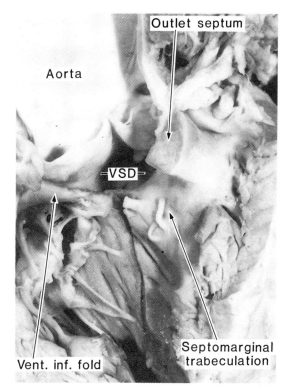

Fig. 12.5 A defect (VSD) with a muscular postero-inferior rim produced by fusion of the posterior limb of the septomarginal trabeculation with the ventriculo-infundibular (vent. inf.) fold.

of the latter is deviation of the outlet septum.[11] The cases with doubly committed defects, nonetheless, are closely related to the tetralogy since, if the septum were to be restored, the anatomical condition of the hearts would be typical. Such doubly committed defects with aortic overriding can be found with aortic–tricuspid valvar continuity or discontinuity, with the attendant implications concerning the conduction tissues. They are much more common in the Far East and in South America than in the Western world.[12, 13]

The various types of outlet defects normally present in Fallot's tetralogy can co-exist with other defects. Inlet defects, when muscular, are particularly important. The combination of an atrioventricular septal defect with tetralogy is also significant, presenting a particular challenge to the surgeon.

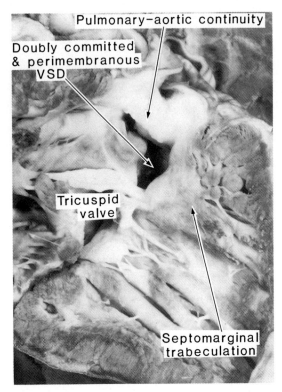

Fig. 12.6 Complete absence of the outlet septum produces a doubly committed subarterial defect (VSD) which in this heart extends to become perimembranous. It is roofed by the aortic and pulmonary valves in fibrous continuity. Although they are often described as examples of the tetralogy, we would not include them because of the absence of the outlet septum.

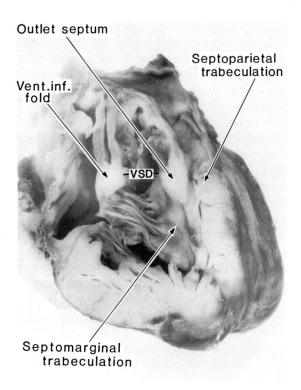

Fig. 12.7 Subpulmonary obstruction is usually due in the greater part to deviation and hypertrophy of the outlet septum. This is exacerbated by other features, particularly hypertrophy of the septoparietal trabeculations (shown in oblique paracoronal cut of the heart).

Pulmonary infundibular stenosis

The subpulmonary stenosis which is an essential part of the tetralogy is due principally to the anterocephalad deviation of the outlet septum. Aortic overriding with valvar pulmonary stenosis in the absence of infundibular septal malalignment should not be categorized as the tetralogy. The anterocephalad deviation produces the larger part of the infundibular stenosis. The anterior component of the obstruction is usually formed simply from hypertrophied septoparietal trabeculations extending onto the ventricular free wall (Fig. 12.7). Additional hypertrophy of the apical trabeculations may produce more proximal stenosis and give the arrangement often described as two-chambered right ventricle. This obstruc-

tion within the body of the right ventricle is superimposed on that occurring at infundibular level. The subpulmonary infundibulum itself can vary considerably in length. Some have stated that hypoplasia of the subpulmonary infundibulum is the essence of the tetralogy,[14] but measurements show that the subpulmonary infundibulum is significantly longer than usual when all cases of the tetralogy are considered as a group.[15] In individual cases, however, the infundibulum may vary from excessive length to extreme hypoplasia.

Aortic overriding

Measurements demonstrate unequivocally that there is true rightward deviation of the aorta in

Fallot's tetralogy.[15,16] The degree of aortic override can vary in different examples from almost exclusive connexion to the right ventricle to almost exclusive connexion to the left ventricle. This has implications for nomenclature. It is our convention to describe hearts in which more than half of *both* great arteries is connected to the right ventricle as having a double outlet ventriculo–arterial connexion. Likewise, when more than half the aortic valve in an example of the tetralogy is connected to the right ventricle we categorize the lesion as having the morphology of tetralogy of Fallot with the ventriculo–arterial connexion of double outlet right ventricle (Fig. 12.8).

Other lesions of the pulmonary circulation

Although the subpulmonary infundibulum is usually the narrowest part of the pulmonary outflow tract in cases of Fallot's tetralogy, other lesions of the outflow tract and pulmonary arteries are also frequent. Pulmonary valvar stenosis is a common accompaniment, due either to unicommissural domed stenosis, to a valve with two leaflets, or to stenosis of a three leaflet valve. When there is valvar stenosis, the lesion at the level of the valve is rarely the major cause of obstruction.

So-called 'absence' of the leaflets of the pulmonary valve is another important condition. The valve is represented by fibrous rudiments, usually accompanied by marked dilatation of the pulmonary trunk (Fig. 12.9). Stenosis of the pulmonary arteries themselves usually occurs at points of branching from the main bifurcation onwards.

Lack of origin of one pulmonary artery (typically the left) from the pulmonary trunk is by no means infrequent. The pulmonary artery concerned is itself almost always present, usually being connected by the arterial duct to some part of the aortic arch system. Rarely, the artery may arise directly from the ascending aorta, and in such cases it tends to be the right pulmonary artery which is anomalously connected. Major systemic–pulmonary collateral arteries are sometimes present in association with Fallot's tetralogy but in such circumstances they

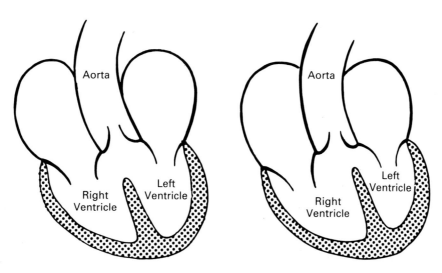

Aorta connected mostly to left ventricle
– concordant vent. –art. connexion

Aorta connected mostly to right ventricle
– double outlet vent. –art. connexion

Fig. 12.8 This diagram shows how the ventriculo–arterial connexion in tetralogy of Fallot can vary from concordant to double outlet right ventricle.

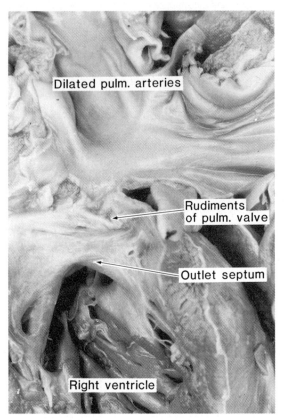

Dilated pulm. arteries

Rudiments of pulm. valve

Outlet septum

Right ventricle

Fig. 12.9 The outflow tract morphology of tetralogy with so-called 'absence' of the pulmonary valve. The valve leaflets are rudimentary and the supravalvar pulmonary arteries are grossly dilated.
Photographed and reproduced by kind permission of
Dr J R Zuberbuhler, Children's Hospital of Pittsburgh, Pittsburgh, Pennsylvania, USA.

co-exist with hilar right and left pulmonary arteries.

Associated anomalies

Many other lesions, such as patency of the oval foramen or an atrial septal defect, can complicate Fallot's tetralogy. A second inlet muscular ventricular septal defect, a common atrioventricular valve and anomalous origin of the anterior descending coronary artery from the right coronary artery are all of major surgical importance. A right aortic arch, though not of functional importance, is common and,

when detected, alerts to the diagnosis of the tetralogy.

TETRALOGY OF FALLOT WITH PULMONARY ATRESIA

There is disagreement on how best to describe this combination of lesions. Some would use the term 'pulmonary atresia with ventricular septal defect', as, indeed, we have on previous occasions,[17] but this phrase describes accurately many more hearts than those in which Fallot's tetralogy co-exists with pulmonary atresia. Thus, hearts with pulmonary atresia and a ventricular septal defect can exhibit the basic features of lesions such as complete transposition (see Ch. 20), congenitally corrected transposition (see Ch. 17), double inlet ventricle (see Ch. 18) or tricuspid atresia (see Ch. 19). A significant number of these hearts have the basic morphology of Fallot's tetralogy, the outlet septum being deviated to the extent that it produces subpulmonary atresia rather than stenosis. It seems reasonable, therefore, to refer to them as Fallot's tetralogy with pulmonary atresia. The atresia may be found at the level of the subpulmonary infundibulum, when it is usually an acquired lesion. More frequently, the atresia is congenital and is then of either muscular (Fig. 12.10a) or valvar nature (Fig. 12.10b). The ventricular septal defect is usually perimembranous but can have a muscular postero-inferior rim. Some such cases are found without any evidence of a subpulmonary infundibulum or an outlet septum. The morphology of the outflow tract is then more reminiscent of the condition of common arterial trunk (see Ch. 22). Although these hearts are usually grouped as examples of Fallot's tetralogy, it is more accurate, because the outlet septum is absent, to consider them as variants of the lesion described above in which there is a doubly committed and juxta-arterial defect with overriding of the aorta (see earlier in this Chapter).[11] In the group as a whole, as with all cases of Fallot's tetralogy, the degree of aortic override can vary markedly. When the aorta is mostly connected to the right ventricle, there is more likelihood

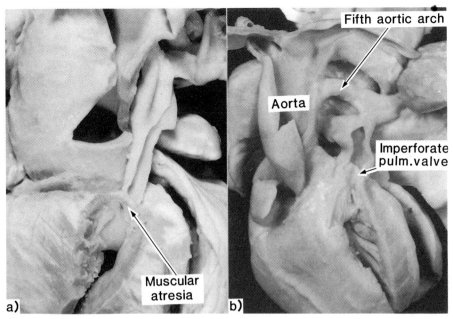

Fig. 12.10 a,b These illustrations show (**a**) muscular and (**b**) valvar pulmonary atresia in hearts with the basic morphology of tetralogy of Fallot.

of a restrictive ventricular septal defect (Fig. 12.11).

When the tetralogy is complicated by pulmonary atresia, the determinant of clinical presentation and of prognosis is the pulmonary arterial blood supply. Self-evidently, this supply must have an extracardiac source in these cases.

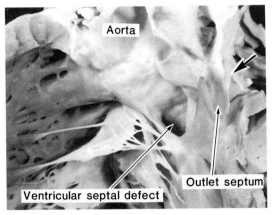

Fig. 12.11 In this heart with tetralogy of Fallot and valvar pulmonary atresia (broad-arrowed), the aorta is connected mostly to the right ventricle and the ventricular septal defect (long arrow) is restrictive.

The two main sources are, first, a persistent arterial duct and, second, major collateral arteries extending from the aorta or its branches to the pulmonary vessels at the hilum of each lung. The arrangement with a persistent arterial duct (Fig. 12.12a) is anatomically much the simplest. Usually, the pulmonary arteries themselves are then confluent and the duct is left-sided, irrespective of whether the aortic arch is left-sided or right-sided. In some cases the pulmonary arteries may be non-confluent, each being supplied by one of a bilateral pair of arterial ducts. The anatomy is much more complex in the presence of systemic–pulmonary collateral arteries. These arteries arise most frequently from the descending aorta and vary in number from two to six (Fig. 12.12b). They may also arise from the brachiocephalic arteries or, rarely, from the coronary arteries.[18,19] Almost always, the collateral arteries co-exist with intrapericardial pulmonary arteries with which they anastomose within the lungs (Fig. 12.13). The 'true' pulmonary arteries, however, do not supply the entirety of the pulmonary parenchyma. Full investigation of such cases requires dissection of both

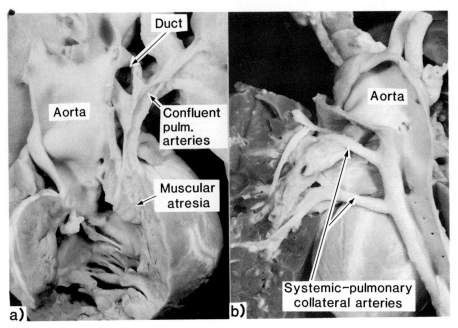

Fig. 12.12 a,b These specimens show the two commonest sources of pulmonary arterial supply in tetralogy of Fallot with pulmonary atresia, namely an arterial duct to confluent pulmonary arteries (**a**) or via major systemic–pulmonary collateral arteries (**b**), seen here from behind.

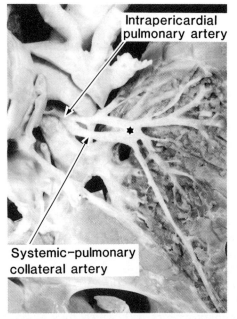

Fig. 12.13 The major systemic–pulmonary collateral arteries anastomose with intraparenchymal pulmonary arteries within the substance of the lung (asterisk).

lungs to establish the area supplied by each collateral artery along with the area supplied by the intrapericardial pulmonary arteries.[20] In some cases in which the pulmonary arteries are non-confluent, those in one lung may be supplied by collateral arteries while those in the other lung are fed through an arterial duct. It is exceedingly rare to find both an arterial duct and major collateral arteries supplying blood to the intraparenchymal pulmonary arteries of the same lung. Although most cases with Fallot's tetralogy and pulmonary atresia will derive their pulmonary arterial supply either from major collateral arteries or from an arterial duct, there are further rarer sources of supply. These may be through an aortopulmonary window, a fistulous communication with the coronary arterial system, a fifth aortic arch or acquired collateral arteries. The acquired collateral supply, which is also frequent, may be derived from bronchial arteries, intercostal arteries or other systemic arteries, including the coronary arteries.

REFERENCES

1. Fallot A. Contribution à l'anatomie pathologique de la maladie bleue (cyanose cardiaque). Marseille Méd 1888; 25: 77–93, 138–158, 207–223, 270–286, 341–354, 403–420.
2. Marquis RM. Longevity and the early history of the tetralogy of Fallot. Br Med J 1956; 1: 819–822.
3. Lev M, Eckner FAO. The pathologic anatomy of tetralogy of Fallot and its variants. Dis Chest 1964; 45: 251–261.
4. Kjellberg SR, Mannheimer E, Rudhe U, Jonsson B. Diagnosis of congenital heart disease. 2nd ed. Chicago: Year Book Medical Publishers, 1959.
5. Keith A. Malformations of the bulbus cordis. An unrecognised division of the human heart. In: Bulloch W, ed. Studies in pathology. Aberdeen, 1906; 55–74.
6. Van Praagh R. What is the Taussig-Bing malformation? Circulation 1968; 38: 445–449.
7. Anderson RH, Becker AE, Van Mierop LHS. What should we call the "crista"?. Br Heart J 1977; 39: 856–859.
8. Goor DA, Lillehei CW. The anatomy of the heart. Congenital malformations of the heart. New York: Grune & Stratton, 1975; 1–37.
9. Titus JL, Daugherty GW, Edwards JE. Anatomy of the atrioventricular conduction system in ventricular septal defect. Circulation 1963; 28: 72–81.
10. Anderson RH, Monro JL, Ho SY, Smith A, Deverall PB. Les voies de conduction auriculo-ventriculaires dans le tétralogie de Fallot. Coeur 1977; 8: 793–807.
11. Griffin ML, Sullivan ID, Anderson RH, Macartney FJ. Doubly committed subarterial ventricular septal defect: new morphological criteria with echocardiographic and angiocardiographic correlation. Br Heart J 1988; 59: 474–479.
12. Ando M. Subpulmonary ventricular septal defect with pulmonary stenosis. Letter. Circulation 1974; 50: 412.
13. Neirotti R, Galindez E, Kreutzer G, Coronel AR, Pedrini M, Becu L. Tetralogy of Fallot with sub-pulmonary ventricular septal defect. Ann Thorac Surg 1978; 25: 51–56.
14. Van Praagh R, Van Praagh S, Nebesar RA, Muster AJ, Sinha SN, Paul MH. Tetralogy of Fallot: underdevelopment of the pulmonary infundibulum and its sequelae. Am J Cardiol 1970; 26: 25–33.
15. Becker AE, Connor M, Anderson RH. Tetralogy of Fallot: a morphometric and geometric study. Am J Cardiol 1975; 35: 402–412.
16. Goor DA, Lillehei CW. Dextroposition of the aorta. Congenital malformations of the heart. New York: Grune & Stratton, 1975; 169–202.
17. Anderson RH, Macartney FJ, Shinebourne EA, Tynan M. Paediatric cardiology, vol. 2. Edinburgh: Churchill Livingstone, 1987; 799–827.
18. Liao PK, Edwards WD, Julstrud PR, Puga FJ, Danielson GK, Feldt RH. Pulmonary blood supply in patients with pulmonary atresia and ventricular septal defect. J Am Coll Cardiol 1985; 6: 1343–1350.
19. Rabinovitch M. Intrapulmonary connections and nonconnections in tetralogy of Fallot with pulmonary atresia. In: Anderson RH, Neches WH, Park SC, Zuberbuhler JR, eds. Perspectives in pediatric cardiology, vol. 1. Mount Kisco, New York: Futura, 1988; 65–80.
20. Haworth SG, Macartney FJ. Growth and development of pulmonary circulation in pulmonary atresia with ventricular septal defect and major aortopulmonary collateral arteries. Br Heart J 1980; 44: 14–24.

Coarctation and interruption of the aortic arch

COARCTATION WITH CLOSED ARTERIAL DUCT

Coarctation, translated literally, means a 'drawing together', a most apt description of this lesion of the aortic arch. When the coarctation is an isolated finding, the wall of the aorta is pinched in waist-like fashion, the ascending and descending portions of the arch tending to expand above and below the site of coarctation. This pattern is seen most frequently in children and adults rather than in infants. In the former group the arterial duct (ductus arteriosus) is closed and, as usual, has been converted into a ligament (ligamentum arteriosum). The constriction of the aorta is then usually at the level of the insertion of the arterial ligament. Almost always, however, there is an additional obstructive lesion within the waist-like aortic segment. The added lesion is a diaphragmatic shelf of fibrous tissue, often with a pin-hole meatus representing the only communication between the ascending and descending aortic segments (Fig. 13.1). This type of coarctation, often described in the past as the 'adult' form,[1] is usually an isolated lesion except for its frequent association with an aortic valve having two leaflets.[2,3] Histology in these cases shows the obstructive shelf to be composed of fibrous tissue.[4] Collateral circulation tends to be well-developed, the intercostal arteries feeding a well-formed anastomotic network, particularly around the scapula. The enlarged intercostal arteries produce the rib notching seen in chest radiographs of older children and adults with this lesion.

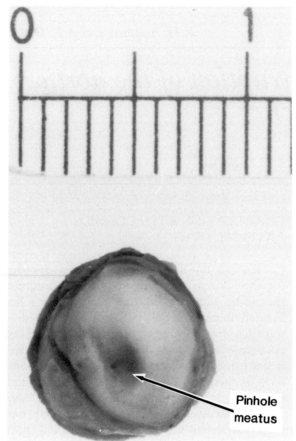

Fig. 13.1 This pin-hole meatus is the lesion excised at surgery from a patient with coarctation and a closed arterial duct.

examination) shows that the tissue making up the shelf is directly continuous with the muscular wall of the duct. In cases observed in infancy, a third obstructive lesion, hypoplasia of the terminal segment (or segments) of the aortic arch, may be superimposed on the waist and shelf anomalies. The hypoplasia may itself be a gradual narrowing down, or extended waisting, from the level of the origin of the left subclavian artery to the site of coarctation. This type of narrowing is usually termed isthmal hypoplasia. Sometimes the narrowing is more uniform and the entire segment of the arch from the subclavian artery to the arterial duct is narrowed, an arrangement described as tubular hypoplasia. Tubular hypoplasia may also affect the segment of arch between the left common carotid and left subclavian arteries (Fig. 13.3). More rarely it may involve the segment between the brachiocephalic and left common carotid arteries. It is this arrangement of tubular hypoplasia which forms the starting point for the spectrum of malformations leading to occlusion of the aortic arch.

RELATIONSHIP OF COARCTATION WITH INTERRUPTION OF THE ARCH

It is an easy matter to appreciate how a hypoplastic tubular segment of the aortic arch can become increasingly narrowed until the lumen is occluded and the arch is ultimately represented by a fibrous strand (Fig. 13.4a). It is then equally easy to envisage how this strand can disappear, resulting in complete interruption of the arch (Fig. 13.4b). This spectrum of hypoplasia, atresia and interruption can be observed both at the isthmus and in the segment of the arch between the left common carotid and subclavian arteries. When interruption is found at these sites, it is often dubbed type A and type B, respectively, following the historical precedent of Patten.[5] Our preference is to avoid alphanumeric categorizations and simply to describe interruption as existing at the isthmus or between the common carotid and left subclavian arteries (Fig. 13.5). Doubt has been expressed concerning the

COARCTATION WITH A PATENT ARTERIAL DUCT

A markedly different arrangement is usually found when coarctation manifests itself in infancy. In these cases the arterial duct is usually open. The obstructive lesion then tends to occur at the junction of the aortic isthmus with the duct and the descending aorta (Fig. 13.2). The obstruction, in some circumstances, may be simply a 'waist' lesion, formed from the infolded aortic wall at the junction with the duct. More usually there is an additional shelf-like lesion within the lumen. The most obvious shelf is found opposite the mouth of the arterial duct, but careful examination (including histological

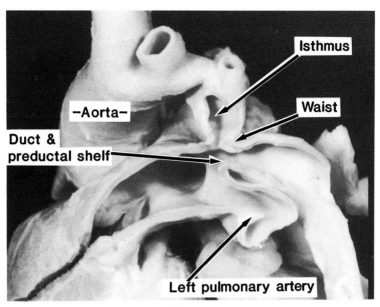

Fig. 13.2 This dissection shows the intimate relationship between the ductal wall and the coarctation lesion found in preductal position when the duct is patent.

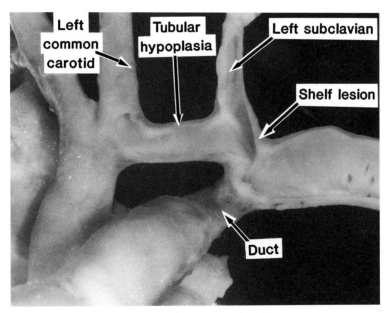

Fig. 13.3 This specimen shows tubular hypoplasia of the segment of aortic arch between the left common carotid and subclavian arteries.

existence of interruption between the brachiocephalic and left common carotid arteries. Well-documented examples of this so-called type C interruption do exist, nonetheless, and we have one such example in our own files.[6] We anticipate the finding, in the fullness of time, of tubular

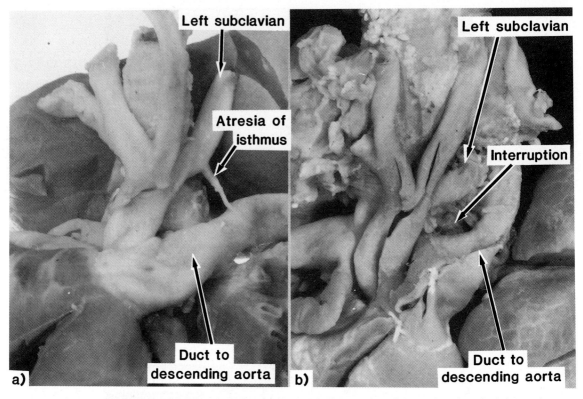

Fig. 13.4 a,b These two hearts show (**a**) atresia of the isthmus and (**b**) interruption of the aortic arch at the isthmus, the descending aorta being supplied through the arterial duct.

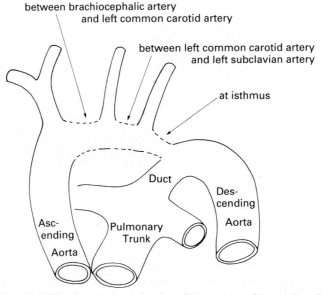

Fig. 13.5 This diagram shows the sites of interruption of the aortic arch.

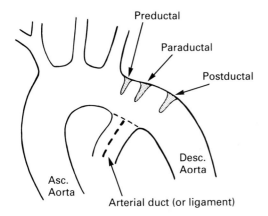

Coarctation – site of lesion

Fig. 13.6 This diagram shows the relationship of the coarctation lesion to the duct when it is open.

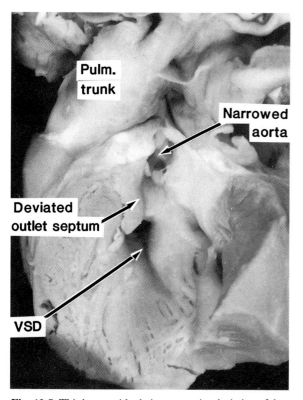

Fig. 13.7 This heart, with obvious posterior deviation of the outlet septum resulting in subaortic stenosis, also exhibited severe preductal coarctation.

hypoplasia and arch atresia at this site in addition to interruption.

POSITION OF THE COARCTATION LESION

Just as interruption and tubular hypoplasia can exist at different sites within the aortic arch, so can discrete coarctation. The major variability in the position of the coarctation lesion is in relation to the aortic junction of the arterial duct. It has become fashionable clinically to describe discrete coarctation lesions as being 'juxtaductal'.[7] If this is meant to indicate a lesion in the environs of the duct, then almost all coarctations are juxtaductal. More usually, this term is employed to indicate lesions *opposite* the mouth of the duct and they, along with those on the descending aortic aspect of the duct, make up only a small minority of coarctations.[3] We believe these are best described, following the approach of Bruins,[8] as paraductal and postductal respectively (Fig. 13.6). The great majority of coarctation lesions are, without question, in the preductal position (Fig. 13.3). Specifically, the shelf-like lesion is located at the isthmal aspect of the junction of the duct with the aorta. Almost always the preductal shelf is an extension of the ductal wall into the lumen.

ASSOCIATED MALFORMATIONS

The commonest anomaly associated with coarctation or interruption of the aortic arch is a patent arterial duct. An aortic valve having two leaflets is also a frequent finding.[3] Associated anomalies of the subclavian arteries are highly significant in the natural history of coarctation. The aortic isthmus itself is defined according to the origin of the left subclavian artery, being the segment of the arch between this origin and the arterial duct. Examination of large numbers of hearts shows marked variability in the length and calibre of this segment. Usually the isthmus is long and in such cases it is often hypoplastic, either as a tapering or as a tubular lesion. Less often the isthmus is very short and in these cases the orifice of the left subclavian artery is itself associated with, and sometimes surrounded by, ductal tissue. On occasions, the segment may be so small as to be considered non-existent. The other significant

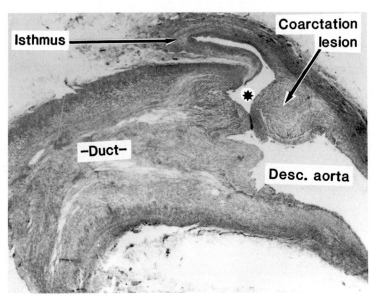

Fig. 13.8 Histological section showing how a severe coarctation lesion is produced by ductal tissue (pale staining) encircling the opening of the isthmus (asterisk).

anomaly of the subclavian arteries is retro-oesophageal origin. The right artery is anomalously attached in this fashion when the aortic arch itself is left-sided, while the left artery takes a retro-oesophageal origin from a right aortic arch (see Ch. 15). Retro-oesophageal origin places the involved subclavian artery beyond the site of the obstruction, with obvious clinical implications for measurements of blood pressure in arms and legs and palpation of the radial pulse. Retro-oesophageal origin is particularly important when there is an interrupted aortic arch, but it can occur with interruption at any site.

Coarctation, irrespective of its site, has a fundamental effect on the left ventricle, producing marked subendocardial fibrosis which increases with age. Although less marked than in congenital aortic stenosis, its presence is likely to affect deleteriously ventricular function.[9] Important malformations occur within the heart in association with coarctation or interruption of the arch. In addition to an aortic valve with two leaflets, lesions of the mitral valve may occur.[10,11] The mitral valve is usually stenotic, either because of fusion and hypoplasia of the papillary muscles or because one papillary muscle is absent and the

corresponding commissure is narrowed. There is also association with a supravalvar stenotic ring within the left atrium.[10] Another frequent associated defect in the heart with concordant segmental connexions is a ventricular septal defect, usually characterized by deviation of the outlet septum into the subaortic outflow tract and by overriding of the pulmonary trunk (Fig. 13.7). In the majority of examples this septal defect is perimembranous and associated with overriding of the aortic valve. The right ventricular margin is often closed or narrowed by tissue tags derived from the tricuspid valve.[12,13] In many cases, however, central ventricular muscular defects are found which do not interfere with aortic flow. Anomalies of chamber connexion are also frequent.[14] Most of these anomalies, but by no means all, have an arrangement which leads to reduced flow through the ascending part of the aorta. The typical lesion is univentricular connexion to a dominant left ventricle (be there double inlet, absent right connexion or absent left connexion) together with a discordant ventriculo–arterial connexion and a restrictive ventricular septal defect (see Chs 18 and 19). Alternatively, there may be a double outlet right ventricle or complete transposition with the pulmonary trunk overriding an outlet ventricular septal defect in the setting of a restrictive subaortic infundibulum (the Taussig–Bing malformation—see Ch. 21). Other associated lesions can be found, but it is exceedingly rare to encounter any which reduce flow through the pulmonary trunk. This is not an absolute rule, however, since coarctation has been reported in association with pulmonary stenosis.[15]

FLOW THEORY VERSUS THE SKODAIC HYPOTHESIS IN THE GENESIS OF COARCTATION

Many years ago, Bonnet[1] suggested that ductal tissue was involved in the production of coarctation. The concept of the aortic wall being 'lassoed' by a circle of ductal tissue as the arterial duct closed subsequently came to be known as the 'Skodaic hypothesis'. The concept tended to lose credibility when Edwards and his colleagues,[4] in a histological study of coarctations from 'adult' cases, showed them to be formed of fibrous rather than recognizably ductal tissue. Persuaded by such studies and by their endorsement by others,[16] Rudolph and his colleagues[7] dismissed the Skodaic theory as being without foundation. Instead, they promoted a concept based on inequality of flow through the aortic and pulmonary pathways during fetal life. They argued that diameters of vessels are proportional to flow through them and further argued that the isthmus was significantly narrower than either the adjacent transverse or descending segments of the aorta. They suggested that any lesion which further reduced aortic flow during fetal life would potentiate the development of significant isthmal hypoplasia. It is, indeed, the case that lesions leading to reduced aortic flow are important in the development of coarctation. But in promoting the importance of flow, the role of the ductal tissue should not be dismissed as insignificant or irrelevant, particularly since many patients with isolated coarctation do not have lesions which would have reduced aortic flow during development. Furthermore, a most important study[17] was ignored by those who dismissed the Skodaic theory.[7] Aortic arches from normal patients, studied microscopically, had been compared with those having coarctation. In the normal arches, the ductal wall had a very discrete junction with the aorta and did not extend around the isthmo–aortic junction. In contrast, in the arches with coarctation, the isthmus was inserted into a luminal sling composed of ductal tissue (Fig. 13.8). These findings were subsequently confirmed by other groups.[18,19] The latter work[19] showed further that, while the coarctation lesion in specimens from children was composed unequivocally of ductal tissue, in the hearts of adults it was made up of fibrous tissue. The inference to be made from this observation is that the shelf lesion becomes converted into fibrous tissue with age. This fact, if correct, reconciles the apparently conflicting observations of those who observed only fibrous tissue in their histological studies of coarctation lesions, and those who found ductal tissue, since the two groups were studying specimens from patients of different ages. Taken together, the overall picture is that both flow and ductal tissue are involved in producing coarctation. One of these features should not be emphasized at the expense of the other.[20]

REFERENCES

1. Bonnet IM. Sur la lésion dite sténose congénitale de l'aorte dans la région de l'isthme. Rev Méd Paris 1903; 23: 108.
2. Reifenstein GH, Levine SA, Gross RE. Coarctation of the aorta: a review of 104 cases of the "adult" type, 2 years of age or older. Am Heart J 1947; 33: 146–168.
3. Becker AE, Becker MJ, Edwards JE. Anomalies associated with coarctation of the aorta. Particular reference to infancy. Circulation 1970; 41: 1067–1075.
4. Edwards JE. Aortic arch system. In: Gould SE, ed. Pathology of the heart and blood vessels. 3rd ed. Springfield, Illinois: Charles C Thomas, 1968; 416–454.
5. Celoria GC, Patton RB. Congenital absence of the aortic arch. Am Heart J 1959; 58: 407–426.
6. Ho SY, Wilcox BR, Anderson RH, Lincoln JCR. Interrupted aortic arch — anatomical features of surgical significance. Thorac Cardiovasc Surgeon 1983; 31: 199–205.

7. Rudolph AM, Heymann MA, Spitznas U. Hemodynamic considerations in the development of narrowing of the aorta. Am J Cardiol 1972; 30: 514–525.

8. Bruins CLD. De arteriele pool van het hart (thesis). Leiden: Groen en Zoon, 1973.

9. Cheitlin MD, Robinowitz M, McAllister H, Hoffman JIE, Bharati S, Lev M. The distribution of fibrosis in the left ventricle in congenital aortic stenosis and coarctation of the aorta. Circulation 1980; 62: 823–830.

10. Shone JD, Sellers RD, Anderson RC, Adams PJ, Lillehei CW, Edwards JE. The developmental complex of "parachute mitral valve", supravalvular ring of left atrium, subaortic stenosis, and coarctation of the aorta. Am J Cardiol 1963; 11: 714–725.

11. Rosenquist GC. Congenital mitral valve disease associated with coarctation of the aorta. A spectrum that includes parachute deformity of the mitral valve. Circulation 1974; 49: 985–993.

12. Anderson RH, Lenox CC, Zuberbuhler JR. Morphology of ventricular septal defect associated with coarctation of the aorta. Br Heart J 1983; 50: 176–181.

13. Smallhorn JF, Anderson RH, Macartney FJ. Morphological characterisation of ventricular septal defects associated with coarctation of aorta by cross-sectional echocardiography. Br Heart J 1983; 49: 485–494.

14. Anderson RH, Ho SY. Aortic coarctation: anatomy of the obstructive and associated lesions. In: Anderson RH, Neches WH, Park SC, Zuberbuhler JR, eds. Perspectives in pediatric cardiology, vol. 1. Mount Kisco, New York: Futura, 1988; 339–346.

15. Wilson N, Fonseka S, Walker D. Severe pulmonary stenosis and duct-dependent coarctation in a neonate. An embryological impossibility. Int J Cardiol 1987; 14: 103–106.

16. Hutchins GM. Coarctation of the aorta as a branch-point of the ductus arteriosus. Am J Pathol 1971; 63: 203–209.

17. Wielenga G, Dankmeijer J. Coarctation of the aorta. J Pathol Bacteriol 1968; 95: 265–274.

18. Ho SY, Anderson RH. Coarctation, tubular hypoplasia and the ductus arteriosus: a histological study of 35 specimens. Br Heart J 1979; 41: 268–274.

19. Elzenga NJ, Gittenberger-de-Groot AC. Localised coarctation of the aorta. An age dependent spectrum. Br Heart J 1983; 49: 317–323.

20. Hoffman JIE, Heymann MA, Rudolph AM. Coarctation of the aorta: significance of aortic flow. In: Anderson RH, Neches WH, Park SC, Zuberbuhler JR, eds. Perspectives in pediatric cardiology, vol. 1. Mount Kisco, New York: Futura, 1988; 347–351.

The arterial duct ('ductus arteriosus')

INTRODUCTION

The arterial duct is a vital part of the normal fetal circulation, conveying the right ventricular output directly to the descending aorta (Fig. 14.1). During development, the normal duct, which is a left-sided structure, has a right-sided counterpart, the developing arterial system being bilaterally symmetrical during early fetal stages. Because of this developmental heritage, a unilateral duct on either side or bilateral ducts can persist and can contribute to the anatomical abnormality of, for example, anomalous pulmonary arterial supply in pulmonary atresia, anomalous aortic supply in aortic atresia or the formation of ring vessels encircling the trachea and oesophagus in the upper part of the mediastinum. Usually the arterial duct becomes closed as part of normal postnatal development and then persists only as the arterial ligament. Postnatal persistence of the duct as a patent structure can be a primary congenital anomaly. This chapter is concerned with the morphology of the closing of the arterial duct and with the persistence of the 'isolated' arterial duct. In recent years it has become evident that the patency of the duct is controllable by certain pharmacological agents, prostaglandins maintaining ductal patency[1,2] and indomethacin and salicylates effecting its closure.[1,3,4] We shall also consider, therefore, the effects of these agents on the duct.

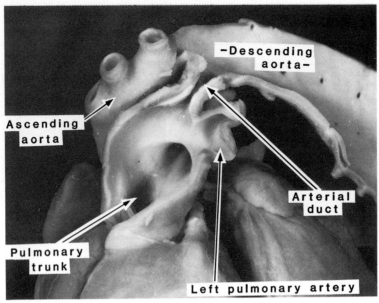

Fig. 14.1 A dissected specimen showing the typical morphological features of a persistently patent arterial duct.

NORMAL CLOSURE OF THE ARTERIAL DUCT

Normally, the arterial duct (the left sixth aortic arch) is closed by the second or third week after birth, the obliterated channel becoming fibrous and forming the arterial ligament. The morphological events which underscore closure are evident histologically several weeks before birth. The normal duct has an intima, an internal elastic lamina, a thick muscular media and an adventitial layer (Fig. 14.2). This mural architecture readily distinguishes the vessel from the fibro-elastic aorta and the pulmonary arteries. By 35 weeks of gestation, the appearance is modified by fragmentation of the internal elastic lamina, formation of intimal cushions and aggregation of mucoid lakes within the inner layer of the media (Fig. 14.3). The prominent intimal cushions have little effect in the distended duct of the late fetus but when, at birth, the duct undergoes muscular contraction, they form an additional resistance to flow and contribute in no small way to functional closure. Thereafter, definitive closure is the consequence of secondary intimal fibrous proliferation.

PREMATURE CLOSURE OF THE ARTERIAL DUCT

Premature closure is an important, albeit rare, finding in neonates and stillborns.[5,6] A duct exhibiting premature closure is distinguished by its diminished external diameter and its narrowed lumen (Fig. 14.4). It should be noted that the duct which is functionally closed can be probed, a procedure that artificially expands its constricted lumen. The passage of a probe through the duct, therefore, should not in itself be taken as evidence of absence of premature closure in functional terms. Additional features will be present and they may be subtle, such as signs of right heart failure. In this respect, the finding of even 5 ml of fluid in the abdominal cavity of a stillborn, even when macerated, is of major significance whereas a similar volume of fluid found in an adult is of no consequence. Minimal dilatation of the right heart cavities may also be seen.

PERSISTENT PATENCY OF THE ARTERIAL DUCT

Persistent ductal patency must be distinguished

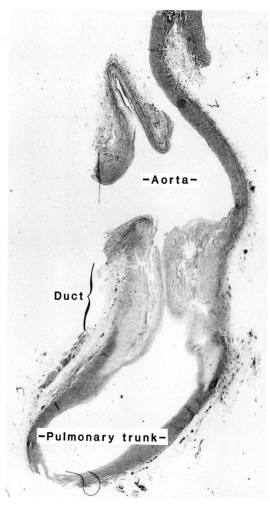

Fig. 14.2 This section of the junctions of the conspicuously muscular arterial duct with the fibromuscular aorta and pulmonary trunk demonstrates the clear histological distinction of their medial structure. Elastica/Van Gieson

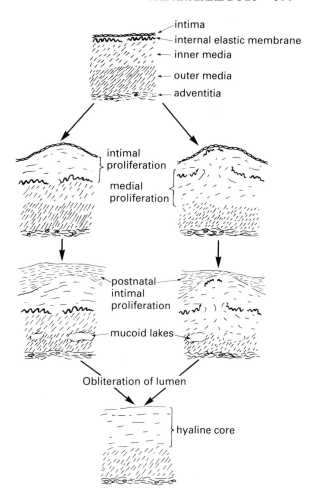

Fig. 14.3 This diagram illustrates the steps involved in the normal process of closure and obliteration of the arterial duct. *Prepared by and reproduced with the kind permission of Dr Siew Yen Ho.*

pathologically from delayed ductal closure. Delayed closure is an expected finding in situations such as prematurity, infants who are 'small-for-dates' and infants born by caesarian section. Such ducts would have been anticipated to close by normal physiological mechanisms if the infant had survived; they should not be interpreted as showing persistent patency. Histological examination is needed to demonstrate the specific pattern of persistent patency.[7,8] The cardinal feature is an intact internal elastic lamina (Fig. 14.5).

Isolated persistent patency of the duct, as opposed to delayed closure, is now an exceedingly rare finding in the autopsy rooms of affluent countries. Edwards has summarized well the changes which may still be pertinent in other societies.[9] Complications of the persistent duct, such as pulmonary vascular disease, bacterial endarteritis or dissecting aneurysm, are also exceedingly rare events in our practice but may be seen in the Third World.

ANEURYSM OF THE ARTERIAL DUCT

Congenital aneurysms of the duct are rare,

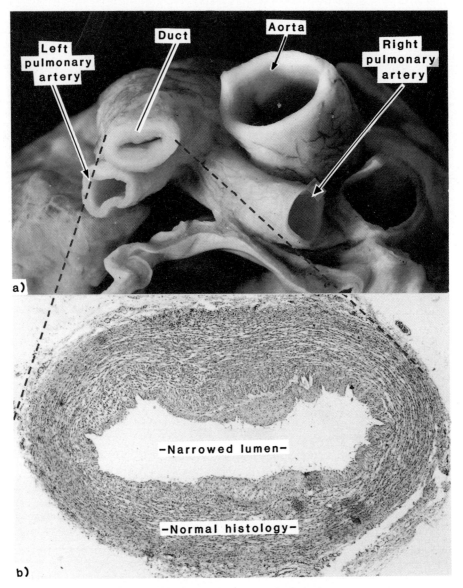

Fig. 14.4 a,b This dissection (**a**) and histological section (**b**) show the gross morphology and histological structure of the arterial duct undergoing premature closure.

although a review[10] has cited more than 70 cases described in the world literature. Most are congenital in that some sort of persistent patency has led to their development. As suggested in another review,[11] they can be categorized in two groups. The first consists of aneurysms having patent aortic and pulmonary ends. Those in the second group are closed at their pulmonary end. All cases seen in infants have been closed at the pulmonary end.[11] Conditions such as rupture, dissection, thrombosis with or without embolism, and infections commonly complicate aneurysmal ducts. Often it is the complications which are the immediate cause of death.

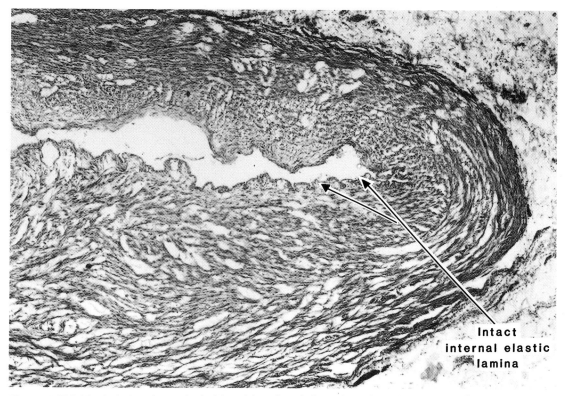

Intact internal elastic lamina

Fig. 14.5 This histological section, stained with a trichromic technique, shows the typical structure of a persistently patent arterial duct, distinguished by the presence of an intact internal elastic lamina.
Prepared and reproduced by kind permission of Dr. Siew Yen Ho.

HISTOLOGICAL MANIFESTATIONS OF THE EFFECTS OF PHARMACOLOGICAL AGENTS ON THE ARTERIAL DUCT

Clinical experience has shown that continuing patency of the duct can be promoted either by administration of prostaglandins or by injection of formalin around the duct. Permanent patency on the basis of prolonged prostaglandin infusion cannot be expected. It seems most likely that, in those cases in which permanent patency is reported, a duct of 'persistent' type has been present from the start. In contrast, functional closure of a duct exhibiting prolonged patency can be achieved by administration of indomethacin, an inhibitor of prostaglandin. Reopening occurs when such a duct, in retrospect, is shown to be of the histologically persistent type.[12]

Examination of a duct which has been kept open by prostaglandins reveals significant morphological changes which are potentially hazardous. Thus, the ductal wall becomes oedematous subsequent to administration of therapeutic amounts of the pharmacological agent; the considerable oedema affects mostly the inner third of the media. Intimal damage and thrombosis have been seen, together with multiple interruptions of the internal elastic lamina and intimal lacerations extending into the media.[13,14] Although some have doubted the significance of the reported changes,[15,16] a careful recent review[17] has shown that detailed study using serial sections will always demonstrate their presence.

REFERENCES

1. Starling MB, Elliot RB. The effect of prostaglandins, prostaglandin inhibition and oxygen on the closure of the ductus arteriosus, pulmonary arteries and umbilical vessels in vitro. Prostaglandins 1974; 8: 187–203.

2. Olley PM, Coceani F, Bodach E. E-type prostaglandins. A new emergency therapy for certain cyanotic congenital heart malformations. Circulation 1976; 53: 728–731.

3. Friedman WF, Hirshklau MJ, Prinz MP, Pitlick PT, Kirkpatrick SE. Pharmacologic closure of patent ductus arteriosus in the premature infant. N Engl J Med 1976; 295: 526–529.

4. Heymann MA, Rudolph AM, Silverman NH. Closure of the ductus arteriosus in premature infants by inhibition of prostaglandin synthesis. N Engl J Med 1976; 295: 530–533.

5. Becker AE, Becker MJ, Wagenvoort CA. Premature contraction of the ductus arteriosus: a cause of foetal death. J Pathol 1977; 121: 187–191.

6. Kohler HG. Premature closure of the ductus arteriosus (P.C.D.A.): a possible cause of intrauterine circulatory failure. Early Hum Dev 1978; 2: 15–23.

7. Gittenberger-de-Groot AC. Persistent ductus arteriosus: probably a primary congenital malformation. Br Heart J 1977; 6: 610–618.

8. Ho SY, Anderson RH. Coarctation, tubular hypoplasia and the ductus arteriosus: a histological study of 35 specimens. Br Heart J 1979; 41: 268–274.

9. Edwards JE. Malformations of the thoracic aorta — patent ductus arteriosus. In: Gould SE, ed. Pathology of the heart and great vessels. 3rd ed. Springfield, Illinois: Charles C. Thomas, 1968; 416–420.

10. Mendel V, Luhmer J, Oelert H. Aneurysma des Ductus arteriosus bei einem Neugeborenen. Herz 1980; 5: 320–323.

11. Falcone HW, Perloff JK, Roberts WC. Aneurysm of the non-patent ductus arteriosus. Am J Cardiol 1972; 29: 422–426.

12. Gittenberger-de-Groot AC, Van Ertbruggen I, Moulaert AJMG, Harinck A. The ductus arteriosus in the preterm infant: histologic and clinical observations. J Pediatr 1980; 96: 88–93.

13. Gittenberger-de-Groot AC, Moulaert AJ, Harinck E, Becker AE. Histopathology of the ductus arteriosus after prostaglandin E1 administration in ductus dependent cardiac anomalies. Br Heart J 1978; 40: 215–220.

14. Gittenberger-de-Groot AC, Sutherland K, Sauer U, Kellner M, Schober JG, Buhlmeyer K. Normal and persistent ductus arteriosus influenced by prostaglandin E1. Herz 1980; 5: 361–368.

15. Silver MM, Freedom RM, Silver MD, Olley PM. The morphology of the human newborn ductus arteriosus: a reappraisal of its structure and closure with special reference to prostaglandin E1 therapy. Hum Pathol 1981; 12: 1123–1136.

16. Park IS, Nihill MR, Titus JL. Morphologic features of the ductus arteriosus after prostaglandin E1 administration for ductus-dependent congenital heart defects. J Am Coll Cardiol 1983; 1: 471–475.

17. Gittenberger-de-Groot AC, Strengers JLM. Histology of the arterial duct (ductus arteriosus) with and without treatment with prostaglandin E1. Int J Cardiol 1988; 19: 153–166.

Anomalies of the great arteries

INTRODUCTION

In this chapter, we will consider the various anomalies of the arterial pathways which can be grouped together as 'vascular rings', including the conditions of right aortic arch and of retro-oesophageal subclavian artery. Although, anatomically, the aorta begins immediately above the aortic valve, anomalies of the ascending aorta such as supravalvar aortic stenosis have already been discussed (see Ch. 11). We will discuss here the aortopulmonary window (or fenestration) and then describe significant malformations of the pulmonary arterial pathways.

RIGHT AORTIC ARCH

A right aortic arch is one which crosses over the right main bronchus and descends to the right side of the vertebral column; it is a 'normal' finding in those who have mirror-image arrangement of their organs. A right-sided aortic arch descending to the right of the vertebral column is also found in patients with usual atrial arrangement and in those with isomerism of their organs (see Ch. 16). The right arch is then considered to be abnormal although, in itself, it produces no clinical problems.

The pattern of the head and arm arteries arising from a right-sided arch may take one of two basic forms. First, there may be mirror-image branching (Fig. 15.1). In this pattern, the first artery to arise from the arch is the brachiocephalic trunk which divides to become the left subclavian

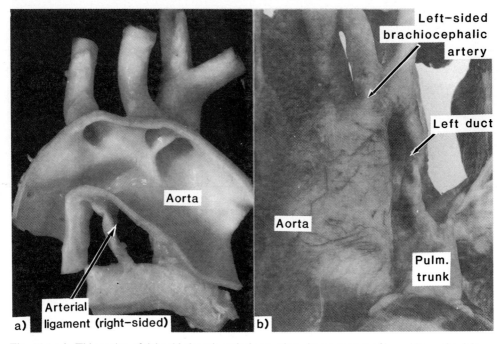

Fig. 15.1 a,b This section of right-sided aortic arch shows mirror-image pattern of branching and a right-sided arterial duct (**a**). This is unusual. More frequently with mirror-image branching, as shown in (**b**), the duct is left-sided, arising from the left-sided brachiocephalic artery.

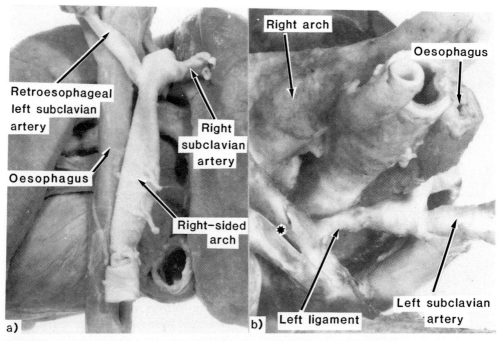

Fig. 15.2 a,b These specimens, photographed from behind (**a**) and from the right (**b**), show a right-sided aortic arch with retro-oesophageal origin of the left subclavian artery. In the example shown in (**b**), the ligament connects the subclavian artery to the left pulmonary artery (asterisk — see Fig. 15.6).

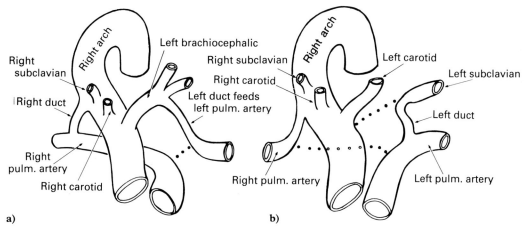

Fig. 15.3 a,b Diagrams explaining the origin of isolation of either the left pulmonary artery (**a**) or left subclavian artery (**b**) in the presence of a right aortic arch.

and left common carotid arteries. This is the usual pattern seen when a right aortic arch is associated with intracardiac malformations.[1] It may be associated with a mirror-image arrangement of the arterial duct (or of the arterial ligament) (Fig. 15.1a) but, more usually, the duct or ligament takes origin from the base of the left-sided brachiocephalic trunk (Fig. 15.1b). The second pattern of origin of the head and arm arteries from a right aortic arch is the one in which the left subclavian artery alone arises as the last branch from the aortic arch, taking a retro-oesophageal course (Fig. 15.2). This type occurs more frequently as an isolated anomaly, unassociated with other intracardiac defects. It is, however, best explained on the basis of a vascular ring (see below). When there are other malformations within the heart, a right aortic arch usually occurs with Fallot's tetralogy (being seen in about 25% of such cases) and common arterial trunk (in up to 50% of these cases).

In a small percentage of cases the aorta may descend to the left of the vertebral column, despite its right-sided origin.[2] This anomaly, known as 'right aortic arch with left-sided descending aorta',[3] is almost always associated with a mirror-image pattern of branching, although rare cases have been described in which an aberrant origin of the left subclavian artery was found.[4] Approximately 25% of these cases occur without any associated cardiac anomaly. A left-

sided descending aorta causes no problems unless it is complicated by formation of the more complex vascular malformation which is known as a vascular ring (see below). Indeed, when the right aortic arch leads to compression of the tracheo-oesophageal pedicle it is almost always part of a vascular ring. A right aortic arch rarely may be part of a complex malformation when it does not produce compression. This is exemplified by the presence of bilateral arterial ducts, the right-sided arch having its own duct connecting to the right pulmonary artery while a left-sided duct arises from the ascending aorta to supply an isolated pulmonary artery (Fig. 15.3a). Alternatively, an isolated subclavian artery may arise from a left pulmonary artery in the presence of a right aortic arch, the connexion between left subclavian and pulmonary arteries representing the left-sided duct and its connexion to the left arch (Fig. 15.3b). Numerous examples of apparent isolation of either the pulmonary arteries or the systemic arteries can be explained by the bilaterally symmetrical arrangement of the aortic arches. This basic pattern of a symmetrical system provides an explanation for the formation of vascular rings.

VASCULAR RINGS

By common consent, the term 'vascular ring'

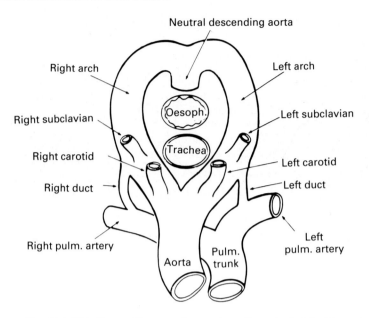

Fig. 15.4 This diagram illustrates the template of hypothetical double aortic arches with a midline descending aorta.

describes a malformation of the aortic arches which interferes with and compresses the trachea and oesophagus. Understanding the genesis of these vascular rings leads to an understanding of 'isolation' of either the pulmonary or systemic arteries. The concept of all these anomalies is based on a hypothetical bilaterally symmetrical system of paired aortic arches.[5] On this template (Fig. 15.4) the descending aorta is displayed in neutral position posterior to the tracheo-oesophageal pedicle, but is connected to the ascending aorta on both right and left sides by a lateral aortic arch. A subclavian artery and a common carotid artery arise from the arch on each side, while a duct on each side connects its arch to its corresponding pulmonary artery. Although the concept is hypothetical, vascular rings are occasionally seen which are remarkably like the template, having separate limbs of comparable size, each limb giving rise to brachiocephalic arteries and encircling the tracheo-oesophageal pedicle to form a descending aorta which is either to the left (Fig. 15.5) or to the right of the vertebral column. Bilateral ducts are not always present in such cases. Perfectly formed double arches, compressing the trachea and oesophagus,

are rare but cases have been reported where the separate limbs of double arches are of unequal diameter, the right usually being the wider.[6] Moreover, a double arch system can produce compression when part of the system is atretic.

When there is focal atresia of part of a double aortic arch, the atretic segment is usually represented by a fibrous cord. Such atresia can affect either the right or the left side of the double arch but almost always the right arch persists as the dominant arch and the atresia then may affect different segments, producing an array of malformations. At its simplest, the atretic segment may represent the most distal part of the arch system between the aortic insertion of the arterial duct and the insertion of the left arch into the descending aorta. Combined with this lesion, the atretic segment may extend to include the arch between the left subclavian artery and the aortic origin of the duct (Fig. 15.6a). As a variant the segment between the left common carotid artery and the left subclavian artery may be atretic (Figs 15.2, 15.6b). Still further possibilities exist, since the left arch may remain dominant while either of these segments may become focally atretic on the right side. On the basis of focal

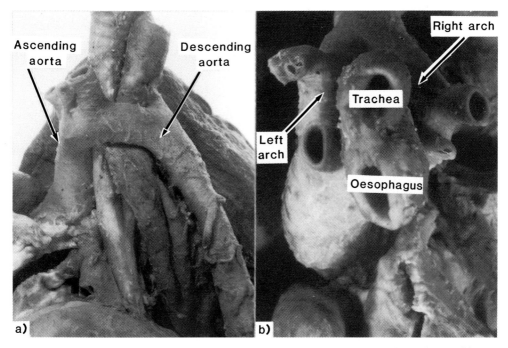

Fig. 15.5 a,b These illustrations show a double aortic arch encircling the trachea and oesophagus with left-sided aorta seen (**a**) from the left and (**b**) from above.

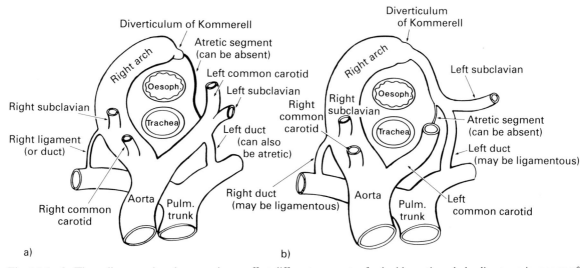

Fig. 15.6 a,b These diagrams show how atresia can affect different segments of a double aortic arch, leading to various sorts of vascular ring. The example shown in (**b**), with complete absence of the atretic segment, is illustrated in Fig. 15.2b.

atresia involving one or other of these segments, which then become fibrous cords, it is possible to account for all the known examples of vascular rings.[5] An atretic segment, however, may not always persist as a fibrous cord but may involve completely and disappear, when the double arch will no longer be a continuous structure. The system of arteries arising from the arches may still

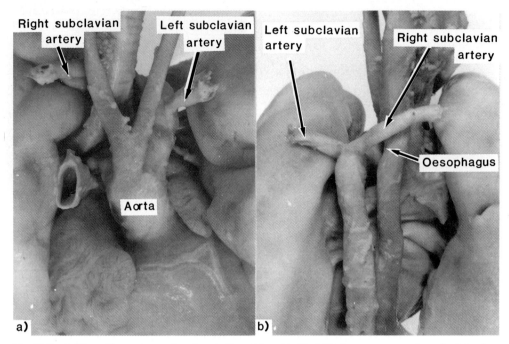

Fig. 15.7 a,b These illustrations, taken from in front (**a**) and behind (**b**) show retro-oesophageal origin of the right subclavian artery. The diagrammatic explanation of this lesion is shown in Fig. 15.8.

partially encircle the oesophagus but an arrangement of this type, with anatomical discontinuity along its length, rarely produces compression. A good example of a discontinuous double arch is represented by retro-oesophageal origin of the subclavian artery which can occur in a right arch (see Fig. 15.2) or else in a left arch, when the right subclavian artery is the fourth branch of an otherwise normal aorta (Fig. 15.7). This anomaly can be explained by the presumption that, initially, a double arch was formed with the right arch supplying the right subclavian artery. Subsequently, if the segment of the right arch between the origin of the right subclavian and the right common carotid arteries became atretic and absorbed, the segment between the descending aorta and the right subclavian artery would be able to migrate cranially, retaining its retro-oesophageal position, to achieve its final position as the fourth branch of a left-sided aortic arch (Fig. 15.8). When double arches are found with atresia or absence of one of their segments, a diverticulum is frequently seen at the site of origin of the atretic segment of the arch.

This feature is known as the diverticulum of Kommerell.

AORTOPULMONARY FENESTRATIONS

Communications between the ascending parts of the aortic and pulmonary trunks, known as aortopulmonary fenestrations, windows or septal defects, produce clinical symptoms similar to those of common arterial trunk (see Ch. 22). Indeed, such anomalies have previously been classified as examples of common arterial trunk.[7,8] We do not recommend this approach since, from the anatomical standpoint, the distinguishing feature of common arterial trunk is the presence of a single arterial valve guarding a common trunk while, almost always, there are separate and discrete aortic and pulmonary valves in hearts with aortopulmonary communications.

The communications, or windows, are found between the ascending portions of the arterial trunks. Rarely, the defects may be circumscribed

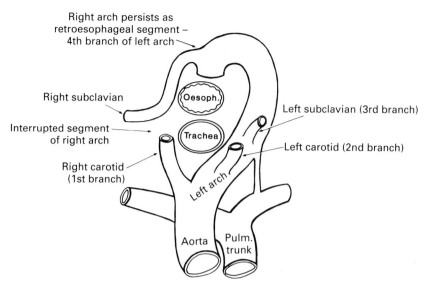

Fig. 15.8 This diagram explains the existence of a retro-oesophageal right subclavian artery as the fourth branch of a left aortic arch, the artery being part of the right arch.

and small but almost always they are large defects, sometimes extending from the sinuses of the great arteries to almost the level of the pulmonary bifurcation (Fig. 15.9). The defect usually represents a simple 'window' in the plane of the conjoined wall of the two great vessels and therefore without the interposition of any conduit between them (Fig. 15.9). Occasionally a tubular conduit is present instead of the simple window: examples have been described with a length of more than one centimetre, enabling their ligation at surgery.[9] Aortopulmonary communications tend to be found in association with other cardiovascular malformations. Thus, about one-third of cases are said to co-exist with at least one other malformation, such as patency of the arterial duct, a ventricular septal defect or a right-sided aortic arch. Anomalous origin of either the right or the left coronary artery from the pulmonary trunk is a relatively frequent accompaniment. Co-existence of an aortopulmonary window with interruption of the aortic arch presents a particular challenge for clinical diagnosis.[10] An aortopulmonary window can also provide an arterial blood supply to the lungs when there is co-existing pulmonary atresia; similarly, it can augment reduced pulmonary flow as, for example, in the tetralogy of Fallot. As with any left-to-right shunt, an aortopulmonary communication also provides the potential for the development of plexogenic pulmonary arteriopathy (see Ch. 26). The frequency of this complication has been greatly reduced where facilities allow for diagnosis and surgical treatment during the first year of life.

MALFORMATIONS OF THE PULMONARY ARTERIAL PATHWAYS

Abnormalities of the pulmonary arteries are most frequently seen in association with pulmonary atresia, particularly when the pulmonary arterial supply is derived via systemic to pulmonary collateral arteries. The complexities of this condition have been described in Chapter 12. The pulmonary arteries can also be abnormal when they are discontinuous and one lung is normally supplied through a pulmonary trunk connected to the right ventricle, or when both lungs have pulmonary arteries connected in normal fashion to the ventricular mass. These last two conditions will be discussed here.

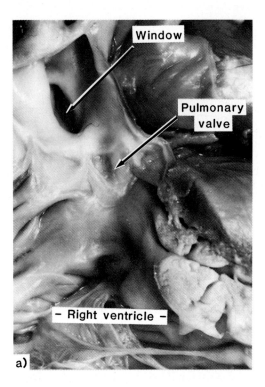

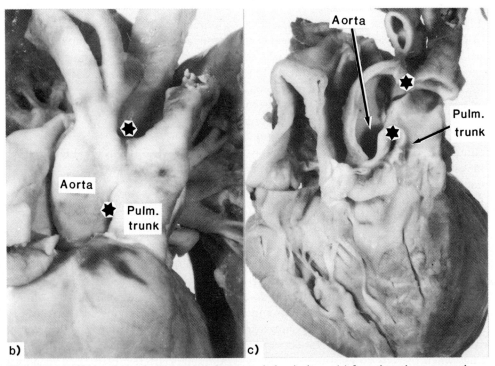

Fig. 15.9 a–c This example of a large aortopulmonary window is shown (**a**) from the pulmonary trunk, (**b**) externally and (**c**) sectioned through both arterial trunks. The extent of the window is shown by the asterisks in (**b**) and (**c**).

Normally connected pulmonary arteries

Anomalies of otherwise normally connected pulmonary arteries make up a diverse group of lesions, all rare, which have been well reviewed by Edwards.[11] Examples are idiopathic pulmonary dilatation, localized pulmonary arterial stenoses, and fistulas between the pulmonary arteries and the cardiac chambers, notably the left atrium. The condition known as 'crossed pulmonary arteries' is a particularly unusual arrangement in which the left pulmonary artery takes origin from the pulmonary trunk to the right of the origin of the right artery (Fig. 15.10). We have seen this arrangement only in association with a common arterial trunk, but it has been described when the pulmonary trunk was concordantly connected.[12] More frequent than crossed pulmonary arteries, and more significant because it produces clinical manifestations, is the so-called 'vascular sling', which is also produced by anomalous origin of one pulmonary artery: the sling (not to be confused with the 'vascular ring' — see above) is produced when the left pulmonary artery arises from the right pulmonary artery and, in its course from right to left hilum, passes between the trachea and the oesophagus (Fig. 15.11). When associated with the arterial ligament or arterial duct, this anomalous pattern may produce a complete ring around the trachea.[13] Vascular slings may be found in otherwise normal hearts or in association with either cardiac or tracheo-bronchial lesions. The eparterial bronchus was found to originate from the trachea ('bronchus suis') in a sixth of one large series of cases.[13]

Anomalous origin of one pulmonary artery

The entire pulmonary artery to one lung may be anomalously connected, or the anomaly may affect one of its branches only. When only part of one lung receives an anomalous vascular supply (pulmonary sequestration), its parenchyma is abnormal and resembles a hamartoma. The commonest variant of sequestration is the 'scimitar syndrome', in which there may not only be abnormal arterial supply from the aorta but also anomalous pulmonary venous drainage, usually to the inferior caval vein, and anomalous bronchial connexions. The complicated patterns are best analysed by considering separately the arterial, venous and bronchial components of the sequestrated segment.[14] It is also usual for the heart to be right-sided in the scimitar syndrome. The name comes from the shadow usually seen

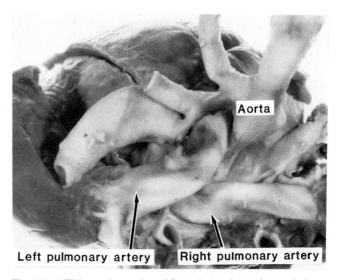

Fig. 15.10 This specimen, viewed from above, shows the rare lesion known as crossed pulmonary arteries, better described as anomalous origin of the right from the left pulmonary artery. There is also aortic coarctation and patency of the arterial duct.

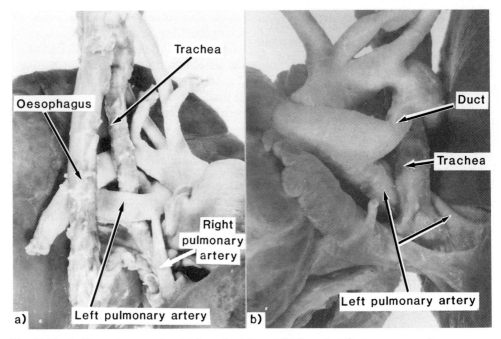

Fig. 15.11 a,b These pictures, taken (**a**) from the right and (**b**) from the left, show an anomalous course of the left pulmonary artery between the trachea and the oesophagus. Note that the arterial duct (arrowed in **b**) is normally located, connecting the pulmonary trunk to the descending aorta and producing a complete ring round the trachea. The right pulmonary artery is hypoplastic.

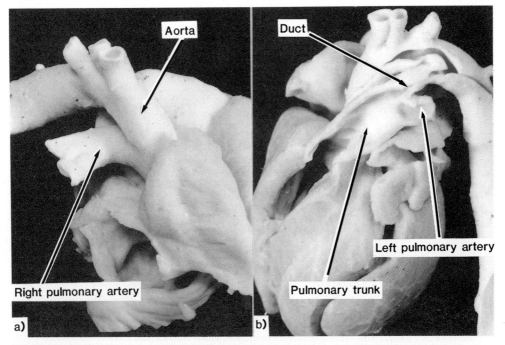

Fig. 15.12 a,b This heart, viewed from right (**a**) and left (**b**) sides, has anatomical origin of the right pulmonary artery from the ascending aorta. The arterial duct is left-sided and patent and, in this case, the aortic arch is also left-sided.

on the chest radiograph, which was said to resemble a Turkish sword.[15]

When one complete pulmonary artery is anomalously connected, the entire blood supply to that lung will be from systemic sources. Although this malformation is frequently described in terms of absence of one pulmonary artery, it is rare for the intrapericardial pulmonary arteries supplying the affected lung to be totally absent, although this can occur. Indeed, in rare circumstances, one entire lung can be totally absent: in such cases there is then compensatory hypertrophy of the other lung and the heart is abnormally located.

Much more common is so-called 'absence' of one pulmonary artery, either the right or the left, when the pulmonary arterial supply to the lung on the affected side is not from the right ventricle but from systemic sources. The supply may be derived from an arterial duct, which itself can be right-sided or left-sided, from systemic–pulmonary collateral arteries, or very rarely from a fifth aortic arch, or the right or left pulmonary artery may take direct origin from the ascending aorta. With such an anomalous origin of one pulmonary artery from the aorta, the other pulmonary artery arises normally from the right ventricle. Most frequently it is the right pulmonary artery which arises anomalously (Fig. 15.12), usually in association with a right aortic arch. The lesion has been called 'hemitruncus', but we do not use this term since the presence of two arterial valves rules out the possibility of a common arterial trunk. In cases of this type it has been said that when the pulmonary supply from the right ventricle is unobstructed, hypertensive pulmonary vascular disease is found in the lung with the normal rather than in that with the anomalous pulmonary vascular supply.[16] This is the consequence of the disproportionately small size of the pulmonary arterial bed when one lung receives the total right ventricular output.

REFERENCES

1. Knight L, Edwards JE. Right aortic arch types and associated cardiac anomalies. Circulation 1974; 50: 1047–1051.
2. Hastreiter AR, D'Cruz IA, Cantez T. Right-sided aorta. Br Heart J 1966; 28: 722–739.
3. Edwards JE. Aortic arch system. In: Gould SE, ed. Pathology of the heart and blood vessels. 3rd ed. Springfield, Ill.: Charles C Thomas, 1968; 416–454.
4. Blieden LC, Schneeweiss A, Deutsch V, Neufeld HN. Right aortic arch with left descending aorta (circumflex aorta). Roentgenographic diagnosis. Pediatr Radiol 1978; 6: 208–210.
5. Stewart JR, Kincaid OW, Edwards JE. An atlas of vascular rings and related malformations of the aortic arch system. Springfield, Ill.: Charles C Thomas, 1964.
6. Neuhauser EBD. The roentgen diagnosis of double aortic arch and other anomalies of the great vessels. Am J Roentgenol 1946; 52: 1–12.
7. Collett RW, Edwards JE. Persistent truncus arteriosus. A classification according to anatomic types. Surg Clin North Am 1949; 29: 1245–1270.
8. Van Praagh R, Van Praagh S. The anatomy of common aortico-pulmonary trunk (truncus arteriosus communis) and its embryologic implications. Am J Cardiol 1965; 16: 406–426.
9. Belcourt CL, Alterman K, Gillis DA, Roy DL. Aortopulmonary window or aortopulmonary communication. Chest 1979; 75: 397–399.
10. Fisher EA, Dubrow IW, Eckner FAO, Hastreiter AR. Aorticopulmonary septal defect and interrupted aortic arch: a diagnostic challenge. Am J Cardiol 1974; 34: 356–359.
11. Edwards JE. Malformations of the pulmonary arteries. In: Gould SE, ed. Pathology of the heart and blood vessels. 3rd ed. Springfield, Ill.: Charles C Thomas, 1968; 455–462.
12. Jue KL, Lockman LA, Edwards JE. Anomalous origins of pulmonary arteries from pulmonary trunk (crossed pulmonary arteries). Am Heart J 1966; 71: 807–812.
13. Jue KL, Raghib G, Amplatz K, Adams P Jr, Edwards JE. Anomalous origin of the left pulmonary artery from the right pulmonary artery. Am J Roentgenol 1965; 95: 598–610.
14. Clements BS, Warner JO, Shinebourne EA. Congenital bronchopulmonary vascular malformations: clinical application of a simple anatomical approach in 25 cases. Thorax 1987; 42: 409–416.
15. Neill CA, Ferencz C, Sabiston DC, Sheldon H. The familial occurrence of hypoplastic right lung with systemic arterial supply and venous drainage: 'scimitar syndrome'. Johns Hopk Med J 1960; 107: 1–15
16. Pool PE, Vogel JHK, Blount SG Jr. Congenital unilateral absence of a pulmonary artery. The importance of flow in pulmonary hypertension. Am J Cardiol 1962; 10: 706–732.

Atrial isomerism

INTRODUCTION

Syndromes have long been recognized in which major malformations are associated with failure or incomplete expression of lateralization of the thoracic and abdominal organs, particularly with abnormalities of the spleen. These syndromes may be approached from different viewpoints determined by the special interest of the pathologist concerned. For example, the gastroenterological pathologist might be most interested in the abnormalities of the gut while an immunologist would be more concerned with those of the spleen. The cardiac pathologist, self-evidently, will focus on the cardiac manifestations. From his point of view, the feature which correlates best with the extremely variable spectrum of malformations is the morphology of the atrial appendages.[1] In this chapter, therefore, these syndromes of visceral heterotaxy will be considered using the morphology of the atrial appendages as the criterion for definition. They will be described in terms of atrial isomerism, the condition in which the atrial appendages both present the morphology of either the usual right-sided appendage or the usual left-sided appendage (right atrial isomerism and left atrial isomerism respectively. Isomerism of the atrial appendages does not, in itself, produce problems. It is the lesions associated with an isomeric arrangement of the appendages which may make description and diagnosis difficult. Recognition of the isomerism, nonetheless, is essential as it is this feature which sets the scene for logical sequential segmental analysis (see Ch. 4).

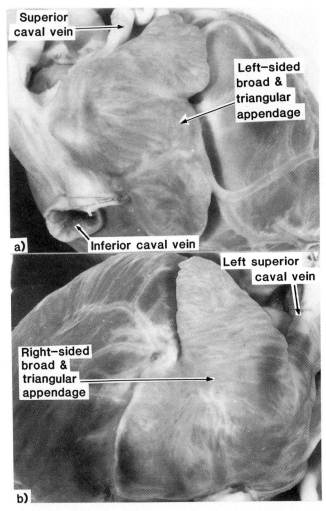

Fig. 16.1 a,b This heart shows bilateral (**a** and **b**) morphologically right atrial (a & b) appendages.

PREVIOUS CATEGORIZATIONS

The fact that certain constellations of cardiac lesions are associated with an unusual arrangement of the organs in the rest of the body has long been recognized. The association of multiple spleens with cardiac malformations was noted by Abernethy.[2] Absence of the spleen had been observed earlier, but it was Martin[3] who first recorded absence of the spleen in association with major cardiac defects. After that, there were many isolated reports of cardiac problems associated with splenic abnormalities. The detailed study by Ivemark[4] established the close link between the

two, and subsequent to his report it became common to describe cardiac lesions in terms of the 'splenic syndromes'. Others then drew attention to the presence of bilateral left-sidedness of the thoracic organs in patients with multiple spleens,[5] and described in detail the isomeric nature of the right atrial appendages and sinus nodes in patients with absence of the spleen.[6] Despite this recognition of an isomeric arrangement of the organs, it became fashionable[7,8] to describe the heart in relation to 'asplenia' or 'polysplenia'. It had also been recognized, however, that not all patients with the cardiac lesions associated with 'asplenia' had absence of their spleen, which led to contradictory descriptions such as 'asplenia syndrome with rudimentary spleen'.[9] Coupled with such semantic aberrations is the fact that clinical recognition of absence or multiplicity of the spleen is difficult. Moreover, the discordances noted between splenic and atrial arrangement have proved to be rather frequent.[10] The best means of identifying these syndromes at autopsy, therefore, is also the most direct — namely, to look at the atrial appendages.[1] The concept of 'splenic syndrome', in this context, could well be dropped.

ANATOMY OF HEARTS WITH ISOMERISM OF THE ATRIAL APPENDAGES

Right atrial isomerism

The cardiac features of right atrial isomerism are dominated by the presence of a morphologically right atrial appendage on both sides, each separated from the midline venous atrial component by bilateral terminal grooves. Sinus nodes are present bilaterally within each of the grooves

in the position anticipated for the normal right atrium (see Ch. 1). This arrangement of the appendages (Fig. 16.1) is present irrespective of whether the superior caval vein is a unilateral or bilateral superior structure. Usually there is a superior caval vein connecting to the atrial roof on each side (Fig. 16.2). When only one vein is present, it may be on the right side or on the left; the other vein is then usually represented by an atretic strand. The inferior caval vein may also be a bilateral structure and drain each side of the liver separately into the midline venous component of the atrial mass; in such cases one of the channels is then in continuity with the distal portion of the inferior caval vein. More usually, the caval vein is a single channel connecting to the atrium, often in a midline position, and issuing from the abdomen in juxtaposition with the descending aorta. At their junction with the atriums, the caval veins are separated internally from the appropriate appendages by bilateral terminal crests, these corresponding with the external terminal grooves. The pectinate muscles arise from these crests all round the atrioventric-

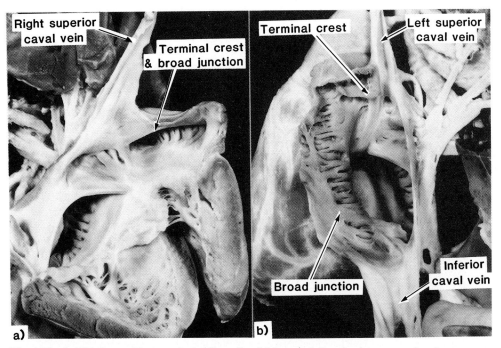

Fig. 16.2 a,b This heart with appendages bilaterally of right morphology has been opened to demonstrate the broad junctions bilaterally and the terminal crest on each side (**a** and **b**).

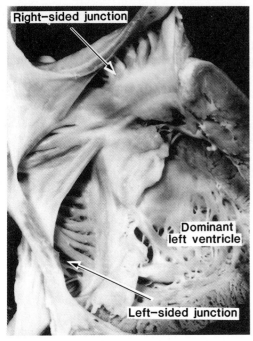

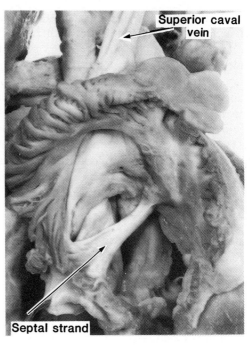

Fig. 16.3 The same heart as shown in Fig. 16.2, with double inlet to a dominant left ventricle through a common valve, has been opened to show the isomeric nature of the pectinate muscles around the right and left sides of the atrioventricular junction (compare with Fig. 16.9).

Fig. 16.4 This specimen shows the typical septal strand spanning the common atrium in a heart with isomerism of the right atrial appendages.

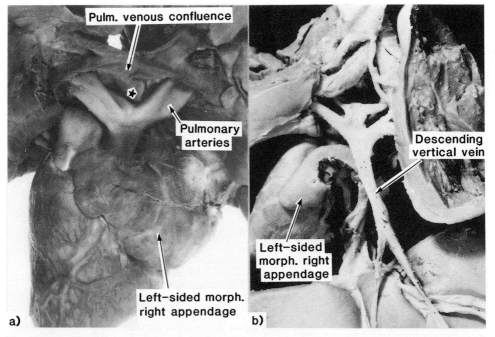

Fig. 16.5 a,b These hearts both have isomerism of the morphologically right appendages and totally anomalous pulmonary venous connexion. In (**a**), the vein draining the pulmonary venous confluence (starred) is in a bronchopulmonary vice. In (**b**), the confluence is connected infradiaphragmatically to the portal venous system.

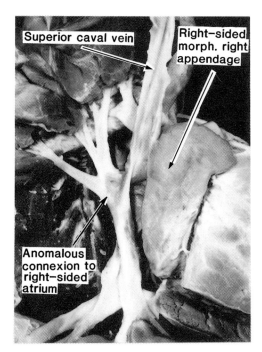

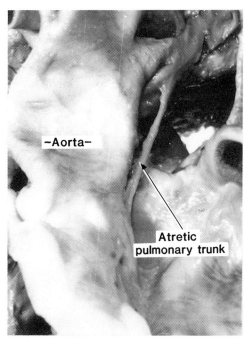

Fig. 16.6 This specimen shows totally anomalous pulmonary venous connexion to the right-sided atrium in a heart with isomerism of the morphologically right appendages.

Fig. 16.7 The thread-like atretic pulmonary trunk seen so frequently in hearts with isomerism of the morphologically right appendages.

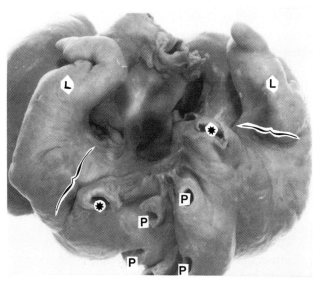

Fig. 16.8 This heart, viewed from above, shows the symmetry of structure seen in hearts with isomerism of morphologically left appendages. The appendages themselves (L) are tubular and have narrow junctions (brackets) with the venous component. Connected to the venous component are bilateral superior caval veins (asterisks) and bilateral pulmonary veins (P). Each caval vein is connected between the appendage and the pulmonary veins.

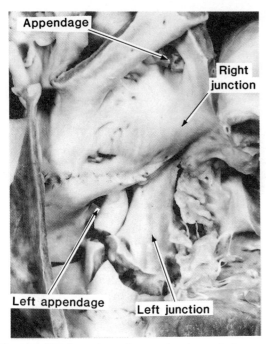

Fig. 16.9 This heart shows the smooth atrioventricular junctions on each side when each appendage is of left morphology (compare with Fig. 16.3).

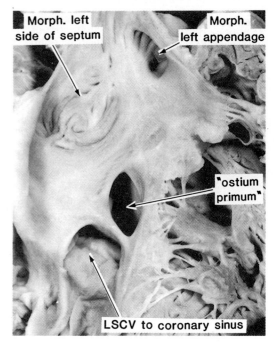

Fig. 16.10 In this heart with appendages bilaterally of left morphology, the right-sided atrium has been opened to show the connexion of a left superior caval vein (LSCV) to the coronary sinus and an interatrial communication of 'ostium primum' type. Note that the atrial septum is roughened, as expected for a morphologically left atrium.

ular junctions (Fig. 16.3). In the majority of hearts, the venous component of the atrial mass located centrally is either unseptate or else crossed only by a septal strand. Both these arrangements effectively produce a common atrium (Fig. 16.4.). In some hearts, the septum is better formed and a muscle bar can be found separating a superior oval fossa from an 'ostium primum' type of defect. Such variations are usually found in association with a double inlet ventricle through a common valve or present a biventricular and ambiguous connexion (see Ch. 4) with an atrioventricular septal defect (see below). Rarely, there may be an intact atrial septum and two separate atrioventricular valves with normal atrioventricular septation. Irrespective of the state of the atrial septum, in all the hearts we have studied with right isomerism there has been absence of the coronary sinus: the coronary venous blood returns to the heart through Thebesian veins. The pulmonary veins, in most cases, have totally anomalous connexions to extracardiac channels (Fig. 16.5) but any mode of pulmonary venous drainage is possible (see Ch. 5). In the minority of cases, the pulmonary veins connect with the atriums, albeit in anomalous fashion. Almost always, such cardiac connexions are to a small midline area of the atrial roof. Often the pulmonary venous sinus thus formed is guarded by valve-like structures within the atrium (Fig. 16.6). In only one instance of right atrial isomerism have we seen all four pulmonary veins connected in approximately normal fashion to an atrium; since this atrium supported an appendage of right atrial morphology, the connexion remained anatomically anomalous.

The atrioventricular connexions in some hearts with right atrial isomerism are biventricular, giving an ambiguous arrangement. This can be found with either right-hand or left-hand topology of the ventricular mass. In about three-quarters of cases, however, there is a double inlet atrioven-

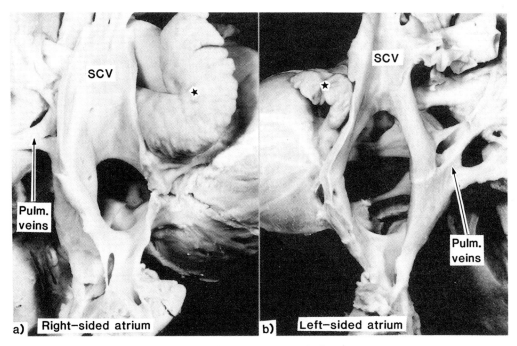

Fig. 16.11 a,b This heart with appendages bilaterally (**a** and **b**) of left morphology (asterisks) shows the typical morphologically left pattern of connexion of both superior caval veins (SCV) to their appropriate atriums.

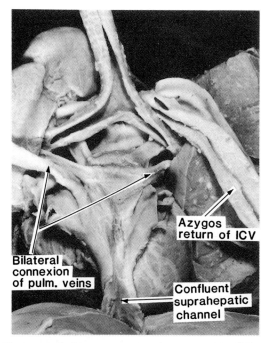

Fig. 16.12 This heart with appendages bilaterally of left morphology has interruption of the inferior caval vein (ICV) with continuation through the azygos vein. The hepatic veins open through a confluence to the venous component of the atriums.

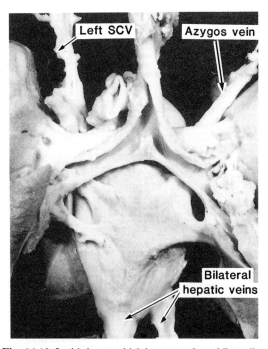

Fig. 16.13 In this heart, which has appendages bilaterally of left morphology, there is interruption of the inferior caval vein with continuation through the right-sided azygos vein; the hepatic veins connect bilaterally to the venous component (compare with Fig. 16.12).

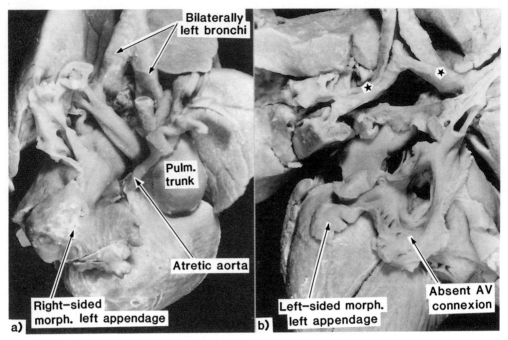

Fig. 16.14 a,b This heart with appendages bilaterally of left morphology and bilateral hyparterial bronchi (arrowed in (**a**) and starred in (**b**)) has aortic atresia (**a**) and absence of the left atrioventricular (AV) connexion (**b**).

tricular connexion, usually through a common atrioventricular valve. The connexion can be to a dominant left or right ventricle or to a solitary and indeterminate ventricle. Absence of one atrioventricular connexion can occur but is very rare. In almost all hearts with right atrial isomerism there is a common atrioventricular junction, associated either with an atrioventricular septal defect or with a double inlet ventricle. The pattern of the ventricular mass is important because it determines the disposition of the atrioventricular conduction axis. With biventricular connexions and right-hand topology, the node and penetrating atrioventricular bundle are located posteriorly within the atrioventricular junction. When biventricular connexions are found with left-hand topology, there is either an anterior node and axis or else a sling of conduction tissue between posterior and anterolateral atrioventricular nodes.[11] The conduction tissue, when there is a double inlet ventricle, is as expected when this connexion occurs with lateralized atrial chambers (see Ch. 18). Thus, an anterolat-

eral node is the rule with a dominant left ventricle. With a dominant right ventricle and a left-sided left ventricle (right-hand topology) there is a posterior atrioventricular node. With a right-sided left ventricle (left-hand topology) there may be an anterolateral node or connexion of the conduction tissues to dual nodes (a 'sling'). Very bizarre patterns of the conduction axis are found in hearts with right isomerism and double inlet to a solitary and indeterminate ventricle.[11] The ventriculo–arterial junction is abnormal in at least 90% of cases of right atrial isomerism. Most have either discordant or double outlet connexions, the latter being either from a right ventricle or a solitary and indeterminate ventricle. Almost always there is a subaortic or a bilateral infundibulum and, most often, the aorta is found anteriorly relative to the pulmonary trunk. Pulmonary atresia or stenosis is found in over half the cases (Fig. 16.7). Almost always an arterial duct is present which augments or totally supplies the pulmonary arterial system.

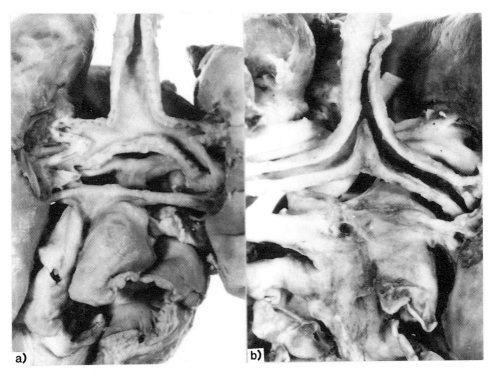

Fig. 16.15 a,b These specimens seen from behind contrast (**a**) the typical bilateral short and eparterial pattern of right bronchial isomerism and (**b**) the long and hyparterial pattern bilaterally of left bronchial isomerism.

Left atrial isomerism

The atrial anatomy of left isomerism is dominated by the presence bilaterally of morphologically left atrial appendages (Fig. 16.8). Both are narrow and tube-like, having a narrow junction with the venous atrium which is not marked on either side by a terminal crest internally or a terminal groove externally. The pectinate muscles within the appendages sometimes spill over to a limited extent into the venous components of the atriums. They never extend posteriorly around the junctions as seen in hearts with bilateral appendages of right morphology (compare Figs 16.3 and 16.9). Because of the absence of the terminal groove, it is difficult to predict the site of the sinus node. Indeed, in most cases of left isomerism, it proved impossible to locate the node.[11] In those in which a structure akin to the node was discovered, it was hypoplastic and found within the anterior interatrial groove close to the atrioventricular junction.[11] Bilateral superior caval veins are found in most cases. Each tends to run down towards the atrioventricular junction in the fashion of the persistent left superior caval vein seen in hearts with usual atrial arrangement (see Ch. 5). In about 50% of cases the left-sided vein then enters the right-sided morphologically left atrium through a coronary sinus (Fig. 16.10), but both veins may drain directly to the atrial roof between the appendage and the pulmonary veins (Fig. 16.11). The pulmonary veins themselves may connect bilaterally to the venous component of the atrium, two on each side, but all four veins tend to connect to one or other atrium in most hearts. Totally anomalous connexion to an extracardiac site has yet to be described in hearts with bilateral appendages of left morphology. The typical venous anomaly of left isomerism is interruption of the inferior caval vein with its continuation via the azygos system (Fig. 16.12). This arrangement may be found on either the left or the right side, but always the azygos vein is situated posteriorly next to the descending aorta. When there is azygos continuation, then in two-thirds of cases the hepatic veins connect separately to the heart. This can occur bilaterally or both veins may drain into one or other atrium (Fig. 16.13). In the remaining one-third of cases, the hepatic veins connect via a common suprahepatic channel to one or other atrium. In a small minority of cases, there is direct connexion of the inferior caval vein to one or other atrium. This can be found with separate connexion of one hepatic vein to the atrium or with both hepatic veins draining via the inferior caval channel.

Atrial septation tends to be much more complete in left than in right isomerism. The atrial septum, therefore, can be well-formed, with the oval fossa having the typically coarse left atrial aspect on both its surfaces but lacking a well-defined rim. Despite this, most cases present with deficient atrioventricular septation. Thus, an 'ostium primum' defect is usually present, most frequently with biventricular and ambiguous atrioventricular connexions and an atrioventricular septal defect. A double inlet connexion can be found or, rarely, absence of the left atrioventricular connexion (mitral atresia) and co-existing aortic atresia (Fig. 16.14). Most cases of left atrial

isomerism, nonetheless, have biventricular atrioventricular connexions (ambiguous) as described above and this can occur with either right-hand or left-hand ventricular topology. Double inlet can also occur, usually to a dominant left ventricle; it is much rarer than in right isomerism. The criteria for prediction of the site of the conduction tissue axis are as described above for right isomerism (see also Ch. 1).

The arrangement of the ventriculo–arterial junction is also much closer to normal than in right isomerism. Severe associated malformations rarely occur, such as aortic atresia. Generally speaking, the ventriculo–arterial connexions are concordant, there is a subpulmonary infundibulum, and the great arteries are normally related. Obstruction to the aortic flow pathways, with either coarctation or interruption of the aortic arch, is found in about two-fifths of autopsied cases.

THE VISCERAL ARRANGEMENT IN ATRIAL ISOMERISM

Isomerism of the atrial appendages is the cardiac manifestation of a general arrangement of bodily symmetry as opposed to lateralization of the organs within the body.[12] In the heart itself, as

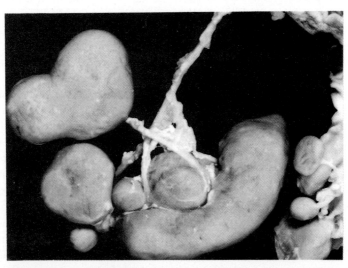

Fig. 16.16 The multiple spleens which are usually, but not always, seen in the presence of isomerism of the left atrial appendages.

described, this symmetry is best expressed in the appendages, is reasonably constant in the veno–atrial connexions but is not seen in the ventricular mass and arterial segments.

In the body in general, the isomeric arrangement is best seen in the thorax. Thus, almost all cases of atrial isomerism will co-exist with a symmetrical arrangement of the bronchial tree.[13,14] This is expressed as bilaterally short and eparterial bronchi with right isomerism and bilaterally long and hyparterial bronchi with left isomerism (Fig. 16.15). In some cases, there is discordance between the bronchial and atrial arrangements.[15] When atrial isomerism is found with one long and one short bronchus, then almost always, in our experience, the heart shows the anticipated cardiac manifestations of isomerism. The lobulation of the lungs is much less constant as a marker of isomerism. Although most cases of right isomerism have bilaterally trilobed lungs and most cases of left isomerism have bilaterally bilobed lungs, this is not nearly as constant an association as the bronchial arrangement. The pattern of the abdominal organs is even less predictable. The liver may be right-sided, central or left-sided in right or left isomerism, as may the stomach and gallbladder. In most cases, particularly in left isomerism, the intestine is malrotated and its mesentery is deficient. Multiple spleens are to be anticipated with appendages bilaterally of left morphology (Fig. 16.16) but, in this respect, it should be noted that there are well-recognized syndromes of multiple spleens with azygos continuation of the inferior caval vein and biliary atresia in which there is usual atrial arrangement.[16] These features serve to emphasize the need, particularly for the pathologist, separately to analyse and record the arrangement of the body organs and the atrial chambers. The heart itself is often malpositioned when there is atrial isomerism. It may be in the right side of the chest, the left side of the chest or midline. The apex may point to the right, to the left or centrally. The finding of an abnormally positioned heart has no predictive value concerning the congenital lesions it may contain.

REFERENCES

1. Sharma S, Devine W, Anderson RH, Zuberbuhler JR. The determination of atrial arrangement by examination of appendage morphology in 1842 autopsied specimens. Br Heart J 1988; 60: 227–231.
2. Abernethy J. Account of two instances of uncommon formations in the viscera of the human body. Philos Trans R Soc Lond 1793; 83: 59–66.
3. Martin G. Observation d'une déviation organique de l'estomac, d'une anomalie dans la situation et dans le configuration du coeur et des vaisseaux qui en partent ou qui s'y rendant. Bull Soc Anat Paris 1826; 1: 40–48.
4. Ivemark BI. Implications of agenesis of the spleen on the pathogenesis of conotruncus anomalies in childhood. An analysis of the heart; malformations in the splenic agenesis syndrome, with 14 new cases. Acta Paediatr Scand [Suppl 104] 1955; 44: 1–110.
5. Moller JH, Nakib A, Anderson RC, Edwards JE. Congenital cardiac disease associated with polysplenia: A developmental complex of bilateral "left-sidedness". Circulation 1967; 36: 789–799.
6. Van Mierop LHS, Wiglesworth FW. Isomerism of the cardiac atria in the asplenia syndrome. Lab Invest 1962; 11: 1303–1315.
7. Van Praagh R. Terminology of congenital heart disease: glossary and commentary. Circulation 1977; 56: 139–143.
8. Van Mierop LHS, Gessner IH, Schiebler GL. Asplenia and polysplenia syndromes. In: Bergsma D, ed. Birth defects: Original Article Series. Baltimore: Williams & Wilkins, 1972; 8(No 5): 36–44.
9. Layman TE, Levine MA, Amplatz K, Edwards JE. "Asplenic syndrome" in association with rudimentary spleen. Am J Cardiol 1967; 20: 136–140.
10. Anderson RH, Sharma S, Ho SY, Zuberbuhler JR, Macartney FJ. Splenic syndromes, "situs ambiguus" and atrial isomerism. Rev Latina Cardiol 1986; 2: 97–110.
11. Dickinson DF, Wilkinson JL, Anderson KR, Smith A, Ho SY, Anderson RH. The cardiac conduction system in situs ambiguus. Circulation 1979; 59: 879–885.
12. Anderson RH, Macartney FJ, Shinebourne EA, Tynan M. Paediatric cardiology, vol. 1. Edinburgh: Churchill Livingstone, 1987; 473–496.
13. Landing BH, Lawrence TK, Payne VC, Wells TR. Bronchial anatomy in syndromes with abnormal visceral situs, abnormal spleen and congenital heart disease. Am J Cardiol 1971; 12: 456–462.
14. Deanfield JE, Chrispin AR. The investigation of chest disease in children by high kilovoltage altered beam radiography. Br J Radiol 1981; 54: 856–860.
15. Caruso G, Becker AE. How to determine atrial situs? Considerations initiated by 3 cases of absent spleen with a discordant anatomy between bronchi and atria. Br Heart J 1979; 41: 559–567.
16. Chandra RS. Biliary atresia and other structural anomalies in congenital polysplenia syndrome. J Pediatr 1974; 85: 649–655.

Discordant atrioventricular connexions

INTRODUCTION

In the past, a group of congenitally malformed hearts has been described under titles such as 'ventricular inversion' or 'l-transposition'. The feature common to these anomalies is discordant atrioventricular connexions, in other words the morphologically right atrium is connected to the morphologically left ventricle while the left atrium is connected to the right ventricle (Fig. 17.1). This particular atrioventricular connexion co-

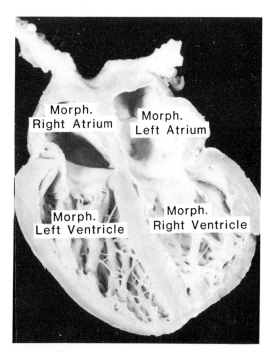

Fig. 17.1 This four chamber section through a heart with congenitally corrected transposition demonstrates the salient features of the discordant atrioventricular connexions.

exists most frequently with discordant ventriculo–arterial connexions. The combination is then appropriately described as 'congenitally corrected transposition'. The discordant atrioventricular connexions can exist in combination with any of the possible ventriculo–arterial connexions, hence the reason for concentrating on the abnormal atrioventricular connexions which unite the group.

SEMANTIC CONSIDERATIONS

Discordant connexions at the atrioventricular junction can exist only when there are both morphologically right and left atriums (as opposed to isomeric atriums — see Ch. 16) and when each atrium is connected to a morphologically inappropriate ventricle (Fig. 17.2). Discordant connexions, therefore, cannot exist in the presence of isomeric atrial chambers or of a univentricular atrioventricular connexion (for example, double inlet left ventricle). The discordant atrioventricular connexion can exist irrespective of the relationship of the ventricles one to the other. Thus, when discordant atrioventricular connexions are found with usual atrial arrangement, the morphologically left ventricle is usually right-sided relative to the right ventricle, the two ventricles tending to be oriented in more side-by-side position than normally anticipated. Similarly, when there is mirror-image atrial arrangement, the left ventricle tends to be left-sided and side-by-side relative to the right ventricle. But this is by no means a universal arrangement. Often there is a supero-inferior obliquity in the orientation of the ventricular mass, with the apex usually shifted rightward with usual atrial arrangement and leftward with the mirror-image variant. The morphologically left ventricle then tends to be the superior ventricle. This positional abnormality is often called the 'superior-inferior' (or 'upstairs-downstairs') heart. Abnormalities of ventricular relationship (Fig. 17.3) may also be found because of rotation around the long axis of the ventricular mass. This means that all or part of the right ventricle achieves a right-sided position in hearts with usual atrial arrangement (or left-sided in those with mirror-image atrial arrangement). This rotational anomaly is called a 'criss-cross heart'.[1]

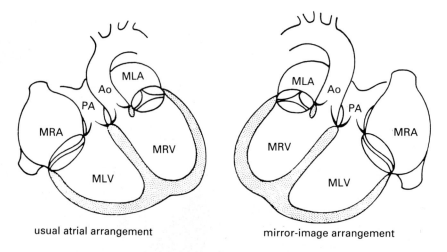

usual atrial arrangement   mirror-image arrangement

Discordant atrioventricular connections
and discordant ventriculo-aterial connections

Fig. 17.2 Congenitally corrected transposition (discordant connexions at both atrioventricular and ventriculo–arterial junctions) can be found with either usual or mirror-image atrial arrangements. Abbreviations: M — morphologically, R — right, L — left, A — atrium, V — ventricle, Ao — aorta, PA — pulmonary trunk.

Usual atrial arrangement, discordant AV and VA connections

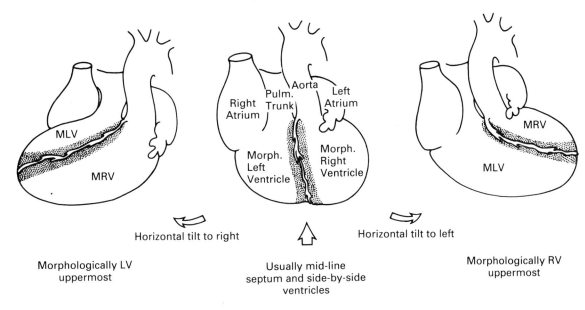

Morphologically LV
uppermost

Horizontal tilt to right

Usually mid-line
septum and side-by-side
ventricles

Horizontal tilt to left

Morphologically RV
uppermost

Fig. 17.3 This diagram shows (middle) the typical side-by-side relationship of the ventricles in hearts with congenitally corrected transposition and (side panels) the tilting in the ventricular long axis which produces supero-inferior ventricles. MLV — morphologically left ventricle, MRV — morphologically right ventricle.

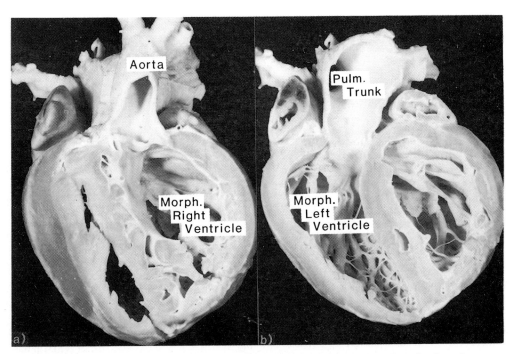

Fig. 17.4 a,b These sections simulating the echocardiographic four chamber views show the discordant ventriculo–arterial connexions in congenitally corrected transposition. The more anterior section (**a**) shows the aorta arising from the morphologically right ventricle (left-sided) while the more posterior section (**b**) shows the pulmonary trunk arising from the right-sided morphologically left ventricle.

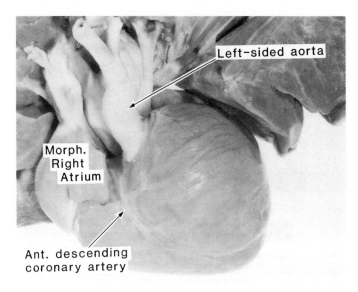

Fig. 17.5 This photograph, taken from the front, shows the anterior and left-sided aorta found in most, but not all, examples of congenitally corrected transposition.

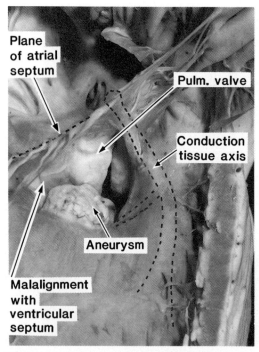

Fig. 17.6 The abnormal course of the atrioventricular conduction axis has been superimposed on a photograph of the right-sided chambers of a case of congenitally corrected transposition with usual atrial arrangement.

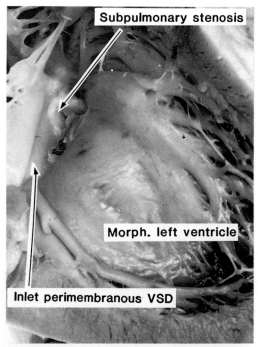

Fig. 17.7 The ventricular septal defect (VSD) in this heart with congenitally corrected transposition is perimembranous (roofed by mitral–tricuspid fibrous continuity) and opens between the ventricular inlets. Note the co-existing shelf-like subpulmonary stenosis.

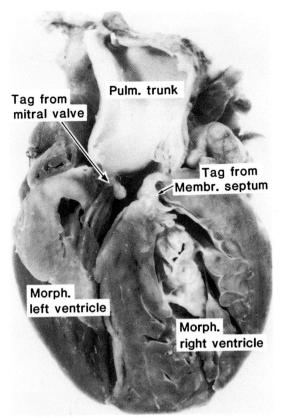

Fig. 17.8 Subpulmonary stenosis in this heart with congenitally corrected transposition, demonstrated by a four chamber section, is due to tissue tags originating from the mitral valve and the remnant of the interventricular component of the membranous septum.

MORPHOLOGY OF CONGENITALLY CORRECTED TRANSPOSITION

When the discordant atrioventricular connexions are accompanied by similar discordant connexions at ventriculo–arterial level, the two discordant connexions, in terms of the pathways of circulation, cancel each other — hence the term 'congenitally corrected'. The arterial trunks spring from morphologically inappropriate ventricles so that the pulmonary trunk arises from the morphologically left ventricle and the aorta from the morphologically right ventricle. Almost always, the pulmonary valve is found in fibrous continuity with the mitral valve while the aortic valve is supported on a complete muscular infundibulum (Fig. 17.4). These infundibular arrangements are also by no means universal. Furthermore, although the aortic valve is usually found in anterior and leftward position relative to the pulmonary trunk (or anterior and rightward in the mirror-image variant), these relationships, while the most common, are not invariable (Fig. 17.5).

The origin of the pulmonary trunk from the morphologically left ventricle has a fundamental effect on septal morphology. In the normal heart, the outflow tract of the left ventricle has a deep posterior recess which produces a plane of cleavage between the mitral valve and the septum. In the heart with discordant atrioventricular connexions, this posterior recess results in marked malalignment between the atrial septum and the inlet part of the ventricular septum. This then has a fundamental effect on the disposition of the conduction tissues.[2] In the normal heart, the atrioventricular node, at the apex of the triangle of Koch, is able to make contact with the branching atrioventricular bundle astride the ventricular septum, the conduction axis penetrating through the atrioventricular component of the membranous septum. A node is still found within the triangle of Koch in corrected transposition, but, because of the marked septal malalignment, it is unable to make contact with the ventricular conduction tissues. Instead, the conduction axis arises anteriorly and encircles the lateral quadrant of the subpulmonary outflow tract, penetrating through the area of fibrous continuity between the pulmonary and mitral valves to reach an atrioventricular node located anterolaterally within the right atrioventricular junction (Fig. 17.6). For some reason, which we are unable to explain, the malalignment gap between the septal structures is much more pronounced in hearts with usual atrial arrangement than in those with the mirror-image variant. For this reason, the conduction axis tends to originate from a regular node in congenitally corrected transposition with mirror-image atrial arrangement.[3,4]

The flow of blood in patients with congenitally corrected transposition is, potentially, entirely normal because, in terms of circulatory pathways, the two discordant connexions cancel each other out. In the absence of associated lesions,

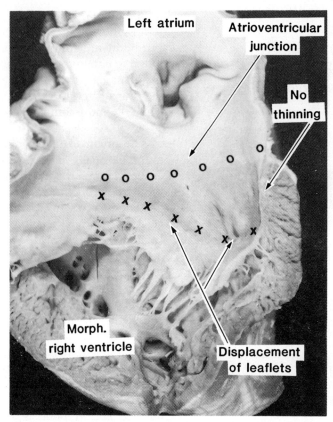

Fig. 17.9 This view of the left-sided chambers in congenitally corrected transposition shows the typical features of Ebstein's malformation but without thinning of the atrialized segment of the right ventricular inlet. The crosses show the attachment of the valve while the circles mark the atrioventricular junction.

therefore, the anatomical arrangement theoretically is capable of supporting life without impediment. Cases are reported in which the lesion has been discovered incidentally as an autopsy finding in the eighth decade of life.[5] It is most unusual, however, to find cases of corrected transposition in which there is not some other lesion elsewhere in the heart. In most instances, these lesions serve to 'uncorrect' the circulatory pattern. Three are sufficiently frequent to be considered an integral part of the anomaly.[6,7] These are a ventricular septal defect, obstruction to the left ventricular outflow tract and malformations of the morphologically tricuspid valve. Concentration on these lesions should not detract from the significance of other anomalies such as subaortic obstruction and coarctation.[8]

Problems of atrioventricular conduction are also frequent, complete heart block occurring in many cases.[2]

THE MAJOR ASSOCIATED LESIONS

A ventricular septal defect is found in about two-thirds of autopsied examples of congenitally corrected transposition.[7] Most frequently, the defect is perimembranous, being roofed by fibrous continuity between the pulmonary, mitral and tricuspid valves and opening primarily between the ventricular inlets (Fig. 17.7). Although the perimembranous defect is seen most frequently, any type of defect can be found with discordant atrioventricular connexions. As in

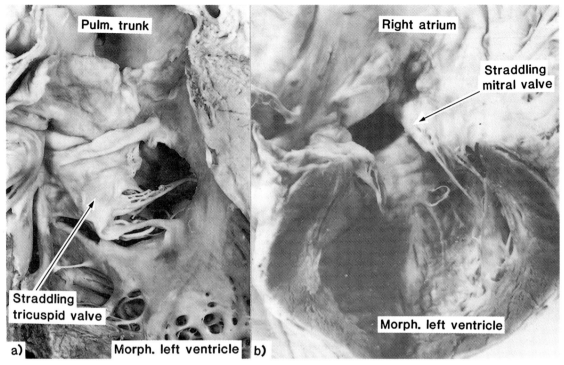

Fig. 17.10 a,b These illustrations show (**a**) the tricuspid valve straddling the inlet part of the septum to open beneath the pulmonary trunk and (**b**) the mitral valve straddling the outlet part of the septum, both viewed from the morphologically left ventricle in hearts with congenitally corrected transposition.

hearts with concordant atrioventricular connexions, the doubly committed and juxta-arterial defect is found most frequently in Far Eastern populations.[9] Muscular defects are rare and atrioventricular septal defects even rarer.

Obstruction to the left ventricular outflow tract can be produced by various lesions, often in association with stenosis at the level of the pulmonary valve.[10] A fibrous shelf is commonly found, producing diaphragmatic obstruction, while fibrous tissue tags are also frequent. The tags can originate from any of the valves in the region of the outflow tract but most frequently are derived from the morphologically tricuspid valve or from the remnant of the interventricular component of the membranous septum (Fig. 17.8). Usually they co-exist with a ventricular septal defect but they may be found with an intact ventricular septum.

Malformations of the morphologically tricuspid valve are, in autopsied hearts, the commonest associated lesions, being observed in up to 90% of all specimens.[7] The most frequent lesion is Ebstein's malformation. As in the setting of concordant atrioventricular connexions, the valve is deformed with respect both to anomalous attachment and dysplasia of its leaflets. Again, as with concordant connexions, it is the mural and septal leaflets which show the greatest degree of distal displacement (Fig. 17.9). Unlike hearts with concordant atrioventricular connexions, however, the malformation when found with discordant connexions is rarely associated with marked thinning and dilatation of the ventricular inlet component. In rare instances, the leaflets can be completely absent and the tricuspid orifice unguarded.[11] Although Ebstein's malformation is the commonest lesion afflicting the tricuspid valve, straddling with or without overriding (see Ch. 9) is probably the most significant abnormality and certainly produces the greatest impediment to surgical correction. When the

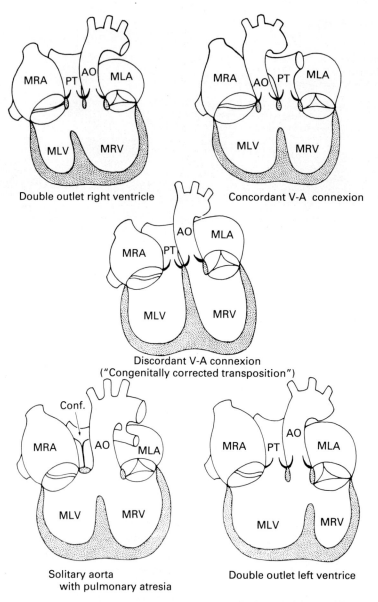

Fig. 17.11 This diagram shows the various ventriculo–arterial connexions which can co-exist with discordant atrioventricular connexions.
AO—aorta; Conf.—confluent pulmonary arteries; MLA—morphologically left atrium; MLV—morphologically left ventricle; MRA—morphologically right atrium; MRV-morphologically right ventricle; PT—pulmonary arterial trunk.

tricuspid valve is afflicted, it straddles and overrides the inlet part of the ventricular septum (Fig. 17.10a), being part of a spectrum of malformations from congenitally corrected transposition to double inlet left ventricle with left-sided rudimentary and incomplete right ventricle. The mitral valve can also straddle and/or override (Fig. 17.10b). It does so across the outlet part of the septum, often in the presence of double outlet right ventricle. The straddling mitral valve is again part of a series of lesions, in this case extending towards double inlet right ventricle with right-sided rudimentary and incomplete left ventricle. Either the mitral valve or tricuspid valve can prolapse in hearts with discordant atrioventricular connexions.[12]

OTHER VENTRICULO–ARTERIAL CONNEXIONS

Although the great majority of patients have discordant connexions at the ventriculo–arterial junction ('congenitally corrected transposition'), any other connexion may be observed and considered (Fig. 17.11). Double outlet right ventricle and single outlet right ventricle co-existing with pulmonary atresia are probably the next most frequent, in that order. As already discussed, the presence of the pulmonary trunk within the right ventricle removes much of the usual malalignment between the atrial and ventricular septal structures. This means that, in double outlet right ventricle, the conduction tissue is more frequently found to originate from a regular atrioventricular node, albeit often with a sling of conduction tissue connecting with the anterolateral node. It was such a sling-like arrangement in the setting of double outlet right ventricle with discordant atrioventricular connexions which Mönckeberg described as long ago as 1913.[13] The ventricular

septal defect which is to be anticipated with double outlet is almost always found in the subpulmonary position. There is no reason why it should not exist in the other known locations for hearts with concordant atrioventricular connexions (subaorctic, non-committed or doubly committed). Pulmonary atresia can be found with an intact ventricular septum and a hypoplastic left ventricle,[14] but more usually it is found with a ventricular septal defect and with the aorta connected to the morphologically right ventricle. The remnant of the pulmonary trunk is then found posteriorly. The pulmonary arterial supply has always, in our experience, been derived via the arterial duct.

The other ventriculo–arterial connexions are much rarer. Concordant ventriculo–arterial connexions are important because their combination with discordant atrioventricular connexions produces the circulatory pattern associated with complete transposition. Double outlet left ventricle, common arterial trunk and single outlet with aortic atresia are all extremely rare.

REFERENCES

1. Anderson RH. Criss-cross hearts revisited. Ped Cardiol 1982; 3: 305–313.
2. Anderson RH, Becker AE, Arnold R, Wilkinson JL. The conducting tissues in congenitally corrected transposition. Circulation 1974; 50: 911–923.
3. Thiene G, Nava P, Rossi L. The conducting tissue in corrected transposition in situs inversus. Eur J Cardiol 1977; 6: 57–70.
4. Wilkinson JL, Smith A, Lincoln C, Anderson RH. The conducting tissues in congenitally corrected transposition with situs inversus. Br Heart J 1978; 40: 41–48.
5. Lieberson AD, Schumacher RR, Chidress RH, Genouese PD. Corrected transposition of the great vessels in a 73 year old man. Circulation 1969; 39: 96–100.
6. Van Praagh R. What is congenitally corrected transposition? N Engl J Med 1970; 282: 1097–1098.
7. Allwork SP, Bentall HH, Becker AE, Cameron H, Gerlis LM, Wilkinson JL, Anderson RH. Congenitally corrected transposition of the great arteries: morphologic study of 32 cases. Am J Cardiol 1976; 38: 910–923.
8. Craig BG, Smallhorn JF, Rowe RD, Williams WG, Trusler GA, Freedom RM. Severe obstruction to systemic blood flow in congenitally corrected transposition (discordant atrioventricular

and ventriculo–arterial connexions): an analysis of 14 patients. Int J Cardiol 1986; 11: 209–217.
9. Okamura J, Konno S. Two types of ventricular septal defect in corrected transposition of the great arteries. Reference to surgical approaches. Am Heart J 1973; 85: 483–490.
10. Anderson RH, Becker AE, Gerlis LM. The pulmonary outflow tract in classically corrected transposition. J Thorac Cardiovasc Surg 1975; 69: 747–757.
11. Brenner JI, Bharati S, Winn WC, Lev M. Absent tricuspid valve with aortic atresia in mixed levocardia (atria situs solitus, L-loop). A hitherto undescribed entity. Circulation 1978; 57: 836–840.
12. Cowley MJ, Coghlan HC, Mantle JA, Soto B. Chest pain and bilateral atrioventricular valve prolapse with normal coronary arteries in isolated corrected transposition of the great vessels. Clinical, angiographic and metabolic features. Am J Cardiol 1977; 40: 458–462.
13. Mönckeberg JG. Zur Entwicklungsgeschichte des Atrioventrikularsystems. Verh Dtsch Pathol Ges 1913; 16: 228–249.
14. Steeg CN, Ellias K, Bransilver B, Gersony WM. Pulmonary atresia and intact septum complicating corrected transposition of the great vessels. Am Heart J 1971; 82: 382–386.

Double inlet ventricle

INTRODUCTION

Understanding of many congenital malformations has been made unnecessarily difficult by the use of illogical terms in their description. Perhaps the hearts to which this most obviously applies are those correctly grouped together because of a double inlet atrioventricular connexion. Although for years it has been conventional to describe these malformations as 'single ventricles', this approach makes little sense since the majority of hearts thus described possess two ventricles, albeit that one is dominant and the other rudimentary and incomplete. For a period this policy was defended by attempts to deny ventricular status to the incomplete ventricle.[1,2] Although serving one of its desired purposes by illustrating the similarity between hearts having double inlet left ventricle and those with classic tricuspid atresia, the approach was cumbersome and proved inadequate for those hearts having straddling and overriding of one atrioventricular valve.[3] In retrospect, it is now easy to recognize that the real problem was the illogical definition of 'single ventricle'.[4,5] Hearts in which both atriums are connected to the same ventricle are not unified because there is only one chamber within their ventricular mass—as stated, most possess in fact two ventricles. They are unified because of their double inlet atrioventricular connexion. If the distinction between the features of ventricular mass and atrioventricular connexions is made, and the hearts are described primarily on the basis of their unifying double inlet atrioventricular connexion, all the apparent problems in recognizing their affinities disappear.[6,7]

THE NATURE OF A DOUBLE INLET ATRIOVENTRICULAR CONNEXION

Double inlet ventricle exists when both atrioventricular junctions are connected in their greater part to the same ventricle. This definition is independent of the nature of the valve or valves guarding the atrioventricular junctions. Thus, both atriums can be connected to the same ventricle when there are two atrioventricular valves or when there is a common atrioventricular valve (Fig. 18.1). The double inlet connexion can also exist when one of two valves is imperforate: obviously it cannot exist when one atrioventricular connexion is absent. On the other hand, atrioventricular valvar atresia, when one valve is imperforate, can rarely co-exist with double inlet: more usually, it constitutes a separate and discrete atrioventricular connexion (see Ch. 19). This definition of double inlet also excludes hearts with huge ventricular septal defects. In the past, it has been customary to consider such hearts, in which an apical rim of septum separates trabecular components of right and left morphology, as 'common ventricles' and to group them along with 'single ventricles'.[4] We prefer to consider such malformations as huge septal defects since it seems to us that, if it is possible to recognize separate right and left ventricular trabeculations, it is more logical to categorize the atrioventricular connexions as concordant, discordant or ambiguous as the case may be. Although excluding huge septal defects, our chosen definition of double inlet does include those hearts with overriding and straddling of an atrioventricular valve. The heart with overriding of one atrioventricular junction will justifiably be catalogued as having a double inlet connexion when the greater part of the overriding junction is connected to the ventricle which also receives the other atrioventricular valve (Fig. 18.2). This also holds for those hearts with an overriding common valve except that, since the common valve guards both atrioventricular junctions, 75% of the overall junction needs to be connected to the dominant ventricle to justify the diagnosis of a double

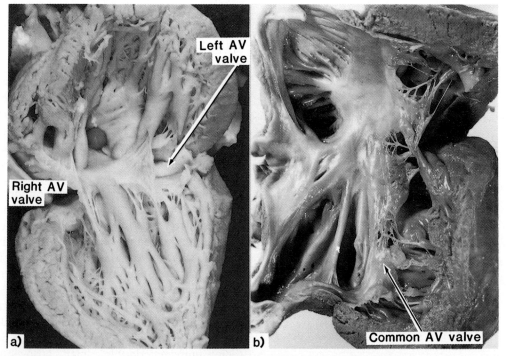

Fig. 18.1 a,b These hearts show how a double inlet connexion (both atriums connected to the same ventricle) can exist when there are two atrioventricular valves (**a**) or a common valve (**b**). The dominant ventricle is of morphologically left pattern in (**a**) but is a right ventricle in (**b**).

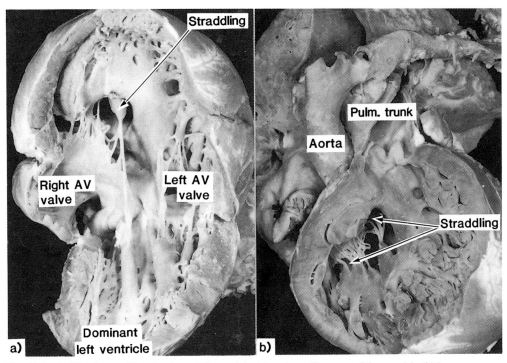

Fig. 18.2 a,b This heart with a dominant left ventricle (**a**) and a rudimentary right ventricle (**b**) has a double inlet atrioventricular connexion although there is straddling and overriding of the right atrioventricular valve.

inlet connexion. When defined in this fashion, double inlet ventricle can be independent of the atrial arrangement, of the morphology of the dominant ventricle, and of the ventriculo–arterial connexion. The combinations of these segmental morphologies produce the variations to be found within the overall group. The most important variable is ventricular morphology.

VENTRICULAR MORPHOLOGY

The atriums in hearts with double inlet connexion may be connected to a morphologically left, a morphologically right or a solitary and morphologically indeterminate ventricle. Most such hearts have the atriums connected to a morphologically left ventricle. Almost always this is found with an incomplete and rudimentary morphologically right ventricle (Fig. 18.3a). Less frequently the dominant ventricle is of morphologically right type, and in this case there is usually an incom-

plete and rudimentary morphologically left ventricle (Fig. 18.3b). The distinction between these two patterns is made according to the apical trabecular patterns of the dominant and rudimentary ventricles. It should be noted that, almost without exception, rudimentary right ventricles are positioned anterosuperiorly relative to dominant left ventricles while rudimentary left ventricles lie postero-inferiorly relative to dominant right ventricles (Fig. 18.3). The indeterminate ventricle is distinguished by having coarser trabeculations than those of the usual morphologically right ventricle (Fig. 18.4). This feature is not always easy to determine. In practice, therefore, indeterminate ventricles are usually diagnosed on the basis of the inability to demonstrate the presence of a second ventricle. When present, the incomplete ventricle is demarcated by descending branches of the coronary arteries which should always be sought for, either on the anterosuperior shoulders or on the postero-inferior diaphragmatic margins of the ventricular

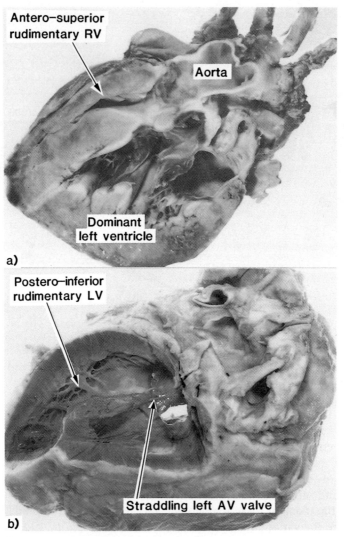

Antero–superior
rudimentary RV

Aorta

Dominant
left ventricle

a)

Postero–inferior
rudimentary LV

Straddling left AV valve

b)

Fig. 18.3 a,b These dissections show the relationship of dominant and
rudimentary ventricles. Rudimentary right ventricles (**a**) are always
located antero-superiorly within the ventricular mass whereas rudimentary
left ventricles (**b**) are positioned postero-inferiorly.

mass. It may still be difficult to exclude the
presence of a second ventricle and, in rare cases,
histological examination may be needed to
demonstrate whether or not there is an incomplete and slit-like chamber.

DOUBLE INLET LEFT VENTRICLE

This is the commonest variant of double inlet

ventricle. It is the malformation which, in the
past, has usually been referred to as 'single
ventricle'. Most often it occurs in hearts
with usual atrial arrangement but it may be found
with all the other atrial arrangements. The
main feature determining variation is the
ventriculo–arterial connexions, which are usually
discordant — that is, with the pulmonary trunk
arising from the dominant left ventricle while the
rudimentary and incomplete right ventricle gives

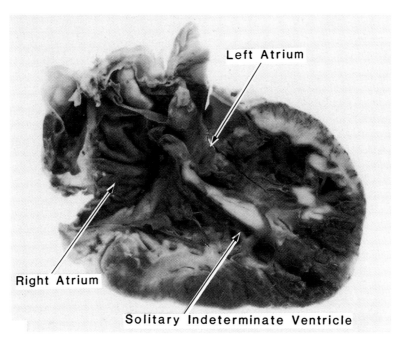

Fig. 18.4 This section through a heart in the long axis ('four chamber') plane shows that both atriums are connected to a solitary ventricle with very coarse apical trabeculations of indeterminate pattern. The apparent septal structure between the valves is simply a muscular ridge between the inlets of the ventricle.

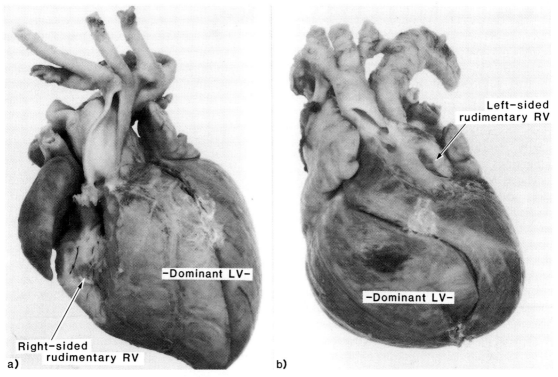

Fig. 18.5 a,b These illustrations show that although rudimentary right ventricles are always located antero-superiorly they can be either right-sided (**a**) or left-sided (**b**) relative to the dominant left ventricle.

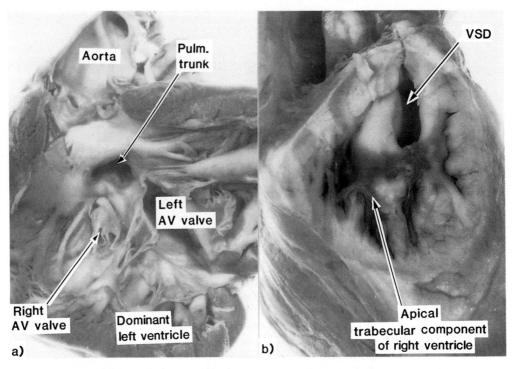

Fig. 18.6 a,b In this heart, with double inlet to and double outlet from a dominant left ventricle (**a**), the rudimentary and incomplete right ventricle (**b**) is represented only by its apical trabecular component.

rise to the aorta. This arrangement may be found in two further variants, with the rudimentary right ventricle positioned to either the right (Fig. 18.5a) or the left (Fig. 18.5b) side of the dominant left ventricle. Although often described in terms of right-hand and left-hand topology ('d and l ventricular looping'), we find it more accurate simply to describe the ventricular relationships directly. Irrespective of the position of the rudimentary ventricle, this pattern tends to be associated with a restrictive ventricular septal defect and, accompanying this feature, coarctation or interruption of the aortic arch. Occasionally, the ventricular septal defect may be non-restrictive and there may be obstruction of the subpulmonary outflow tract from the dominant left ventricle. This is most often due to posterior deviation of the outlet septum, but the stenosis may be caused by tissue tags derived from adjacent fibrous structures or by anomalous attachment of the leaflets of the atrioventricular valves. Subpulmonary stenosis is then usually accompanied by additional stenosis at valvar level,

the valve often having only two leaflets. If deviation of the outlet septum is extreme, both great arteries may be connected in their greater parts (or, rarely, exclusively) to the dominant left ventricle. In this circumstance, the rudimentry right ventricle is represented only by its apical trabecular component (Fig. 18.6). Double outlet co-existing with double inlet left ventricle is a rarity.

The second commonest ventriculo–arterial connexion is a concordant one whereby the aorta arises from the dominant left ventricle and the pulmonary trunk from the rudimentary right ventricle. This is called the 'Holmes heart',[8] of which there are two variants. The more typical has the apical trabecular component of the rudimentary right ventricle in right-sided position and the outlet component supporting the pulmonary trunk in left-sided position (Fig. 18.7). The great arteries then spiral as they ascend from the heart, giving the pattern usually described as 'normal relations'. The less frequent variant has the rudimentary right ventricle exclusively in left-

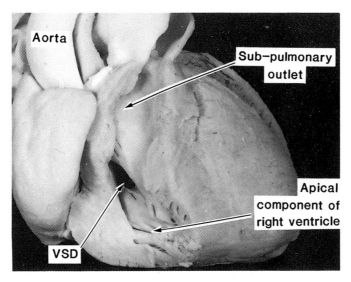

Fig. 18.7 This illustration shows the typical morphology of the rudimentary right ventricle in hearts with double inlet left ventricle and concordant ventriculo–arterial connexions ('Holmes heart').

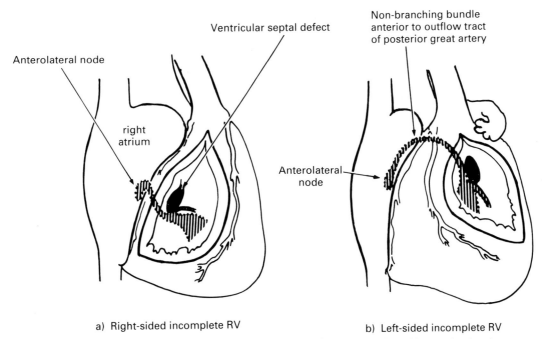

a) Right-sided incomplete RV

b) Left-sided incomplete RV

Fig. 18.8 a,b This diagram illustrates the more extensive course of the long non-branching conduction tissue bundle in double inlet left ventricle when the rudimentary right ventricle is in left-sided (**b**) as opposed to right-sided (**a**) position. The relation of the bundle to the ventricular septal defect, however, is the same in both patterns.

sided position and the arterial trunks ascend in parallel fashion as they course towards the mediastinum.[9] Both of these arrangements may be found either with two atrioventricular valves or

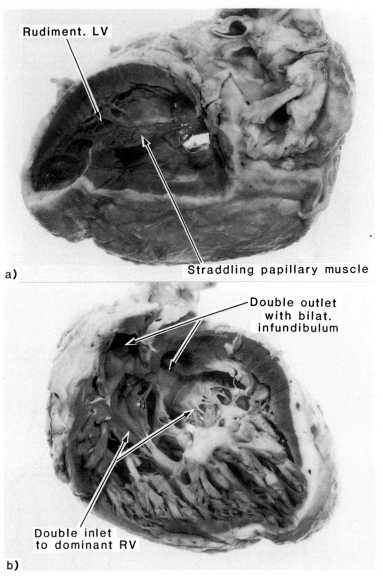

Fig. 18.9 a,b These illustrations show the typical pattern of hearts with double inlet to and double outlet from a dominant right ventricle (**b**). The incomplete and rudimentary left ventricle (**a**), in this case retaining one papillary muscle of the left atrioventricular valve, is effectively made up of only the apical trabecular component.

with a common valve guarding both right and left atrioventricular junctions.

The cardinal diagnostic feature of double inlet left ventricle is that the ventricular septum is located anterosuperiorly within the ventricular mass and that there is total lack of any inlet septal structures (Fig. 18.3a). It is this feature which

determines the anomalous course of the atrioventricular conduction axis.[10-12] Because of the lack of any inlet septal structures, it is not possible for the regular atrioventricular node, found within the triangle of Koch, to give rise to a penetrating atrioventricular bundle to make contact with the ventricular conduction tissues. These tissues,

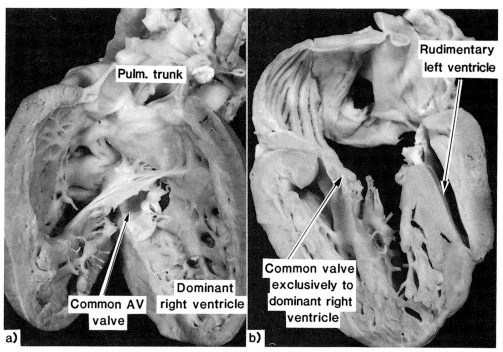

Fig. 18.10 a,b This heart, with double inlet to a dominant right ventricle (**a**), has a common atrioventricular valve and concordant ventriculo–arterial connexions. Although it can be considered as the extreme form of an atrioventricular septal defect with right ventricular dominance, the 'four chamber' section (**b**) shows that the atriums are connected exclusively to the dominant right ventricle.

located astride the apical trabecular septum, are situated anterosuperiorly. An anomalous atrioventricular node also lies anterosuperiorly within the right atrioventricular junction. From this node arises the penetrating atrioventricular bundle which, having reached the ventricles, becomes the long non-branching bundle. This bundle always descends towards that part of the apical trabecular septum closest to the right atrioventricular valve (presuming usual atrial arrangement). The only difference when the rudimentary right ventricle is left-sided rather than right-sided is that the bundle must cross the outflow tract from the dominant left ventricle when the incomplete ventricle is left-sided (Fig. 18.8). The conduction tissue axis never runs through the outlet septum. In some cases, however, the ventricular septal defect itself is crossed by muscle bundles. The exact relationship of the axis to these anomalous muscle bars has yet to be established.

DOUBLE INLET RIGHT VENTRICLE

Theoretically, it is possible for double inlet right ventricle to exist with all possible atrial arrangements and with any ventriculo–arterial connexion. In practice, there are two common patterns. Most frequently, there is double inlet to and double outlet from the morphologically right ventricle, the rudimentary left ventricle being represented by only its apical trabecular component (Fig. 18.9). This malformation is often found with straddling of the mitral valve in cases with either usual atrial arrangement or right atrial isomerism. Usually there are two atrioventricular valves, but a common valve may be found, particularly with double inlet right ventricle when the ventriculo–arterial connexions are concordant (Fig. 18.10). This pattern can be considered as the extreme form of right ventricular dominance accompanying an atrioventricular septal defect. Indeed, the distinction between

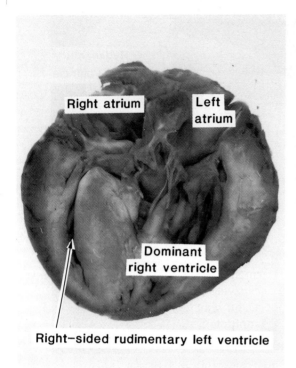

Fig. 18.11 This example of double inlet right ventricle with two atrioventricular valves has a right-sided rudimentary and incomplete left ventricle (left-hand topology) with minimal straddling of the right-sided morphologically mitral valve. The heart has been sectioned in 'four chamber' fashion.

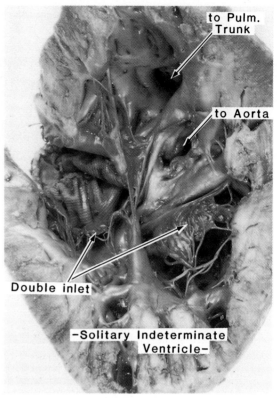

Fig. 18.12 This heart has double inlet to and double outlet from a solitary and indeterminate ventricle. The 'four chamber' section of the heart is shown in Fig. 18.4.

these two malformations, on occasions, may be difficult. On the other hand, in extreme cases there is no doubt that the common valve may be exclusively connected to the dominant right ventricle (unequivocal double inlet connexion—Fig. 18.10). The outflow tract from the rudimentary left ventricle to the aorta is usually compromised in this combination by either severe coarctation or interruption of the aortic arch.

Most examples of double inlet right ventricle occur when the rudimentary left ventricle is left-sided. Rarely, the rudimentary ventricle may be right-sided, in which case the heart has much in common with congenitally corrected transposition (see Ch. 17). These cases with right-sided rudimentary ventricles usually have two atrioventricular valves, often with straddling and overriding by the right-sided mitral valve, and double outlet from the dominant right

ventricle with the aorta in left-sided position (Fig. 18.11).

The anatomy of the conduction tissues in examples of double inlet right ventricle varies according to the location of the rudimentary and incomplete left ventricle. When the latter is left-sided, although the apical trabecular septum is not positioned between the ventricular inlets, it does approximate to the crux of the heart. Because of this, the normally located atrioventricular node is able to penetrate through the atrioventricular insulating plane to reach the ventricular conduction tissues carried astride the apical septum. The conduction axis, therefore, follows the normal course. When, however, the rudimentary left ventricle is right-sided, there is left-hand ventricular topology. This is accompanied, as in congenitally corrected transposition, by either an anomalous anterolateral node or a 'sling' of conduction tissue between a normally sited and an anterior atrioventricular node.[13]

DOUBLE INLET SOLITARY AND INDETERMINATE VENTRICLE

This is the rarest variant of double inlet ventricle and, as described above, is often the hardest to diagnose with certainty. The patterns of the apical trabeculations are much coarser than those of the usual right ventricle and, usually, the apex of the ventricle is crossed by prominent trabeculations which support the tension apparatus of one or both atrioventricular valves (Fig. 18.12). A further distinguishing feature is the lack of any structure resembling the septomarginal trabeculation of the morphologically right ventricle. Such a heart usually has two atrioventricular valves and can only have either double or single outlet from the solitary ventricle. Since, by definition, the heart does not possess any apical septal structures, there cannot be straddling of either atrioventricular valve. In contrast, the heart possesses an outlet septum and this can be deviated to produce either subpulmonary or subaortic stenosis.

The conduction tissues in double inlet solitary ventricle are most bizarre.[13,14] The conduction axis is usually a single strand which descends from an anomalously located node and disperses in the lateral wall of the ventricular mass. We have also seen cases in which the conduction axis descended in a prominent trabeculation from a regular node[13] and cases with most unusual slings from dual nodes in the presence of right atrial isomerism[14].

REFERENCES

1. Anderson RH, Becker AE, Wilkinson JL, Gerlis IM. Morphogenesis of univentricular hearts. Br Heart J 1976; 38: 558–572.
2. Anderson RH, Tynan MJ, Freedom RM et al. Ventricular morphology in the univentricular heart. Herz 1979; 4: 184–197.
3. Brandt PWT. Cineangiography of atrioventricular and ventriculo-arterial connexions. In: Godman MJ, ed. Paediatric cardiology, vol. 4. Edinburgh: Churchill Livingstone, 1981; 199–220.
4. Van Praagh R, Ongley PA, Swan HJC. Anatomic types of single or common ventricle in man: morphologic and geometric aspects of sixty necropsied cases. Am J Cardiol 1964; 13: 367–386.
5. Edwards JE. Discussion. In: Davila LC, ed. 2nd Henry Ford Hospital International Symposium on Cardiac Surgery. New York: Appleton-Century-Crofts, 1977; 242.
6. Anderson RH, Becker AE, Tynan M, Macartney FJ, Rigby ML, Wilkinson JL. The univentricular atrioventricular connection: getting to the root of a thorny problem. Am J Cardiol 1984; 54: 822–828.
7. Anderson RH, Crupi G, Parenzan L. Double inlet ventricle. Anatomy, diagnosis and surgical management. Tunbridge Wells: Castle House Publications, 1987.
8. Holmes AF. A case of malformation of the heart. Trans Med Chir Soc Edinb 1824; 1: 252–259.
9. Anderson RH, Lenox CC, Zuberbuhler JR, Ho SY, Smith A, Wilkinson JL. Double-inlet left ventricle with rudimentary right ventricle and ventriculoarterial concordance. Am J Cardiol 1983; 52: 573–577.
10. Anderson RH, Arnold R, Thaper MK, Jones RS, Hamilton DI. Cardiac specialized tissues in hearts with an apparently single ventricular chamber. (Double inlet left ventricle.) Am J Cardiol 1974; 33: 95–106.
11. Bharati S, Lev M. The course of the conduction system in single ventricle with inverted (L) loop and inverted (L) transposition. Circulation 1975; 51: 723–730.
12. Wenink ACG. The conduction tissues in primitive ventricle with outlet chamber: two different possibilities. J Thorac Cardiovasc Surg 1978; 75: 747–753.
13. Essed CE, Ho SY, Shinebourne EA, Joseph MC, Anderson RH. Further observations on conduction tissues in univentricular hearts—surgical implications. Eur Heart J 1981; 2: 87–96.
14. Dickinson DF, Wilkinson JL, Anderson KR, Smith A, Ho SY, Anderson RH. The cardiac conduction system in situs ambiguus. Circulation 1979; 59: 879–885.

Atrioventricular valvar atresia

INTRODUCTION

Atresia is the term used to describe total congenital occlusion of a naturally occurring channel of the body. At the level of the atrioventricular junction, this can be produced by two quite discrete mechanisms. The first, and by far the commoner, is for one of the normal atrioventricular junctions to be totally lacking. The floor of the affected atrium is then muscular and is separated by the fibrofatty tissue of the atrioventricular groove from the ventricular mass (Fig. 19.1). The other mechanism is for the atrioventricular junction to be formed, albeit usually in hypoplastic fashion, but to be blocked completely by an imperforate valve (Fig. 19.2). Although generally believed to be the usual form of atrioventricular valvar atresia, this second pattern is relatively rare. Both types are usually described in terms of either tricuspid or mitral atresia but this convention leads to problems in classification. Thus, absence of the right atrioventricular connexion is by far the commonest variant of tricuspid atresia, a terminology that implies that, had the right valve been formed, it would have been of tricuspid morphology. The anatomical arrangement of most hearts with tricuspid atresia supports this presumption. But some hearts with absence of the right atrioventricular connexion, in which the systemic venous atrium ends blindly, have their left atrium connected to a dominant right ventricle in the presence of a right-sided rudimentary and incomplete left ventricle.[1] This pattern is strongly suggestive of left-hand ventricular topology and, in this arrangement, it is likely that, had the

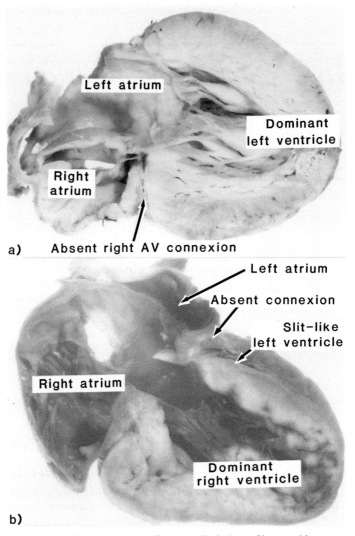

Fig. 19.1 a,b These sections in 'four chamber' plane of hearts with atrioventricular valvar atresia show the essential anatomy of absence of (**a**) the right and (**b**) the left atrioventricular connexion.

right atrioventricular valve been formed, it would have been of mitral morphology. Yet most observers would understand by 'mitral atresia' a blockage of the pulmonary venous atrium and it would be potentially confusing to describe this variant with a blind-ending right atrium as 'mitral atresia'. Equally, it would be anatomically inaccurate to describe it as 'tricuspid atresia'. The same problem exists in hearts in which there is usual atrial arrangement and absence of the left

atrioventricular connexion, and in which the right atrium is connected to a dominant left ventricle in the presence of a left-sided incomplete and rudimentary right ventricle.[2] Functionally, such hearts have 'mitral atresia', yet anatomically, had the left valve formed, it would almost certainly have been of tricuspid morphology. Fortunately, such hearts are relatively rare. Our approach is to give a full segmental description and then account for absence of either the right-sided or

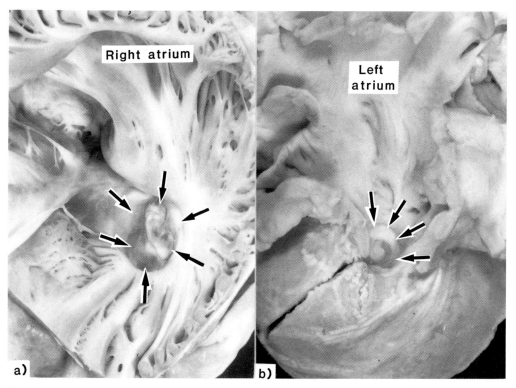

Fig. 19.2 a,b In these hearts, tricuspid atresia (**a**) and mitral atresia (**b**) are produced by the much rarer lesions of an imperforate valve membrane, indicated by the arrows.

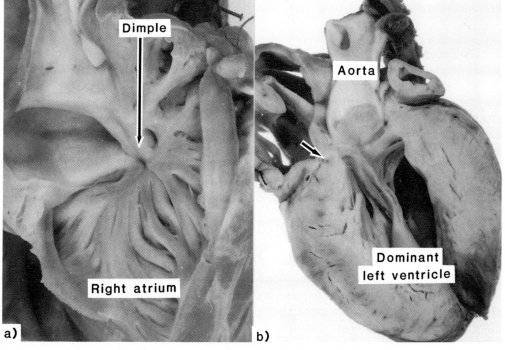

Fig. 19.3 a,b The section (**b**), in 'four chamber' plane, through a heart with classic tricuspid atresia, has passed through the dimple (arrowed). The gross morphology is shown in (**a**). The dimple lies above the atrioventricular component of the membranous septum and 'points' to the dominant left ventricle.

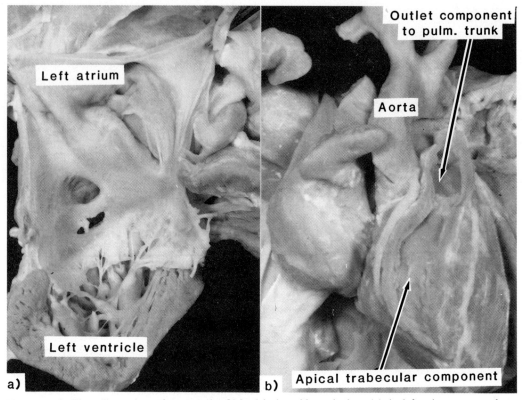

Fig. 19.4 a,b These illustrations of an example of 'classic' tricuspid atresia show (**a**) the left atrium connected to the dominant left ventricle and (**b**) the rudimentary and incomplete right ventricle giving rise to the pulmonary trunk.

left-sided connexion, rather than describing the condition as 'mitral' or 'tricuspid' atresia.[3] Such hearts will be described in this fashion in this chapter. We are concerned more with the morphology of classic mitral and tricuspid atresia. The variants will, therefore, be described according to the physiological disorder they produce rather than by their presumed embryogenesis.

TRICUSPID ATRESIA

As indicated above, this lesion can be produced either by absence of the right atrioventricular connexion or by an imperforate tricuspid valve. Probably 90% of cases coming to the attention of the pathologist will have the classic lesion,

absence of the atrioventricular connexion.[1] The floor of the morphologically right atrium is entirely muscular. If a dimple is seen, often thought to represent the atretic valve, it overlies the atrioventricular component of the membranous septum and 'points' towards the outflow tract of the dominant left ventricle (Fig. 19.3). This suggests that, had the valve been formed, it would have been in the arrangement of a double inlet ventricle rather than concordant connexions.[4] This feature also highlights the marked similarity between the ventricular mass in hearts with 'classic' tricuspid atresia and those with a double inlet left ventricle.[4,5] The systemic venous output crosses the interatrial communication, which rarely may be restrictive, and enters the left atrium. All the venous return crosses the mitral valve to enter the dominant left ventricle (Fig. 19.4a) and the pathways of the circulation

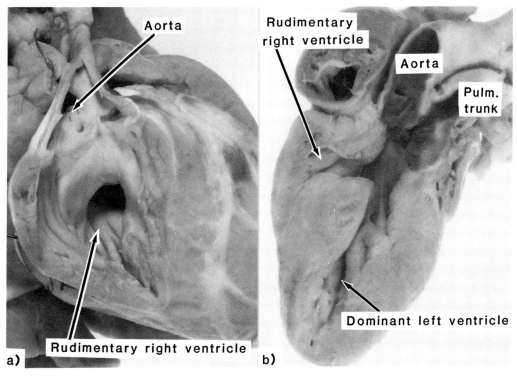

Fig. 19.5 a,b These hearts with tricuspid atresia show (**a**) discordant ventriculo–arterial connexions and (**b**) double outlet from the dominant left ventricle, the rudimentary right ventricle being represented only by its apical trabecular component.

depend upon the ventriculo–arterial connexion. Most cases have concordant connexions, with the aorta arising from the dominant left ventricle and the pulmonary trunk from the rudimentary right ventricle (Fig. 19.4b). The rudimentary ventricle is almost always arranged with its apical component to the right and the outlet component to the left ('normal relations'), although in a rare variant the entire incomplete and rudimentary right ventricle may be right-sided and the pulmonary trunk parallel to a left-sided aorta ('anatomically corrected malposition'[6]). With the more usual variant, there is typically a restrictive ventricular septal defect which produces subpulmonary stenosis. Further stenosis may then be found between the apical trabecular and outlet components of the rudimentary right ventricle. Less frequently, the ventricular septal defect may be unrestrictive or, in contrast, there may be pulmonary atresia. These features, combined with

the nature of the ventriculo–arterial connexion, are often used in alphanumeric fashion to describe the overall lesion.[7] We prefer to avoid such cryptic classifications and simply describe directly what is found.

The second commonest ventriculo–arterial connexion is a discordant one, when the usually restrictive ventricular septal defect is associated with subaortic stenosis and either aortic coarctation or interruption (Fig. 19.5a). This variant is associated with parallel arterial trunks, usually with the aorta to the right but rarely with a left-sided aorta arising from an anteriorly located rudimentary right ventricle. The arrangement with discordant ventriculo–arterial connexions may also be found with subpulmonary stenosis, usually the consequence of posterior deviation of the outlet septum but, as with double inlet left ventricle, sometimes due to fibrous tissue tags or anomalous attachment of the tension apparatus of

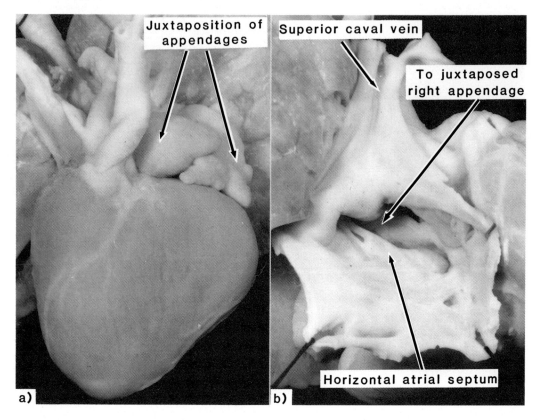

Fig. 19.6 a,b These illustrations show (**a**) left-sided juxtaposition of the atrial appendages in a heart with tricuspid atresia and (**b**) the influence of this lesion on the atrial septal morphology.

the left atrioventricular valve. The least common ventriculo–arterial connexion is double outlet, either from the dominant left ventricle, when the rudimentary ventricle is represented only by its apical trabecular component (Fig. 19.5b), or from the rudimentary ventricle itself. Single outlet from the heart via a common trunk has been described in association with tricuspid atresia but is exceedingly rare.

Associated defects may be found in any part of the heart. The valve of the inferior caval vein (Eustachian valve) is frequently prominent, but is of no functional significance since the flow of right atrial blood is to the left atrium. The left superior caval vein may persist and open through an enlarged coronary sinus. The most significant atrial malformation is juxtaposition of the atrial appendages which distorts the atrial anatomy,

the anticipated site of the oval fossa being occupied by the mouth of the juxtaposed right appendage (Fig. 19.6). The other major associated defects in such cases are subarterial stenosis and ventricular septal defect as described above.

Not all examples of tricuspid atresia are of this 'classic' pattern. Very rarely, hearts may be encountered in which a sizeable imperforate tricuspid valve blocks the morphologically right side of concordant atrioventricular connexions (Fig. 19.2a). More usually, when the atrioventricular connexions are concordant and the tricuspid valve is imperforate, it is either a hypoplastic structure in a heart with co-existing pulmonary atresia, or it is a structure of near normal size in a heart with Ebstein's malformation (Fig. 19.7). Another lesion closely

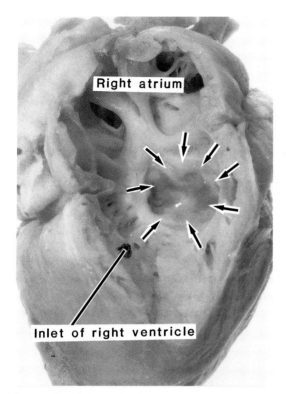

Fig. 19.7 In this heart with Ebstein's malformation and concordant atrioventricular connexions, the displaced valve is imperforate (arrowed), thus producing tricuspid atresia.

include absence of the right atrioventricular connexion with the left atrium connected to a dominant right ventricle, the rudimentary and incomplete left ventricle being right-sided and the morphologically tricuspid valve overriding the septum between the ventricles (Fig. 19.8). This malformation is difficult to classify precisely. Morphologically, the heart exhibits left-hand ventricular topology and, therefore, had the right atrioventricular valve formed it would certainly have been of mitral morphology. Yet the physiological derangement is that usually described as tricuspid atresia and, in terms of right atrial morphology, the lesion is indistinguishable from the 'classic' malformation (compare Figs 19.3a and 19.8a). The best solution to this dilemma, considering the rarity of such

related to Ebstein's malformation, and which produces the haemodynamic effects of tricuspid atresia, is when the morphologically right ventricle is divided into two discrete components, an imperforate muscular partition separating the two. In this pattern, the right atrium is connected concordantly to the inlet component of the ventricle while the distal component, made up of the apical trabecular and outlet components, is fed through a ventricular septal defect as in classic tricuspid atresia.[8] In essence, the lesion represents congenital unguarding of the tricuspid orifice but, as indicated, it produces the functional derangement of 'tricuspid atresia'. An imperforate right atrioventricular valve producing the effect of tricuspid atresia may also be found in hearts with double inlet ventricle, usually double inlet left ventricle. Rarer lesions may produce the same functional effects: they

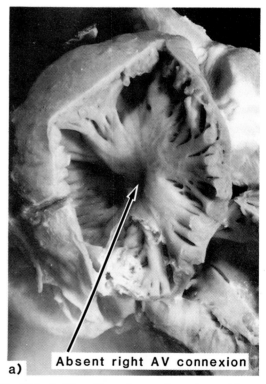

Fig. 19.8 a,b These illustrations are from a heart with absence of the right atrioventricular connexion (**a**) in which the left atrium is connected to both ventricles. As seen in (**b**), the left ventricle is incomplete and rudimentary but right-sided, suggesting left-hand ventricular topology. Had the right valve been formed, it would have been of mitral morphology. The haemodynamics, nonetheless, are those usually associated with tricuspid atresia.

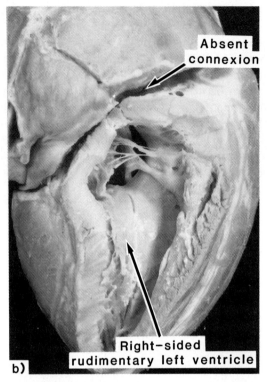

Fig. 19.8 b
[The caption is on the preceding page.]

anomalies, is to describe their full segmental morphology.

MITRAL ATRESIA

Mitral atresia, in its 'classic' form, produces complete blockage of the outflow tract of the morphologically left atrium. Because the normal mitral valve 'belongs' to the left ventricle, problems of classification may arise, as discussed above, in distinguishing between anatomical and physiological disturbances produced by 'mitral' atresia. In the majority of cases the atresia is found as an integral part of the so-called 'hypoplastic left heart syndrome'. The morphological arrangement in such cases may be either absence of the left atrioventricular connexion, when the left ventricle is incomplete and rudimentary (Fig. 19.1b), or an imperforate valve, when the left ventricle is

normally constructed but grossly hypoplastic. The commoner arrangement is absence of the connexion. Imperforate mitral valves in hearts with concordant atrioventricular connexions are more frequently encountered when the aortic root is patent (Fig. 19.9), either when the ventriculo–arterial connexions are concordant and there is a ventricular septal defect or when there is a double outlet from the right ventricle, again usually with a ventricular septal defect.[9,10] An imperforate left atrioventricular valve may also be found with a double inlet left ventricle and, although we have not seen it, must be expected to occur with all variants of double inlet atrioventricular connexion.

Absence of the left atrioventricular connexion may also be found in another relatively common pattern. This is when the right atrium is connected to a dominant left ventricle which is, in turn, connected to the pulmonary trunk.[2] The

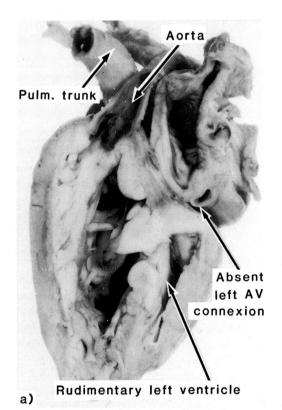

Fig. 19.9 a,b These hearts show mitral atresia with a patent aorta (**a**) arising from the right ventricle along with the pulmonary trunk and (**b**) (next page) arising from a hypoplastic left ventricle.

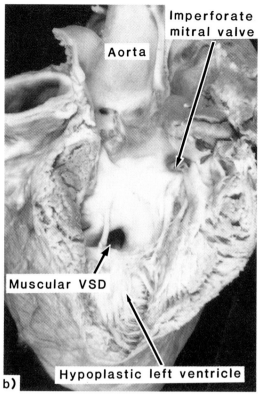

Fig. 19.9 b
[The caption is on the preceding page.]

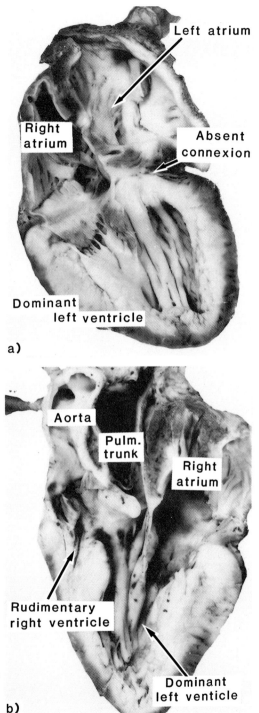

rudimentary and incomplete right ventricle gives rise to the aorta and is left-sided (Fig. 19.10). This malformation is difficult to classify accurately. Anatomically, the heart shows strong evidence of left-hand ventricular topology and, had the left valve formed, it would almost

Fig. 19.10 a,b In this heart with absence of the left atrioventricular connexion (**a**), the right atrium is connected to a dominant left ventricle. As seen in the long axis plane at right angles to the atrial septum (**b**), there is a rudimentary and incomplete right ventricle in anterosuperior position with a discordant ventriculo–arterial connexion. Although embryologically this heart can be thought to show tricuspid atresia, the haemodynamics are those of mitral atresia (compare with Fig. 19.8).

certainly have been of tricuspid morphology. The physiological derangement, nonetheless, is that of classic mitral atresia with a patent aortic root.

Again, the least ambiguous way of classifying the anomaly is to give a full segmental description of the lesions present.

REFERENCES

1. Scalia D, Russo P, Anderson RH et al. The surgical anatomy of hearts with no direct communication between the right atrium and the ventricular mass—so-called tricuspid atresia. J Thorac Cardiovasc Surg 1984; 87: 743–755.

2. Tandon R, Marin-Garcia J, Moller JH, Edwards JE. Tricuspid atresia with l-transposition. Am Heart J 1974; 88: 417–424.

3. Anderson RH, Rigby ML. The morphologic heterogeneity of 'tricuspid atresia'. Int J Cardiol 1987; 16: 67–73.

4. Anderson RH, Wilkinson JL, Gerlis LM, Smith A, Becker AE. Atresia of the right atrioventricular orifice. Br Heart J 1977; 39: 414–428.

5. Deanfield JE, Tommasini G, Anderson RH, Macartney FJ. Tricuspid atresia: an analysis of the coronary artery distribution and ventricular morphology. Br Heart J 1982; 48: 485–492.

6. Freedom RM, Harrington DP. Anatomically corrected malposition of the great arteries. Report of 2 cases, one with congenital asplenia; frequent association with juxtaposition of atrial appendages. Br Heart J 1974; 36: 207–215.

7. Edwards JE, Burchell HB. Congenital tricuspid atresia: a classification. Med Clin North Am 1949; 33: 1117–1119.

8. Zuberbuhler JR, Allwork SP, Anderson RH. The spectrum of Ebstein's anomaly of the tricuspid valve. J Thorac Cardiovasc Surg 1979; 77: 202–211.

9. Watson DG, Rowe RD, Coren PE, Duckworth JWA. Mitral atresia with normal aortic valve. Report of 11 cases and review of the literature. Pediatrics 1960; 25: 450–467.

10. Mickell JJ, Mathews RA, Anderson RH et al. The anatomical heterogeneity of hearts lacking a patent communication between the left atrium and the ventricular mass ('mitral atresia') in presence of a patent aortic valve. Eur Heart J 1983; 4: 477–486.

Complete transposition

INTRODUCTION

A well-recognized group of cardiac malformations presents common haemodynamic and clinical features because the morphologically right atrium is connected to the morphologically right ventricle which then gives rise to the aorta (Fig. 20.1a) while the morphologically left atrium is connected to the morphologically left ventricle which supplies the pulmonary trunk (Fig. 20.1b). The result of this morphological arrangement is that, in the absence of other associated defects, the systemic and pulmonary blood streams circulate in parallel rather than in series, as is the usual arrangement. When described in this fashion, the basic anatomy of such hearts is straightforward and easily understood. Attempts to clarify the different categories within the group by using various nominative terminologies have engendered no little controversy.[1,2]

We find it most satisfactory to describe the arrangement in which the aorta springs from the morphologically right ventricle and the pulmonary trunk from the left ventricle as discordant ventriculo–arterial connexions.[3] But this ventriculo–arterial connexion can exist with various atrioventricular connexions, such as a discordant one, an ambiguous one, a double inlet ventricle or absence of one atrioventricular connexion.[4] We prefer to describe the specific combination of discordant ventriculo–arterial connexions accompanied by concordant atrioventricular connexions as complete transposition. Complete transposition so defined may be found with usual or mirror-image atrial arrangement (Fig. 20.2). The condition cannot exist in hearts

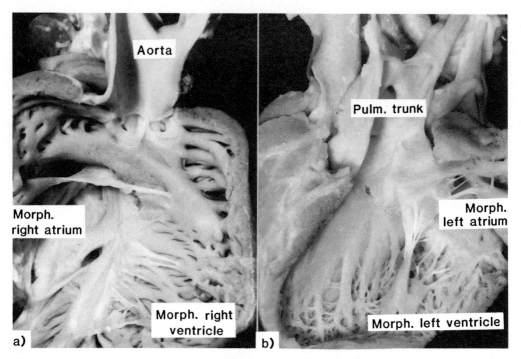

Fig. 20.1 a,b In hearts with complete transposition, the morphologically right ventricle (**a**), connected to the right atrium, gives rise to the aorta. The morphologically left ventricle (**b**), receiving blood from the left atrium, gives rise to the pulmonary trunk.

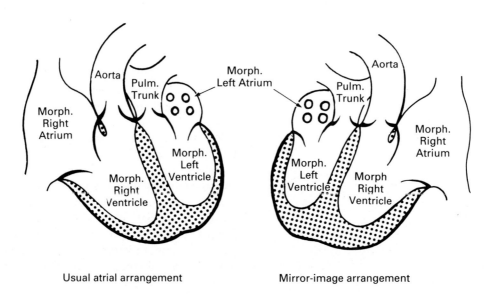

Usual atrial arrangement   Mirror-image arrangement

COMPLETE TRANSPOSITION

Concordant atrioventricular connexion
and discordant ventriculo-arterial connexion

Fig. 20.2 We use the term 'complete transposition' to describe only the specific connexions of segments shown in this diagram.

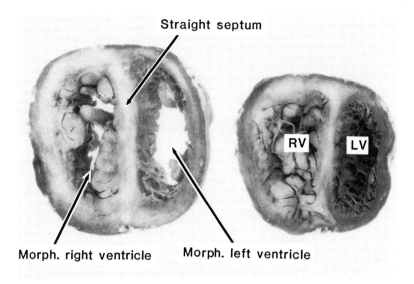

Straight septum

RV   LV

Morph. right ventricle   Morph. left ventricle

Fig. 20.3 As shown in these sections across the ventricular mass, the ventricular septum is a relatively straight structure in the presence of complete transposition (RV— morphologically right ventricle, LV—morphologically left ventricle).

having isomeric atriums, and the term is inappropriate for hearts with other atrioventricular connexions.

RELATIVELY CONSTANT FEATURES OF COMPLETE TRANSPOSITION

The atrial morphology of hearts with complete transposition can be virtually normal, although often there is a deficiency of the floor of the oval fossa permitting an interatrial communication. When there has been no natural interatrial communication it is usual nowadays for balloon septostomy to be performed when facilities for clinical diagnosis and treatment are available: if the case comes to autopsy the septum will not then be seen in its natural state but will have been rent asunder by the procedure.

The ventricular morphology is dominated by the discordant ventriculo–arterial connexions. In the majority of cases, this reflects the fact that the aorta springs in an anterior and rightward position from the morphologically right ventricle with its valve supported by a completely muscular infundibulum (Fig. 20.1a). The pulmonary trunk, in contrast, lies posteriorly and leftward and its

valve is usually in fibrous continuity with the mitral valve (Fig. 20.1b). These are by no means constant features but they are seen in the great majority of cases. When found in this typical arrangement, the ventricular septum is virtually straight and the arterial trunks arise in parallel fashion, markedly different from the way they originate from the normally constructed heart with concordant ventriculo–arterial connexions (Fig. 20.3).

Other features relatively constant in complete transposition are the disposition of the coronary arteries and the conduction tissues. There are three important aspects pertaining to the coronary arteries: their origin from the aortic sinuses, their courses relative to the pedicles of the arterial trunks, and the origin and course of the artery supplying the sinus node. The epicardial course of the arteries within the ventricular mass is virtually normal, with the anterior interventricular artery running within the anterior interventricular groove and the right coronary and circumflex arteries within their respective atrioventricular grooves. As in the normal heart, the posterior interventricular branch can originate either from the right coronary artery or from the circumflex artery. With regard to the origin of the coronary

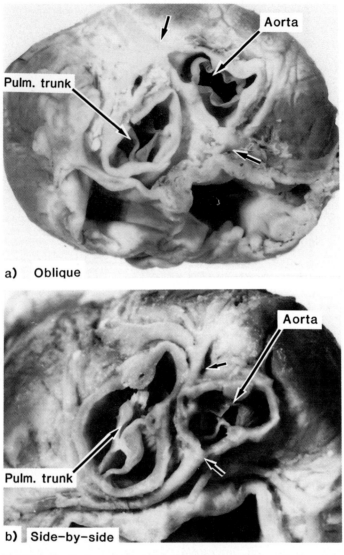

Fig. 20.4 a,b As shown in these two dissections of the short axis viewed from above, the coronary arteries (short arrows) arise from those sinuses of the aorta which face the pulmonary trunk irrespective of the relationship of the arterial trunks to one another, (**a**) oblique or (**b**) side-by-side.

arteries from the aortic sinuses, in our experience they have originated always from one or other (more usually both) of the sinuses adjacent to the pulmonary trunk (the facing sinuses—Fig. 20.4). Origin from facing sinuses is found irrespective of the relationship of the aorta to the pulmonary trunk within the overall anatomy of the heart. We describe these sinuses simply as being to the right hand or the left hand. Potentially, any of the three coronary arteries can arise from either of the

facing sinuses. Usually the anterior descending and circumflex coronary arteries arise by a common stem from the right-hand facing sinus while the right coronary artery takes origin from the left-hand facing sinus. This pattern occurs in perhaps two-thirds of all examples of complete transposition.[5–8] The second commonest pattern is for the right and circumflex coronary arteries to originate from the left-hand sinus, the circumflex artery then running a retropulmonary course

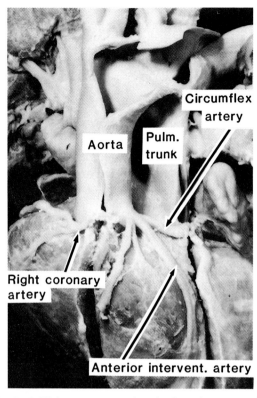

Fig. 20.5 All the coronary arteries arise from the same aortic sinus in this heart with complete transposition.

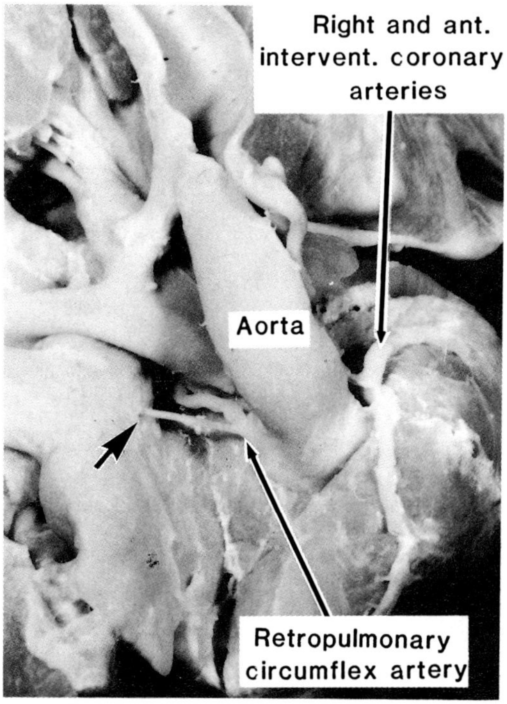

Fig. 20.6 The left circumflex coronary artery, arising from the left-hand facing sinus in this heart with complete transposition, passes through the transverse sinus to reach the left atrioventricular groove. Note the origin of the artery to the sinus node (arrowed).

through the transverse sinus, while the anterior interventricular artery takes origin in isolation from the right-hand sinus. Any combination is possible. On occasion, all three coronary arteries arise from the same sinus, by one or more orifices (Fig. 20.5). The major variability in course relative to the arterial pedicles occurs when one of the arteries, usually the circumflex, extends through the inner curvature of the heart (Fig. 20.6). The right coronary, if arising from the right-hand sinus, may also cross anteriorly relative to the subaortic infundibulum. The artery to the sinus node, in most cases, arises from the proximal segments of either the right coronary artery or the circumflex artery or, rarely, takes a direct origin from a facing aortic sinus. A significant variation is seen in, perhaps, 10% of cases when the artery crosses the lateral wall of the right atrial appendage (Fig. 20.7) or the dome of the left atrium. More usually, the artery ascends

through the interatrial groove; taking this course it may burrow deeply through the atrial wall as it ascends towards the sinus node.

The course and disposition of the conduction tissues are virtually normal in hearts with complete transposition. Thus, the sinus node lies in the terminal groove, usually lateral to the crest of the atrial appendage; occasionally it is draped across the crest in horseshoe fashion. The sinus impulse is distributed through the plain working myocardium of the atrial walls to reach the atrioventricular junction. The preferential route of conduction through these walls is determined by their geometry and by the anisotropic orientation of the muscle fibres within the walls. As discussed elsewhere (see Ch. 1), there are no insulated or 'specialized' tracts of conduction tissues running through the atrial walls. The atrioventricular specialized junctional area, as in the normal heart, is contained exclusively within

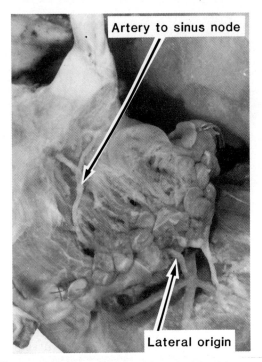

Fig. 20.7 This dissection shows a lateral origin of the artery to the sinus node from the right coronary artery in a heart with complete transposition.

the triangle of Koch (see Ch. 1). The conduction axis penetrates the atrioventricular septum to reach the subpulmonary outflow tract. The bundle branches are then related to the ventricular septum as in the normal heart, with the right bundle branch surfacing on the posterior limb of the septomarginal trabeculation, usually in relation to the medial papillary muscle.

ASSOCIATED MALFORMATIONS

The preceding account of complete transposition has been concerned exclusively with the consequences of the discordant ventriculo–arterial connexions. When there are no associated lesions to complicate the anomaly the arrangement is often described as 'simple' complete transposition. Many would include within the 'simple' grouping cases having lesions such as an atrial septal defect within the oval fossa or patency of the arterial duct. Other lesions, however, would be considered sufficiently major to make the entity 'complex'. These include particularly a ventricular septal defect or obstruction at some level within the left ventricular outflow tract, but other malformations may also occur and should be borne in mind.

Ventricular septal defect

An interventricular communication may exist at

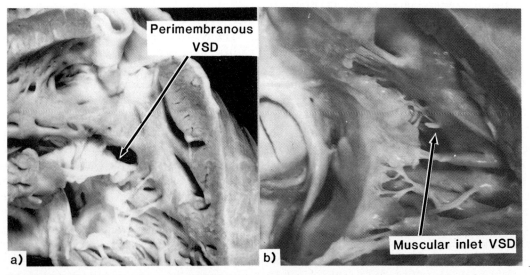

Fig. 20.8 a,b These hearts with complete transposition have (a) a perimembranous and (b) a muscular inlet ventricular septal defect.

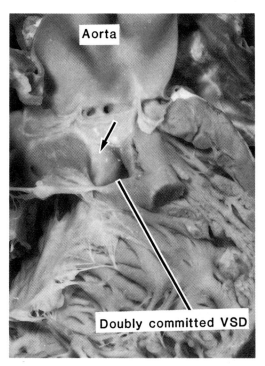

Fig. 20.9 The ventricular septal defect in this heart with complete transposition and a posterior aorta is doubly committed and juxta-arterial. Note that its roof (short arrow) is formed by fibrous continuity between the aortic, mitral and pulmonary valves.

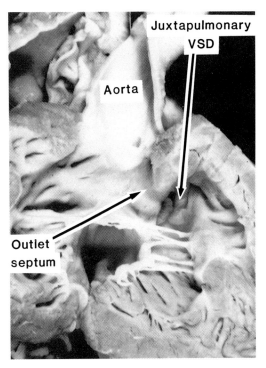

Fig. 20.10 This heart with complete transposition, viewed from the right ventricle, has a juxtapulmonary ventricular septal defect, the outlet septum being malaligned relative to the rest of the ventricular septum.

any of the sites expected for hearts with concordant ventriculo–arterial connexions (see Ch. 8), remembering that the anatomy is subtly altered when the pulmonary trunk instead of the aorta is connected to the morphologically left ventricle. Thus, the defect may be perimembranous (Fig. 20.8a) or it may have exclusively muscular borders (Fig. 20.8b). Defects may also extend to be bordered by the fibrous continuity between the arterial valves (Fig. 20.9). Such doubly committed and juxta-arterial defects are rare but are seen in two specific circumstances when the muscular outlet septum is completely absent. The first is when the aorta is posteriorly located and to the right of the pulmonary trunk (so-called 'normal relations') although connected to the morphologically right ventricle. The other situation is when the aorta is anteriorly located but is to the left of the pulmonary trunk.[9]

Perimembranous or muscular defects may extend so as to open to the inlet or apical trabec-

ular parts of the right ventricle. Alternatively both may open centrally into the ventricle immediately beneath the ventriculo-infundibular fold. Perhaps the most characteristic type of defect is the one which opens to the outlet of the right ventricle in association with malalignment of the outlet septum and overriding of the pulmonary trunk (Fig. 20.10). Depending on the extent of overriding of the pulmonary trunk, there is a spectrum between the extremes of discordant ventriculo–arterial connexions and double outlet right ventricle, the Taussig–Bing heart. An important part of the complex is deviation of the outlet septum: this tends to compromise the subaortic outflow tract with the consequence that coarctation or interruption of the aortic arch is a frequent finding while straddling and overriding of the mitral valve is by no means uncommon.[10] In the presence of a ventricular septal defect, the outlet septum may also be malaligned within the left ventricle. This variation may also occur with

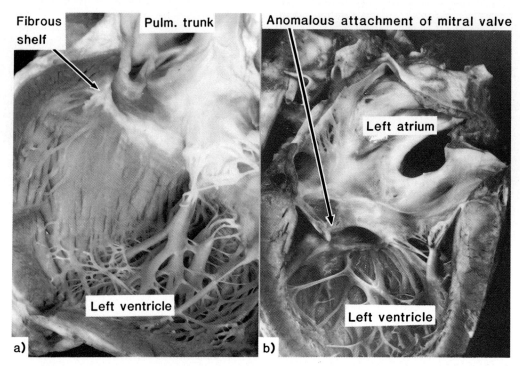

Fig. 20.11 a,b Both these hearts with complete transposition have subpulmonary obstruction, produced (**a**) by a fibrous shelf and (**b**) by anomalous attachment of the mitral valve in association with a fibrous shelf.

muscular or perimembranous defects, resulting in significant subpulmonary stenosis (see below). The rules for the disposition of the conduction tissues in the presence of a ventricular septal defect are as for hearts with concordant atrioventricular and ventriculo–arterial connexions (see Ch. 8).

Obstruction of the left ventricular outflow tract

Any of the lesions which, in the normally constructed heart, produce subaortic obstruction can produce subpulmonary obstruction in complete transposition. Thus, the obstruction can be found at supravalvar, valvar or subvalvar levels, the last being the most significant. The subvalvar obstruction may be muscular when due to hypertrophy of the ventricular septum or it may be a dynamic event due to bulging of the septum. Overt subvalvar obstruction in the setting of an intact ventricular septum may be produced by a fibrous shelf (Fig. 20.11a), by anomalous tissue

tags or by an anomalously attached tension apparatus of the mitral valve (Fig. 20.11b). Subpulmonary obstruction in the presence of a septal defect is usually due to posterior malalignment of the outlet septum (Fig. 20.12).

Other associated lesions

Any congenital lesion may be found in the heart with complete transposition but some are especially associated with this segmental combination. Coarctation is particularly important and is usually found with a restrictive subaortic outflow from the right ventricle. Straddling and overriding of either the mitral or tricuspid valves may be found. Atrioventricular septal defects are exceedingly rare and, if seen, they should arouse the suspicion of atrial isomerism, as should the finding of anomalous pulmonary or systemic venous connexions. Any of these lesions rarely may be found in hearts with otherwise 'simple' complete transposition. Another important associated lesion is juxtaposition of the atrial

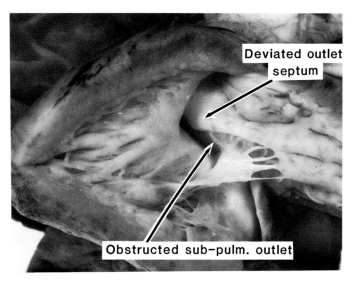

Fig. 20.12 This heart with complete transposition has subpulmonary obstruction due to posterior deviation of the outlet septum.

appendages. Complete transposition may occur with an abnormally located heart or with a right-sided aortic arch but perhaps the most significant malposition is when the segmental combination is in its complete mirror-image format (so called 'situs inversus').

Other morphological variations in complete transposition

Thus far, attention has been directed to the segmental morphology and the associated lesions. Major variations may also be found in terms of arterial relationships and infundibular morphology which distort the basic anatomy of complete transposition without altering the segmental arrangement. In the majority of affected hearts the aorta is located anteriorly and to the right of the pulmonary trunk but in a significant number it may be directly anterior to the pulmonary trunk, or anterior and to the left of the latter, or side-by-side with it. The left-sided aorta is the rule when complete transposition is found in its mirror-image format but it is seen also with some frequency when there is usual atrial arrangement.[11] Side-by-side arteries are found most frequently in association with a ventricular septal defect and are indicators of abnormal coronary arterial patterns. Perhaps the rarest arterial relationship, although of major diagnostic importance, is when the aorta is posterior and to the right of the pulmonary trunk (so-called 'normal relations'). Infundibular morphology may also vary. Usually there is a complete subaortic infundibulum and valvar continuity between the leaflets of the pulmonary and mitral valves. The discordant ventriculo–arterial connexions, however, are not disturbed by the rare finding of a bilateral infundibulum nor even when there is aortic–mitral fibrous continuity through the roof of a doubly committed and juxta-arterial ventricular septal defect (Fig. 20.9).

REFERENCES

1. Van Praagh R. Transposition of the great arteries. II. Transposition clarified. Am J Cardiol 1971; 28: 739–741.
2. Van Mierop LHS. Transposition of the great arteries. Clarification or further confusion? Editorial. Am J Cardiol 1971; 28: 735–738.
3. Becker AE, Anderson RH. How should we describe hearts in which the aorta is connected to the right ventricle and the pulmonary trunk to the left ventricle? A matter for reason and logic. Am J Cardiol 1983; 51: 911–912.

4. Tynan MJ, Anderson RH.Terminology of transposition of the great arteries. In: Godman MJ, Marquis RM, eds. Paediatric cardiology, vol. 2. Disease in the newborn. Edinburgh: Churchill Livingstone, 1979; 341–349.
5. Rowlatt UF. Coronary artery distribution in complete transposition. JAMA 1962; 179: 269–278.
6. Elliott LP, Neufeld HN, Anderson RC, Adams P, Edwards JE. Complete transposition of the great vessels. I. An anatomic study of sixty cases. Circulation 1963; 27: 1105–1117.
7. Shaher RM, Puddu GC. Coronary arterial anatomy in complete transposition of the great arteries. Am J Cardiol 1966; 17: 355–361.
8. Smith A, Arnold R, Wilkinson JL, Hamilton DI, McKay R, Anderson RH. An anatomical study of the patterns of the coronary arteries and sinus nodal artery in complete transposition. Int J Cardiol 1986; 12: 295–304.
9. Lincoln C, Hasse J, Anderson RH, Shinebourne E. Surgical correction in complete levotransposition of the great arteries with an unusual subaortic ventricular septal defect. Am J Cardiol 1976; 38: 344–351.
10. Kitamura N, Takao A, Ando M, Imai Y, Konno S. Taussig–Bing heart with mitral valve straddling: case reports and post-mortem study. Circulation 1974; 49: 761–767.
11. Carr I, Tynan MJ, Aberdeen E, Bonham-Carter RE, Graham G, Waterston DJ. Predictive accuracy of the loop rule in 109 children with classical complete transposition of the great arteries. (Abstract.) Circulation 1968; 38: VI: 52.

Double outlet ventricle

INTRODUCTION

Our approach to hearts with a double outlet ventricle is simple and straightforward. We consider the lesion to represent what the phrase suggests—a ventriculo–arterial connexion.[1] We describe double outlet ventricle, therefore, whenever more than half of both arterial valves is connected to the same ventricle, whether the latter be of right, left or indeterminate morphology. In this chapter, we will describe the specific variations which are to be found with a double outlet from the morphologically right or left ventricle. Double outlet indeterminate ventricle, because of the solitary ventricular chamber, was described briefly in Chapter 18. Some, who have a more traditional approach to cardiac morphology, would disagree with the definition given above on the grounds that double outlet right ventricle has been defined in the past in terms of a bilateral infundibulum ('aortic–mitral discontinuity'[2,3]). To us, it makes little sense to define one feature of the heart (the ventriculo–arterial connexion) in terms of another (the infundibular morphology). Indeed, how should the heart in which both great arteries arise exclusively from the morphologically right ventricle in the absense of a bilateral infundibulum sensibly be described except as double outlet right ventricle?

DOUBLE OUTLET RIGHT VENTRICLE

Self-evidently, our chosen definition of a double outlet connexion takes account of the morphology in only a very small part of the heart, namely the ventriculo–arterial junction. There are also formidable and numerous abnormalities of atrial arrangement and atrioventricular connexions, any of which can be associated with the abnormal ventriculo–arterial connexion. When present, these anomalies, such as atrial isomerism or discordant or double inlet atrioventricular connexions, dominate the picture and are described in the appropriate chapters. In this chapter, we are concerned with only the largest subset of double outlet right ventricle, that with usual atrial arrangement and concordant atrioventricular connexions. There are many anatomical variants within this subset: the most important variable feature is the location of the ventricular septal defect.[4]

With an intact ventricular septum

Very rarely, double outlet right ventricle is found in the presence of an intact ventricular septum (Fig. 21.1). Almost always, in such circumstances the features suggest intra-uterine or postnatal closure of a pre-existing ventricular septal defect.[5, 6]

With a subaortic ventricular septal defect

In the commonest group of hearts with double outlet right ventricle the septal defect, which is the primary outlet from the left ventricle (Fig. 21.2), is located beneath the outflow tract supporting the aortic valve (Fig. 21.3). The septal defect is always (in our experience) positioned between the limbs of the septomarginal trabeculation ('septal band'), this prominent muscular structure reinforcing the right ventricular aspect of the ventricular septum. In this setting, the leaflets of the aortic valve often override the crest of the ventricular septum and there can be doubt about which ventricle the aorta is most connected to, particularly when the morphology of the tetralogy of Fallot is also present (see Ch. 12). Our solution to this dilemma is to quantitate the degree of override by constructing, in the ventricular short axis, the arc of the circle of the aortic circumference subtended by the ventricular septum (Fig. 21.4). If this geometrical construction shows that the aortic valve is mostly connected to the

right ventricle, we diagnose the ventriculo–arterial connexion as double outlet, irrespective of the presence or absence of the morphology of the subpulmonary outflow tract indicative of the tetralogy of Fallot. It should be noted in this respect that we do not use the inclination of the ventricular septum when trying to determine the degree of aortic override (Fig. 21.4). As indicated, overriding is seen most frequently in association with the tetralogy of Fallot; in these circumstances, there is almost always fibrous continuity between the aortic and mitral valves and often with the tricuspid valve. In the more 'classic' variant, with a subaortic defect, there is usually a complete subaortic muscular defect: this pattern is usually found with both arterial valves exclusively connected to the right ventricle (Fig. 21.3). Then, although there is discontinuity between the aortic valve and both atrioventricular valves, it is still the rule to find fibrous continuity between the mitral and tricuspid valves—that is, for the septal defect to be perimembranous. This feature is of surgical importance, since it indicates that the atrioventricular conduction axis, being closely related to the margin of the interventricular communication in its postero-inferior rim, is in danger of being interrupted at operation. Only rarely with a subaortic interventricular communication is there discontinuity between the mitral and tricuspid valves.

Irrespective of the infundibular morphology, the interventricular communication in double outlet right ventricle is the only direct outlet from the left ventricle. Therefore, stenosis of the interventricular communication (Fig. 21.5) effectively produces subaortic obstruction although there is, of course, free access to the aortic outflow tract from the right ventricle. In the majority of cases, however, the subaortic outflow tract is widely patent from both ventricles, and the outlet septum, exclusively a right ventricular structure (Fig. 21.3), is deviated in anterocephalad direction to produce subpulmonary obstruction. This associated malformation can exist either in the setting of a bilateral infundibulum, with the aorta exclusively connected to the right ventricle, or with aortic overriding and aortic–mitral–tricuspid continuity. The latter, of course, is the morphology of the tetralogy of Fallot which, as

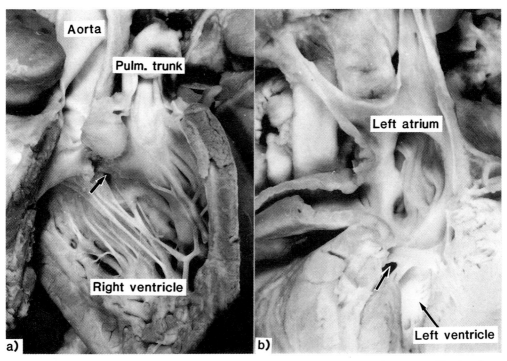

Fig. 21.1 a,b This heart with double outlet right ventricle (**a**) has an intact ventricular septum. The site of a septal defect initially present but subsequently spontaneously closed (arrowed) is seen from both the right (**a**) and left (**b**) ventricles.

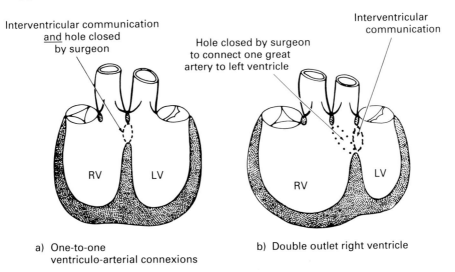

Fig. 21.2 a,b Diagram illustrating the functional nature of the interventricular communication in hearts with (**a**) one-to-one ventriculo–arterial connexions and (**b**) double outlet right ventricle.

we have described (see Ch. 12), can be found with concordant or double outlet ventriculo–arterial connexions.

Almost always the arterial trunks are found in spiral orientation ('normal relations') when the interventricular communication is subaortic, or

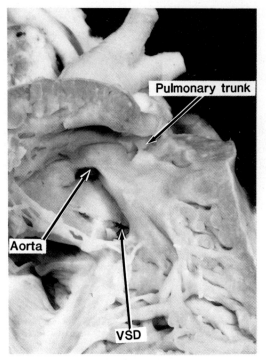

Fig. 21.3 This heart, seen from the apex of the right ventricle, has a double outlet right ventricle with a subaortic ventricular septal defect and a completely muscular subaortic infundibulum.

side-by-side with the aorta to the right. In one rare variant, however, the aorta can be anterior and to the left of the pulmonary trunk (with usual atrial arrangement and concordant atrioventricular connexions).[7,8] Although the ventricular septal defect is almost always in subaortic position with this rare pattern, making it possible in most cases for the surgeon to connect the aorta directly to the left ventricle, the septal defect can rarely occupy the locations to be described below when the aorta is left-sided.

With subpulmonary ventricular septal defect

The second most frequent pattern of double outlet right ventricle is for the arterial trunks to be parallel, with the aorta to the right and slightly or markedly anterior (Fig. 21.6). With this arrangement, the ventricular septal defect is between the limbs of the septomarginal trabeculation (Fig. 21.6) but in subpulmonary rather than subaortic location (compare Figs 21.3 and 21.6). It is the orientation of the outlet septum, exclu-

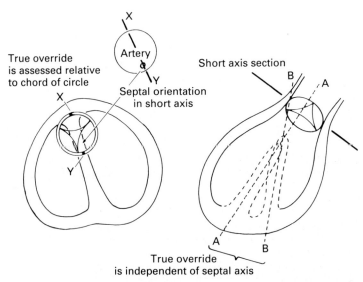

Fig. 21.4 In the presence of overriding arterial valves, the commitment of the valve to the ventricles is made according to the relation of the chord of its circle (X – Y) subtended relative to the ventricular septum in short axis. The relation of the plane of the septum in long axis (A – B) is not a good criterion.

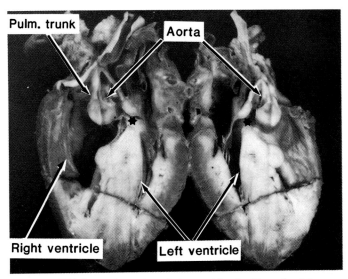

Fig. 21.5 This long axis section of a heart with a double outlet right ventricle and a subaortic ventricular septal defect shows how obstruction of the defect results in subaortic stenosis. The asterisk is on the outlet septum.

sively a right ventricular structure, which is the key feature, and the resulting lesion is usually

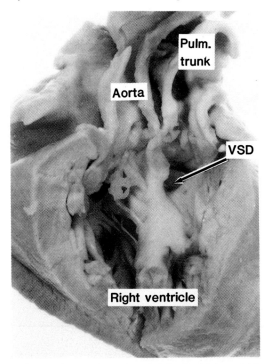

Fig. 21.6 The ventricular septal defect in this heart with double outlet right ventricle is in subpulmonary position. There is a completely muscular subpulmonary infundibulum.

described as the Taussig–Bing heart. There is argument, however, as to whether the original Taussig–Bing heart exhibited a double outlet[9] or discordant ventriculo–arterial connexions.[10] In reality, such hearts exhibit a spectrum of malformation determined by the precise connexion of the overriding pulmonary valve. Our preference is to refer to the entire spectrum as the Taussig–Bing anomaly. Then, as with the tetralogy of Fallot, we describe either a double outlet or one-to-one ventriculo–arterial connexions depending on the degree of override.[11] The original Taussig–Bing heart possessed a bilateral infundibulum but we would make the diagnosis of a double outlet with a subpulmonary defect irrespective of the presence or absence of pulmonary to mitral fibrous continuity (Fig. 21.7). In most cases, nonetheless, there is mitral to tricuspid discontinuity so that the defect has a muscular postero-inferior rim. Rightward deviation of the outlet septum producing subaortic obstruction is also frequent, as is concomitant aortic coarctation. Straddling and overriding of the mitral valve is the other malformation frequently associated with this pattern of double outlet right ventricle.[12]

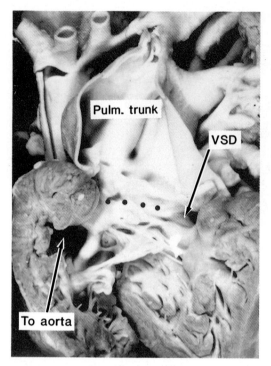

Fig. 21.7 This heart, again with unequivocal double outlet and a subpulmonary ventricular septal defect, has fibrous continuity between the leaflets of the pulmonary and mitral valves (dotted line).

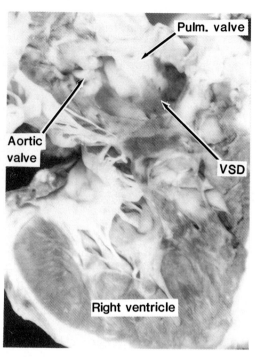

Fig. 21.8 The ventricular septal defect in this case has a muscular postero-inferior rim but the outlet septum is lacking, fibrous continuity being present between the leaflets of the aortic and pulmonary valves.

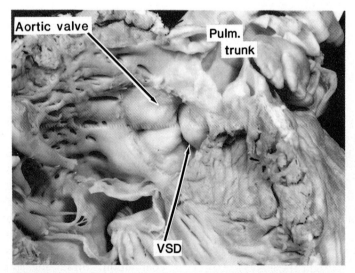

Fig. 21.9 In this heart with an overriding aortic valve connected mostly to the right ventricle, the pulmonary valve is hypoplastic and stenotic. There is again fibrous continuity between the leaflets of the aortic and pulmonary valves.

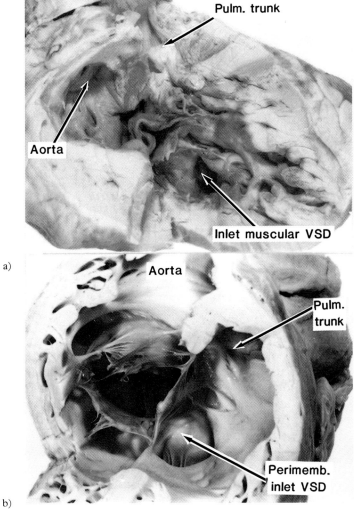

Fig. 21.10 a,b In both of these hearts with double outlet right ventricle, the ventricular septal defect is non-committed. There is a muscular inlet defect in the upper panel (**a**) and a perimembranous defect opening to the inlet of the right ventricle in the lower (**b**).

With doubly committed juxta-arterial ventricular septal defect

The major feature of this variant is complete absence of the muscular outlet septum so that there is fibrous continuity between the facing leaflets of the aortic and pulmonary valves. The large interventricular communication is then located immediately beneath both arterial valves, which have a marked tendency to override (Fig. 21.8). Some would term this lesion 'double

outlet both ventricles',[13] an acceptable descriptive term but lacking precision. Our preference is to assign the overriding valves to one or other ventricle, only diagnosing a double outlet connexion when the greater part of each valve is committed to one ventricle, be it morphologically right or left.[14] The defect can be perimembranous (mitral–tricuspid continuity) or have a muscular postero-inferior rim. Often the raphe between aortic and pulmonary valves is deviated in antero-cephalad direction to produce pulmonary stenosis

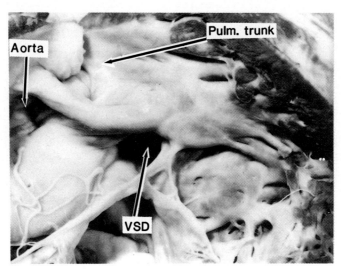

Fig. 21.11 In this heart with double outlet right ventricle and a long subaortic infundibulum, it is arguable whether the defect is subaortic or non-committed.

with overriding of the aortic valve (Fig. 21.9). Some would diagnose this as a variant of the tetralogy of Fallot but we prefer to describe the defect as being doubly committed and juxta-arterial and then to give an account of the ventriculo–arterial connexion.[15]

With non-committed ventricular septal defect

Pathologists working in centres where excellent results are achieved with corrective surgery are now more likely to see, and be called upon to recognize, the more complex and lethal variants of each particular malformation. With regard to double outlet right ventricle, these will be the examples with a non-committed ventricular septal defect. Rarely, the defect may be non-committed because it is within the inlet or apical trabecular components of the muscular septum (Fig. 21.10a). These variants are likely to defeat all but the most heroic attempts at surgical correction. More often the defect is non-committed because it is perimembranous and opens into the right ventricle beneath the septal leaflet of the tricuspid valve   (Fig. 21.10b), or because the tension apparatus of the atrioventricular valves interposes between the margins of the defect and

the subarterial outflow tracts. To this extent, there is a conflict between the anatomical and functional definitions of a non-committed defect. What is anatomically a committed defect may be rendered non-committed functionally because of the interposition of vital structures, usually a valvar tension apparatus, between the defect and the arterial valves. The pathologist must take account of all these features, and must also use his judgement, on occasions arbitrarily, to decide when a defect is non-committed or subarterial (Fig. 21.11).

DOUBLE OUTLET LEFT VENTRICLE

This is a much rarer form of ventriculo–arterial connexion and, as with double outlet from the right ventricle, it can be found with any atrial arrangement and any atrioventricular connexion.[16] Again, as with double outlet right ventricle, when it is found with abnormal atrioventricular connexions, such as double inlet or discordant connexions, it will be the arrangement at the atrioventricular junction which will determine the clinical and pathological picture. When found with usual atrial arrangement and concordant atrioventricular connexions, most

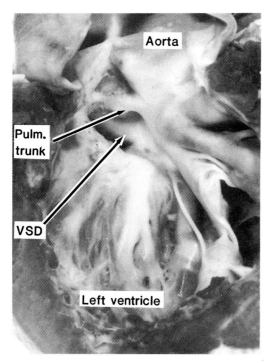

Fig. 21.12 In this heart, seen from the left ventricle, both great arteries are connected exclusively to the left ventricle. The subpulmonary outflow tract is stenotic.

cases have a doubly committed and juxta-arterial defect (Fig. 21.12). There is complete absence of the outlet septum, presumably permitting both arterial valves to ride posteriorly into the left ventricle so that the major part of the circumference of each valve is supported by left ventricular structures.[17] As stated above, these are the hearts which some would call 'double outlet both ventricles'[13] but our preference is to reach a decision as to whether the valves are connected mostly to right or to left ventricular structures. Usually there is fibrous continuity between both arterial valves and both atrioventricular valves (bilaterally deficient infundibulum) but this is by no means a constant finding. Indeed, when large numbers of cases are analysed,[16,17] just as much variation is seen in terms of arterial relationships, infundibular morphology, and morphology and location of the interventricular communication, as has been described for double outlet right ventricle, including cases with an intact ventricular septum.[18] This merely serves to emphasize the anatomical heterogeneity of hearts grouped together on the basis of only one of their anomalous features, in this case a ventriculo–arterial connexion.

REFERENCES

1. Anderson RH, Becker AE, Wilcox BR, Macartney FJ, Wilkinson JL. Surgical anatomy of double-outlet right ventricule—a reappraisal. Am J Cardiol 1983; 52: 555–559.
2. Van Praagh S, Dick M, DeLisle G, Van Praagh R. Ventricule droit à double issue. Constatations necropsiques sur 45 cas et applications diagnostiques et chirurgicales. [Double outlet right ventricle. Necropsy findings in 45 cases and diagnostic and surgical applications.] Coeur 1973; 319–321.
3. Baron MG. Radiologic notes in cardiology: angiographic differentiation between tetralogy of Fallot and double outlet right ventricle. Circulation 1971; 43: 451–455.
4. Lev M, Bharati S, Meng CCL, Liberthson RR, Paul MH, Idriss F. A concept of double-outlet right ventricle. J Thorac Cardiovasc Surg 1972; 64: 271–281.
5. Ainger LE. Double outlet right ventricle: intact ventricular septum and blind left ventricle. Am Heart J 1965; 70: 521–525.
6. MacMahon HE, Lipa M. Double outlet right ventricle with intact ventricular septum. Circulation 1964; 30: 745–748.
7. Van Praagh R, Perez-Trevino C, Reynolds JL et al.

Double outlet right ventricle [S,D,L] with subaortic ventricular septal defect and pulmonary stenosis. Report of six cases. Am J Cardiol 1975; 35: 42–53.
8. Lincoln C, Anderson RH, Shinebourne EA, English TAH, Wilkinson JL. Double outlet right ventricle with l-malposition of the aorta. Br Heart J 1975; 37: 453–463.
9. Van Praagh R. What is the Taussig–Bing malformation? Circulation 1968; 38: 445–449.
10. Hinkes P, Rosenquist GC, White RI Jr. Roentgenographic re-examination of the internal anatomy of the Taussig–Bing heart. Am Heart J 1971; 81: 335–339.
11. Stellin G, Zuberbuhler JR. Anderson RH, Siewers RD. The surgical anatomy of the Taussig–Bing malformation. J Thorac Cardiovasc Surg 1987; 93: 560–569.
12. Kitamura N, Takao A, Ando M, Imai Y, Konno S. Taussig–Bing heart with mitral valve straddling: case reports and post-mortem study. Circulation 1974; 49: 761–767.
13. Brandt PWT, Calder AL, Barratt-Boyes BG, Neutze JM. Double outlet left ventricle. Morphology, cineangiography, diagnosis and surgical treatment. Am J Cardiol 1976; 38: 897–909.

14. Ueda M, Becker AE. Classification of hearts with overriding aortic and pulmonary valves. Int J Cardiol 1985; 9: 353–360.

15. Griffin ML, Sullivan ID, Anderson RH, Macartney FJ. Doubly committed subarterial ventricular septal defect: new morphological criteria with echocardiographic and angiocardiographic correlation. Br Heart J 1988; 59: 474–479.

16. Anderson RH, Shinebourne EA. The anatomy of congenital heart disease. In: Weatherall DJ, Ledingham JGG, Warrell DA, eds. Oxford textbook of medicine, 2nd ed. Oxford: Oxford University Press, 1987; 2: 13.233–13.246.

17. Otero Coto E, Quero Jimenez M, Castaneda AR, Rufilanchas JJ, Deverall PB. Double outlet from chambers of left ventricular morphology. Br Heart J 1979; 42: 15–21.

18. Paul MH, Sinha SN, Muster AJ, Cole RB, Van Praagh R. Double outlet left ventricle. Report of an autopsy with an intact ventricular septum and consideration of its developmental implications. Circulation 1970; 41: 129–135.

Common arterial trunk and single outlet of the heart

INTRODUCTION

The term 'single outlet' describes the ventriculo–arterial connexion (see Ch. 4) in which only one arterial trunk can, with certainty, be traced to become continuous with the ventricular mass. This definition encompasses four discrete arrangements (Fig. 22.1). By far the most frequent is when the arterial trunk is a common one, supplying directly the systemic and coronary arteries and at least one pulmonary artery, the arterial orifice being guarded by a common valve. In two of the remaining arrangements there are two arterial trunks but one is atretic, and the atretic vessel cannot be traced with certainty to its ventricular origin. Thus, there may be a solitary aortic trunk connected to the ventricular mass with pulmonary atresia, or a solitary pulmonary trunk with aortic atresia. These two categories are rarely diagnosed by the pathologist since, when a thread-like atretic trunk is observed, it is almost always possible to trace its ventricular origin (Fig. 22.2). They are more likely to be employed in a clinical context since, often, the techniques of investigation are insufficiently precise to delineate the origin of thread-like trunks. These two arrangements will not be discussed further in this chapter. A fourth category occurs when there is complete absence of the intrapericardial pulmonary arteries or when the pulmonary arteries themselves are confluent but there is no evidence of the pulmonary trunk. In this setting it is not possible to tell what the origin of the pulmonary trunk would have been had it existed. Theoretically, the trunk that is present could have been either an aorta or a common trunk (Fig. 22.3). Since there is no way of resolving this conundrum, the solution is to describe a solitary arterial trunk.[1] In this chapter, therefore, we are concerned with the description of hearts having either a common or a solitary arterial trunk.

COMMON ARTERIAL TRUNK

When a given structure is described as a common trunk, it follows that the trunk must supply directly the coronary, systemic and pulmonary arterial systems and must be guarded by a common arterial valve.[2] Such vessels are often described in embryological terms as 'persistent truncus arteriosus'; however, such terms can give rise to problems in definition and our preference, therefore, is for the more descriptive term 'common arterial trunk'. Hearts having a common arterial trunk can vary in several significant ways. They may exist with any atrial arrangement, but almost always they are found with the usual arrangement. Similarly, they may

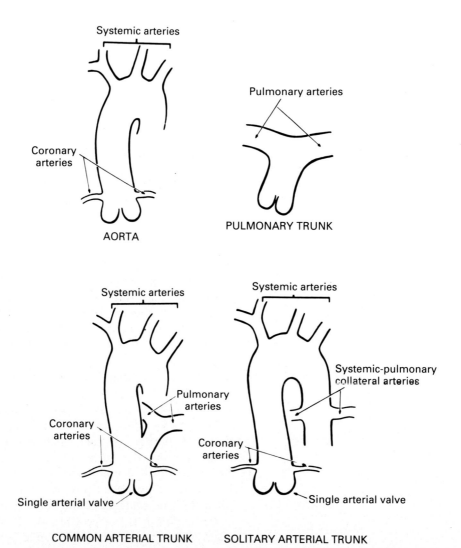

Systemic arteries

Coronary arteries

AORTA

Pulmonary arteries

PULMONARY TRUNK

Systemic arteries

Coronary arteries

Pulmonary arteries

Single arterial valve

Systemic arteries

Systemic-pulmonary collateral arteries

Coronary arteries

Single arterial valve

COMMON ARTERIAL TRUNK   SOLITARY ARTERIAL TRUNK

Fig. 22.1 The types of arterial trunk designated according to their pattern of branching. Only one (bottom, left) is a common trunk.

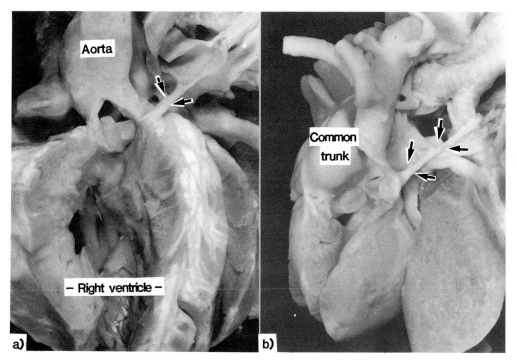

Fig. 22.2 a,b These dissections show two hearts in which, clinically, it may seem that there is a solitary trunk, since it may not prove possible in life to identify the thread-like pulmonary trunk (arrows). The pathologist, however, can show that in (**a**) the trunk is connected to the ventricle, so that, potentially, there is a concordant ventriculo–arterial connexion. In (**b**), in contrast, the atretic pulmonary vessel is connected to the arterial trunk, indicating that this vessel was, originally, a common trunk.

be found with any atrioventricular connexion but cases with other than concordant connexions at atrioventricular level are exceedingly rare. Thus, the significant variations in hearts with a common trunk are found with respect to the ventricular

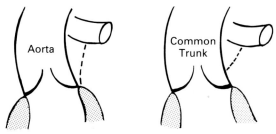

Fig. 22.3 The reason that we use the term 'solitary' trunk is that, when the intrapericardial arteries are totally lacking, there is no way of knowing whether, had they been present, they would have connected to the heart, making the patent trunk an aorta (left-hand diagram), or to the trunk itself, making it a common vessel (right-hand diagram). As shown in Fig. 22.2, these possibilities are not hypothetical.

origin of the trunk, the nature of the juxtatruncal ventricular septal defect, the morphology of the common truncal valve, the anatomy of the pulmonary arterial pathways, and the arrangement of the aortic arch and its branches. These variations are considered in the following paragraphs.

Ventricular origin of the trunk

Almost always the common trunk overrides the septum so as to be connected, more or less equally, to both right and left ventricles (Fig. 22.4). In our experience of such cases, fibrous continuity between the leaflets of the truncal valve and the mitral valve is invariably present. In a minority of cases, the trunk may be exclusively connected either to the right or to the left ventricle. When the trunk arises exclusively from the right ventricle, its valve may be supported by a complete muscular infundibulum.

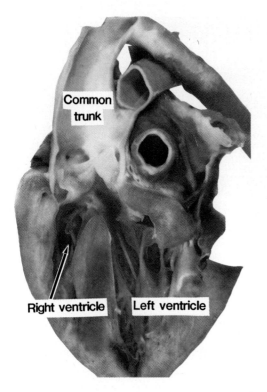

Fig. 22.4 This oblique section shows the overriding origin of a common arterial trunk.

The ventricular septal defect, the only outlet from the left ventricle in this circumstance, may then be restrictive (Fig. 22.5).

The morphology of the ventricular septal defect

The ventricular septal defect is typically in immediately juxtatruncal position although additional septal defects may be found elsewhere within the muscular ventricular septum.

Sometimes the leaflets of the truncal valve abut directly on the crest of the ventricular septum during diastole (Fig. 22.6), a pattern which some have suggested represents absence of the septal defect.[3] With this arrangement, the space between the limbs of the septomarginal trabeculation is closed when the leaflets are themselves closed during diastole; in contrast, in most cases, there is a gap between the septal crest and the leaflets throughout the cardiac cycle. Because of this persistent space between the septal crest and the attachments of the overriding truncal valve, even when the leaflets abut the crest, we question the wisdom of describing the septum as intact in this circumstance.

The major variability in the defect is found in the morphology of its postero-inferior corner. Usually, at this site, the posterior limb of the

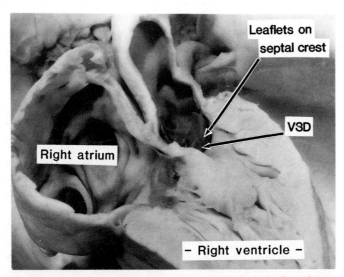

Fig. 22.5 In this heart with a common arterial trunk, the leaflets of the truncal valve coapt on the crest of the ventricular septum. When the leaflets open, they leave a typical juxtatruncal ventricular septal defect.

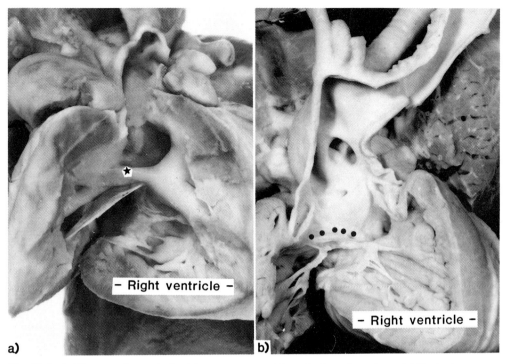

Fig. 22.6 a,b These specimens, both with a common arterial trunk, show the major variability in the morphology of the juxtatruncal ventricular septal defect. It can have (**a**) a muscle bar separating the truncal and tricuspid valves (asterisk) or (**b**) fibrous continuity between these valves (dotted line).

septomarginal trabeculation fuses with the ventriculo-infundibular fold so that there is discontinuity between the attachments of the tricuspid and truncal valves (Fig. 22.6a). In a minority of cases, the leaflets of the tricuspid and truncal valves are in fibrous continuity so that the defect is not only juxtatruncal but also perimembranous (Fig. 22.6b). Some hearts show transitional patterns where the muscular tissue is almost, but not quite, attenuated. The muscle bar is important when surgery is undertaken because, when present, it protects the atrioventricular conduction axis from possible damage.

The truncal valve

In most cases the truncal valve has three leaflets but it may possess two, four or even more leaflets. It has been suggested that a valve with three leaflets is an aortic valve rather than a common truncal valve and that, in reality, 'truncus' is no more than pulmonary atresia with complete absence of the subpulmonary infundibulum.[4] If that were the case, the coronary arteries would be expected to arise from the truncal sinuses facing the anticipated site of the presumptive subpulmonary outlet. In fact, the coronary arteries arise from the common trunk in a pattern most unlike the usual origin of normal coronary arteries from the aorta.[2] Most frequently at least one of the coronary arteries takes a high origin at or above the sinutruncal bar. The anatomy, therefore, does not support the notion that the valve with three leaflets is aortic. Very frequently the truncal valve, irrespective of the number of its leaflets, is grossly dysplastic and stenotic.[5] It may also be incompetent.[6]

The pulmonary arterial pathways

Conventionally, the pattern of the pulmonary arteries has been used to categorize hearts with a common arterial trunk.[7] Four patterns were originally described, one of which is exceedingly rare

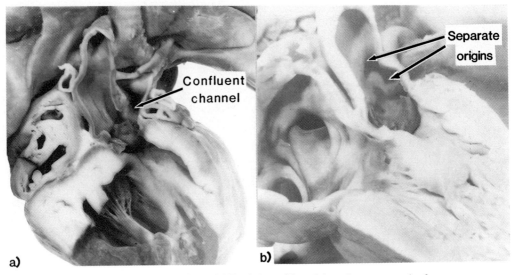

Fig. 22.7 a,b These hearts show the major variability in branching of the pulmonary arteries from a common trunk. There may be a common pulmonary channel (**a**) or separate origins from the trunk (**b**).

(so-called type III) while another (so-called type IV) is not, in fact, an example of a common arterial trunk. Distinction between the other two types is often not clear-cut, while still other patterns are found which cannot be accommodated in the original categorization.[8] It is our preference, therefore, simply to describe the arrangement of the pulmonary arteries as they arise from the common trunk. In a proportion of cases, a common channel arises immediately above the sinuses from the left lateral margin of the trunk. This common channel then divides into the left and right pulmonary arteries (Fig. 22.7a). It is unusual for the channel to be long, and frequently the right and left arteries arise together from the trunk, so that it is difficult to decide with certainty whether they have common or separate origins (Fig. 22.7b). In some cases the origins are clearly separated one from another, but it is rare to find them arising from opposite walls of the common trunk (so-called type III). Occasionally, the origin of the pulmonary arteries, either separately or together, is more from the posterior or rightward aspect of the trunk. Some have likened this to 'transposition with a common trunk',[9] but we cannot support this notion. Very rarely the pulmonary arteries may arise from unusual sites of the arch, such as the case we

encountered with a common origin from the underside of the transverse segment.[8] All the patterns described above have the origin of both pulmonary arteries directly from the common trunk. An important variation is found when the pulmonary arteries are discontinuous and one arises from an alternative site, such as an arterial duct. This arrangement is sometimes called 'hemitruncus', but it must then be distinguished from other cases described in this way in which there is an anomalous origin of the right pulmonary artery from the ascending aorta while the left pulmonary artery takes origin from the pulmonary trunk, the latter vessel being connected to the right ventricle (see Ch. 15). This pattern is not, of course, an example of a common arterial trunk and because of the potential confusion our preference is to avoid the use of the term 'hemitruncus'.

The aortic pathways and the arterial duct

Traditionally, as discussed, hearts with a common arterial trunk have been categorized according to the morphology of the pulmonary arterial pathways.[7] This should not detract attention from important variations in the aortic pathways. The most significant of these lesions is complete inter-

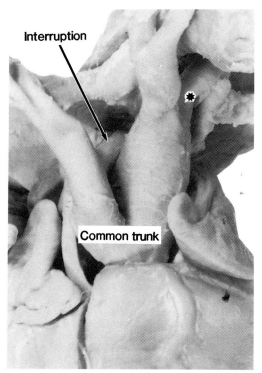

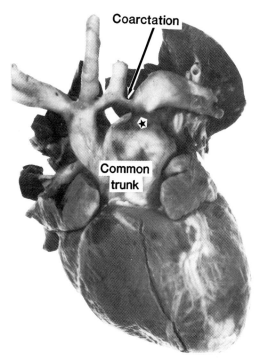

Fig. 22.8 This heart with a common arterial trunk has interruption of the aortic arch between the left common carotid and left subclavian arteries. An arterial duct (asterisk) supplies the distal part of the aorta.

Fig. 22.9 This heart with a common arterial trunk has isthmal hypoplasia, coarctation and patency of the arterial duct (asterisk) to the descending aorta.

ruption of the aortic arch, the proximal aorta arising directly from the common trunk and the distal aorta being fed through persistence of the arterial duct (Fig. 22.8). Interruption can occur at any site (see Ch. 13) but is most frequent either at the isthmus or between the left common carotid and left subclavian arteries. As with any form of interruption, these malformations can be associated with an anomalous retro-oesophageal origin of one subclavian artery, often the left, since a right aortic arch is a frequent finding in hearts with a common arterial trunk.

Although interruption is the most frequent anomaly of the aortic pathways to be associated with a common arterial trunk, others that may be found include isthmic hypoplasia, discrete coarctation and an arterial duct linking the common trunk to the descending aorta (Fig. 22.9). Other than in this circumstance, and in the presence of aortic interruption or discontinuous pulmonary arteries, it is exceedingly rare (if it ever occurs) to find an arterial duct co-existing with a common arterial trunk.

SOLITARY ARTERIAL TRUNK

In rare instances, it is possible to find hearts in which, despite careful dissection, no evidence can be found of any intrapericardial pulmonary arteries (Fig. 22.9). The total pulmonary blood supply in such circumstances is derived either from systemic–pulmonary collateral arteries or through an arterial duct. In clinical terms, such hearts have most features in common with tetralogy of Fallot and pulmonary atresia (see Ch. 12), and the arterial trunk in such a setting is usually presumed to be an aorta.[2] The problem with this concept, however, is that it presumes that, if the pulmonary trunk had been present and thread-like, it would have been connected to the outflow tract of the right ventricle (Fig. 22.3). As reported elsewhere,[1] there is no reason why the atretic pulmonary trunk could not be considered to have arisen from the trunk itself, and we have recently encountered a case which supports this hypothesis.[10] Since it cannot be stated with certainty where the non-existent pulmonary trunk would have originated, it is reasonable to describe this arrangement as a solitary arterial trunk. It is a safe assumption that such solitary trunks exist, with exclusive pulmonary arterial supply from systemic–pulmonary collateral arteries, with bilateral arterial ducts, or with a duct combined with collateral arteries, or with confluent pulmonary arteries in the absence of a thread-like pulmonary trunk.[2]

REFERENCES

1. Thiene G, Anderson RH. Pulmonary atresia with ventricular septal defect. Anatomy. In: Anderson RH, Macartney FJ, Shinebourne EA, Tynan M, eds. Paediatric cardiology, vol. 5. Edinburgh: Churchill Livingstone, 1983; 80–101.
2. Crupi G, Macartney FJ, Anderson RH. Persistent truncus arteriosus. A study of 66 autopsy cases with special reference to definition and morphogenesis. Am J Cardiol 1977; 40: 569–578.
3. Carr I, Bharati S, Kusnoor VS, Lev M. Truncus arteriosus communis with intact ventricular septum. Br Heart J 1979; 42: 97–102.
4. Van Praagh R, Van Praagh S. The anatomy of common aortico-pulmonary trunk (truncus arteriosus communis) and its embryologic implications. Am J Cardiol 1965; 16: 406–426.
5. Becker AE, Becker MJ, Edwards JE. Pathology of the semi-lunar valve in persistent truncus arteriosus. J Thorac Cardiovasc Surg 1971; 62: 16–26.
6. Gerlis LM, Wilson N, Dickinson DF, Scott O. Valvar stenosis in truncus arteriosus. Br Heart J 1984; 52: 440–445.
7. Collett RW, Edwards JE. Persistent truncus arteriosus: a classification according to anatomic types. Surg Clin North Am 1949; 29: 1245.
8. Rubay JE, Macartney FJ, Anderson RH. A rare variant of common arterial trunk. Br Heart J 1987; 57: 202–204.
9. Angelini P, Verdugo AL, Illera JP, Leachman RD. Truncus arteriosus communis. An unusual case associated with transposition. Circulation 1977; 56: 1107.
10. Schofield DE, Anderson RH. Common arterial trunk with pulmonary atresia. Int J Cardiol 1988; 20: 290–294.

Congenital anomalies of the endocardium, myocardium and epicardium and of the conduction tissues and coronary arteries

INTRODUCTION

In this chapter, we will give an account of congenital lesions of the muscular mass of the heart along with its endocardial and epicardial coverings. We will include also some details of congenital malformations of the impulse-producing and conducting system and of the coronary arteries. Although not exhaustive, the account will cover those conditions which, in our opinion, are most likely to be encountered by the pathologist.

THE ENDOCARDIUM

The most frequently encountered congenital lesion of the endocardial lining of the heart is that produced by deposition within it of fibroelastic tissues, a process termed fibroelastosis. The pearly white layer produced in this fashion can also be the result of acquired change and can then affect any of the cardiac chambers. When seen as a congenital lesion, it is usually restricted to the left ventricle and then, when the mitral valve is patent, it is an integral part of the so-called hypoplastic left heart syndrome (see Ch. 10). Although present at birth, the fibroelastosis seen in this combination is almost certainly a secondary rather than a primary lesion. A condition that is referred to as primary prenatal fibroelastosis does exist but is much rarer: it is believed to be a consequence of other conditions, particularly virus-induced myopathy occurring during intrauterine life.[1,2] It has been observed

287

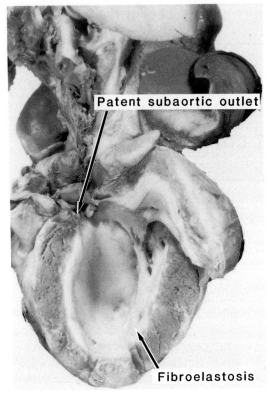

Fig. 23.1 This left ventricle shows the primary contracted form of endocardial fibroelastosis with a patent subaortic outflow tract.

also in siblings,[3,4] although this fact, in itself, offers no direct clue to its pathogenesis. Morphologically, primary fibroelastosis occurs in two discrete forms, the first variant being associated with a hypoplastic left ventricle.[5] Differentiation of this type from the secondary lesions seen in the hypoplastic left heart syndrome is difficult but the fact that some cases have a relatively hypoplastic ventricle, lined with a thick fibroelastotic layer in the absence of significant aortic stenosis (Fig. 23.1), points to the contracted variant of primary fibroelastosis as a distinct entity.[6] The commoner variant is the dilated type in which the cavity of the left ventricle is enlarged and the papillary muscles of the mitral valve seem to take a 'high' origin (Fig. 23.2). A similar picture is seen in congenital dilated cardiomyopathy, suggesting a link between the two. In the cases with a hyperplastic endothelial layer, however, histology fails to reveal any abnormalities within the myocardium.

THE MYOCARDIUM

By the very nature of their deformed anatomy,

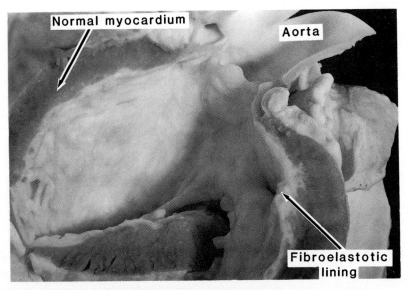

Fig. 23.2 In this heart with primary endocardial fibroelastosis, the left ventricle is dilated, producing a picture similar to that of dilated cardiomyopathy (see Fig. 23.4).

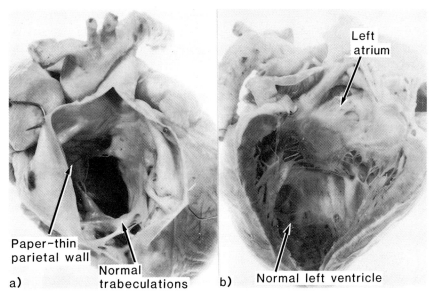

Left
atrium

Paper-thin
parietal wall

a)   Normal
             trabeculations

b)   Normal left ventricle

Fig. 23.3 a,b These illustrations show congenital absence of the myocardium of the parietal wall of the right ventricle (**a**) with a normally formed septum and left ventricle (**b**). This is Uhl's anomaly.

most of the hearts described in previous chapters have congenital lesions of the myocardium. These are not the lesions we are concerned with in this chapter; here we are dealing with those problems produced by congenital malformations of the myocardium itself in an otherwise normally structured heart. A good example is congenital absence of the myocardium of the right ventricle. This is the very rare disease first described by Uhl.[7] The essence of the lesion is that, in an otherwise normal heart, the parietal segments of the right ventricular muscle mass are totally lacking, the endocardium being adherent to the epicardium with the production of a 'parchment' wall (Fig. 23.3). Although many hearts have been placed in Uhl's category subsequent to the original description, relatively few have congenital absence of the myocardium.[8] Most have acquired thinning of the ventricular wall, as occurs, for example, in pulmonary atresia with an intact septum and a congenitally unguarded tricuspid orifice or Ebstein's malformation. Alternatively, the muscle of the ventricular wall is thinned as a consequence of fatty infiltration, a process that is becoming increasingly recognized as an important putative cause of right ventricular dysplasia and, with its attendant arrhythmias, carrying the risk of

sudden death;[9] clearly, this condition is not Uhl's anomaly.

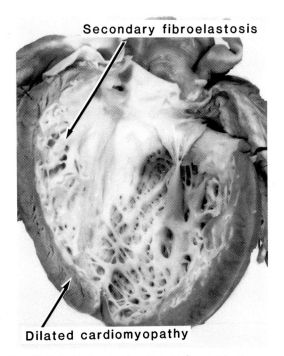

Secondary fibroelastosis

Dilated cardiomyopathy

Fig. 23.4 In this heart with a dilated left ventricle, the problem is myocardial, that is dilated cardiomyopathy, and the fibroelastosis is a secondary phenomenon.

Congenital cardiomyopathy

The most obvious lesions of the myocardium seen by the paediatric pathologist are, perhaps, the cardiomyopathies. It is questionable, however, whether these lesions are truly congenital or are the result of acquired disease during childhood. For example, dilated cardiomyopathy is readily recognized when seen in children (Fig. 23.4), but it is difficult, if not impossible, for the pathologist to determine whether the changes derive from congenital disease. The same uncertainty used to surround idiopathic hypertrophic cardiomyopathy. When encountered as a cause of subaortic stenosis in patients with concordant ventriculo–arterial connexions or of subpulmonary stenosis in those with discordant connexions, its morphology is unmistakable (Fig. 23.5). Again, it remains problematical whether the lesion, or its precursor, has been present from birth or whether the change represents acquired disease. Increasing experience with fetal echocardiography leads to the conclusion that the morphological derangement is present during fetal life and the hearts studied in such cases have all the classic features of hyper-

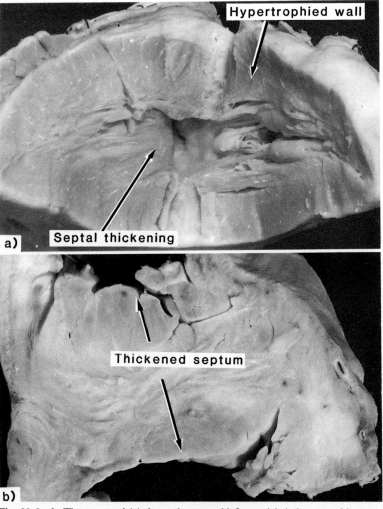

Fig. 23.5 a,b The top panel (**a**) shows the opened left ventricle in hypertrophic cardiomyopathy. The bottom panel (**b**) is a section across the hypertrophied septum, showing the gross evidence of myocardial disarray.

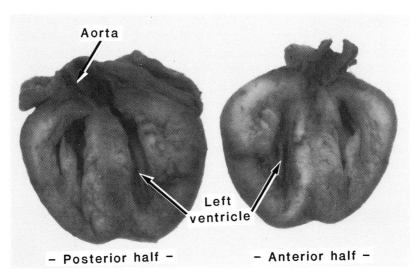

Fig. 23.6 This section across the ventricles of a fetal heart in four chamber plane shows the typical features of hypertrophic cardiomyopathy.

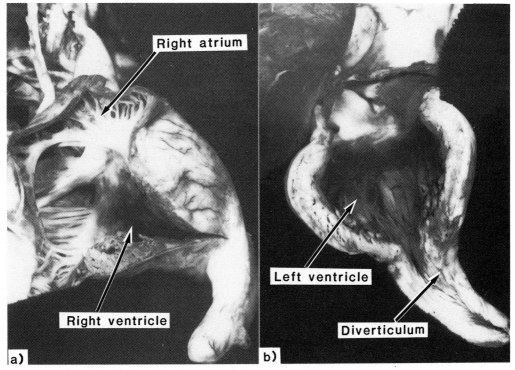

Fig. 23.7 a,b This heart has a ventricular apical diverticulum (**a**), made up predominantly from the left ventricular wall (**b**).

trophic cardiomyopathy (Fig. 23.6). In some cases, then, the lesion is certainly congenital, but in the majority the disease is one of adult life.

The whole subject of the cardiomyopathies is dealt with in greater detail in Part B of this volume.

Congenital diverticulums

Congenital diverticulums of the myocardium are appropriately considered here with other myocardial disorders. Typically, they involve the ventricular apices and are seen most frequently as part of a syndrome of midline dysraphism known as the pentalogy of Cantrell.[10] The extreme form of this abnormality is an extrathoracic heart (ectopia cordis); in less severe forms, the ventricular apices

are herniated through pericardial and sternal deficiencies. Either the right ventricle can be involved, or else the tips of both ventricles are extruded in spout-like fashion (Fig. 23.7). Often there are associated intracardiac defects but the diverticulums can be found as the only cardiac malformation. Other types of diverticulums are found, some involving the fibrous tissues of the ventricular walls.[11] They can also affect the atriums.

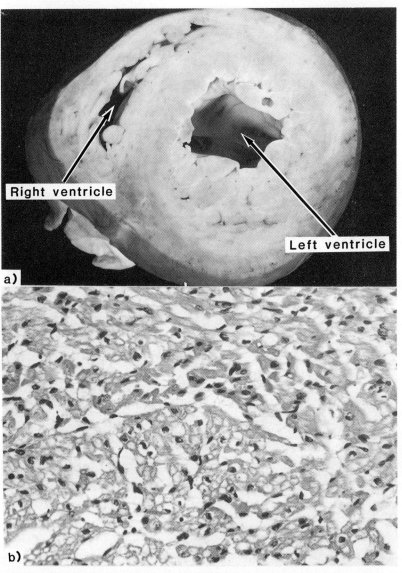

Fig. 23.8 a,b This heart shows thickening of the left ventricular walls (**a**), the cells having a foamy appearance (**b**). This is the so-called histiocytoid change.

Congenital tumours and miscellaneous lesions

Some cardiac tumours are undoubtedly present at birth, particularly rhabdomyomas and teratomas,[12,13] which differ in no way from those seen in adults. They, too, are described in greater detail in Part B of this volume. Here, however, we must comment upon a peculiar type of myocardial lesion which presents because of rhythm problems within the first two years of life. Considered by some to be a cardiomyopathy,[14,15] it has been described under various names, including foamy myocardial transformation of infancy[16] and histiocytoid change.[17] It has been suggested also that the lesion is diffuse, involving the peripheral ramifications of the conduction system (the Purkinje fibres)[18] and clinical evidence increasingly supports this notion. Morphologically, the involved heart is either of normal size or shows hypertrophy of the ventricular walls (Fig. 23.8a). Where thickened, the myocardium may have fibroelastosis of its lining. Histologically, the myocytes are swollen and have a slightly granular, eosinophilic and abundantly vacuolated cytoplasm (Fig. 23.8b). This appearance accounts for their description as 'foamy', 'lipoid' or 'histiocytoid' cells. There is usually no evidence of inflammation or ischaemia although collagen may be deposited between affected regions. The changes may be found anywhere within the myocardium but, in most cases, they have a predilection for the subendocardial layers; rarely, foam cells may be found within the valves.

An interesting congenital lesion that requires histological examination for its demonstration is cell death. Extensive areas of dead myocardium, often calcified, have been discovered by all who have examined carefully the myocardium of newborns with various congenital defects.[19–21] The full significance of these changes remains to be established, as does their extent in hearts from infants and neonates without congenital malformations.

THE EPICARDIUM AND PERICARDIUM

Malformations of the pericardium, which of course includes the epicardium (the inner layer of the serous pericardium), are discussed in this section. Congenital malformations of either the serous or the fibrous layer of the pericardium are infrequent; the commonest is deficiency or

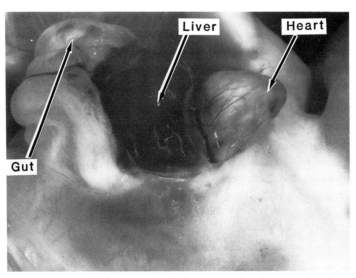

Fig. 23.9 This fetus has an extrathoracic heart which lacks any pericardial covering. The gut and liver are also herniated through the midline deficiency of the abdominal wall.

absence of the fibrous pericardium. Absence of the pericardium is part of the syndrome of midline defects referred to above as the pentalogy of Cantrell. A pericardial covering is lacking in most, but not all, cases of extrathoracic heart (ectopia cordis).[22] When the fibrous pericardium is absent, survival is most unlikely (Fig. 23.9). Partial degrees of pericardial deficiency can be small or large;[23] when large, they tend to be asymptomatic and are discovered as incidental autopsy findings. Paradoxically, small pericardial defects provide the potential for herniation of part of the heart, usually the left atrial appendage, and this can lead to strangulation and functional impairment. Narrowing of the anterior interventricular artery has also been observed beneath the edge of a partial pericardial defect.[23]

Another very rare congenital malformation involving the pericardium is the formation of cysts or diverticulums. These tend to be found incidentally at autopsy (Fig. 23.10); when large, they have been noted in life to be associated with palpitation, venous obstruction or compression of the lungs.

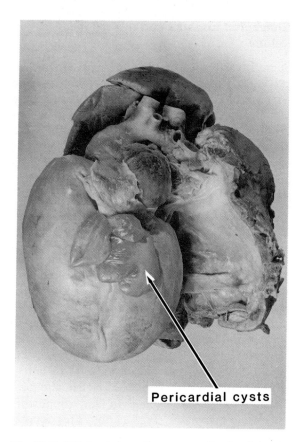

Pericardial cysts

Fig. 23.10 This heart shows the presence of pericardial cysts which were an incidental finding at autopsy.

MALFORMATIONS OF THE CONDUCTION SYSTEM

The system of specialized myocardial fibres which generates and conducts the cardiac impulse comprises the sinus node and the atrioventricular conduction axis. There are remnants of atrioventricular-node-like structures to be found, scattered around the atrial aspects of the atrioventricular junctions,[24] which in the normal heart, have no functional significance. It is crucial to the proper coordination of the normal cardiac contraction, however, that the atrial myocardium is separated from the ventricular muscle mass at all points except where the atrioventricular conduction axis penetrates the junction of the two. The structures separating the atrial and ventricular muscle masses, therefore, although not a part of the specialized conduction system, are essential for normal conduction. As described in Chapter 1, there is no evidence for the existence of specialized tracts coursing through the atrial walls to connect the sinus node to the atrioventricular node. Many of the congenital malformations discussed in previous chapters may involve parts or the whole of the conduction tissues and these have been highlighted at the appropriate points in the text. Over and above these abnormalities, which are a direct consequence of the anatomical derangement of the heart, there are other intrinsic lesions to be discussed in this section.

It is becoming increasingly evident that many of the atrial arrhythmias which affect infants and neonates have a structural basis involving either hypoplasia or excessive fibrosis of the sinus node and its adjacent atrial myocardium.[25] The extent and incidence of these changes will only be discovered when more pathologists undertake the investigation of the conduction system in neonates and infants, a perfectly feasible procedure.[26]

The major lesion involving the atrioventricular junctional area, producing congenitally complete heart block, is discontinuity of the conduction axis at some point along its length. Histological studies of the atrioventricular junction are somewhat more complicated than those of the sinus node, requiring serial section techniques. When this is done, three different patterns can be discerned (Fig. 23.11). The commonest is when the atrioventricular node itself, along with the muscular base of the atrial septum, is replaced by fibrofatty tissue so that the conduction axis starts as a blind structure within the central fibrous body. This pattern, known as discontinuity between the atrial myocardium and the conduction axis,[27] is now established as being the consequence of maternal collagen disease.[28] Much rarer is the variant in which the atrioventricular node is normal in formation but separated by the atrioventricular insulation mechanism from the branching atrioventricular bundle. The rarest pattern is that in which the ventricular bundle branches are insulated by fibrous tissue from the ventricular segment of the conduction axis. Although of interest concerning the way in which the conduction pathways are formed during development, these various patterns are of little functional significance.

The other significant congenital lesions involving the conduction system are concerned with the arrhythmia known as ventricular pre-excitation. The function of the specialized atrioventricular junctional area in the normal heart is to delay the cardiac impulse so that the ventricles have time to fill with blood prior to ventricular systole. This delay occurs primarily in the atrioventricular node but an increment of delay is added as the impulse passes through the ventricular conduction pathways before exciting the ventricular myocardium. Any anomalous muscular connexions, either between atrial and ventricular muscle masses or between the conduction axis and the ventricular myocardium, which short-circuit this normal pathway of conduction, can result in ventricular pre-excitation. The importance of the anomalous connexions is not so much that they pre-excite the ventricles but that they provide the circuit for reciprocating tachycardias (arrhythmias in which the impulse circulates round a pathway to produce a very rapid heart rate). There are several hypothetical pathways which can serve as part of such circuits (Fig. 23.12). The ones of which most is known morphologically and pathologically are those which are associated with the classic Wolff–Parkinson–White variant of pre-excitation. These are tiny bundles of working atrial myocardium which connect the atrial and ventricular muscle masses at some point outside the specialized junctional area (Fig. 23.13). They can be left-sided, right-sided or situated within the area of the atrioventricular septum, and may be multiple. For the most part, they traverse the atrioventricular fibrofatty groove on the epicardial aspect of the fibrous tissues supporting the leaflets of the atrioventricular valves (Fig. 23.13). Rarely they can originate in those remnants of atrioventricular nodal tissue known to exist in the atrial aspect of the atrioventricular junctions, particularly the tricuspid junction.[29] Histological identification of these pathways is difficult and is the domain of the specialized laboratory. Ideally, the entire atrioventricular junctional area should be studied using serial section techniques. Because of the time and effort involved, it is probably best to reserve such studies for cases which have been fully investigated electrophysiologically. Much less is known about the detailed morphology of other lesions responsible for pre-excitation. Most laboratories equipped to carry out studies of the conduction system are usually delighted to receive such specimens for study should they be encountered.

The other major area in which detailed studies of the conduction system may be necessary is in the investigation of sudden death in infancy. Those carrying out such studies should be cautious in their interpretation. It has been suggested that lesions of the conduction system account for many of these fatalities.[30] The studies we have carried out, however, indicate that the changes postulated to produce the substrate for the sudden infant death syndrome are normal maturational changes to be found in all hearts.[31] This is not to deny that, in certain cases, a malformation of the conduction tissues may be respon-

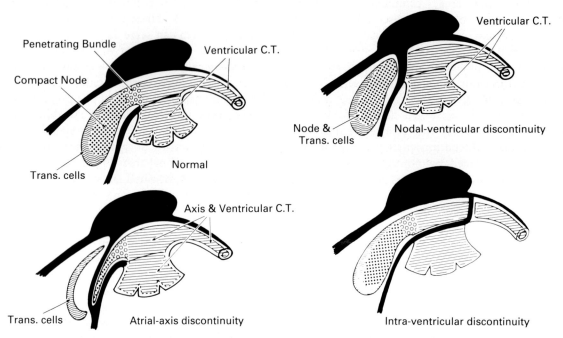

Fig. 23.11 These diagrams show the normal arrangement of the atrioventricular conduction axis contrasted with the different histological patterns of congenitally complete heart block. Black = central fibrous body and atrioventricular 'insulation' arrangement, Trans. = transitional, C.T. = conduction tissue.

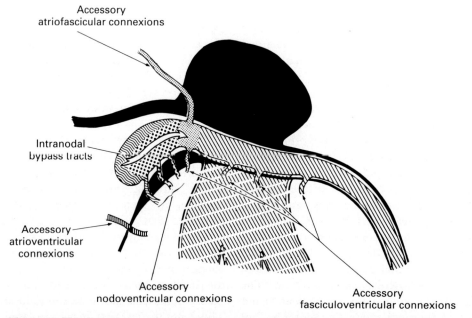

Fig. 23.12 This diagram shows the potential anomalous substrates for ventricular pre-excitation. The black area is the central fibrous body with 'insulation' arrangement.

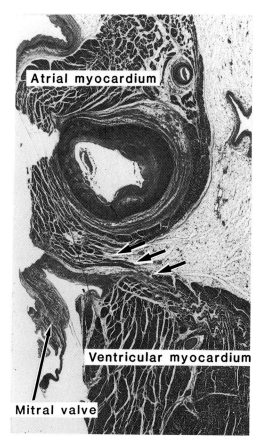

Fig. 23.13 This section across the left atrioventricular junction shows the morphology of a characteristic accessory muscular atrioventricular connexion (short arrows).

sible for sudden death in infancy. Indeed, the very first case of this type we examined had a grossly abnormal structure of the atrioventricular node which could have caused pre-excitation.[32] Since then, we have not encountered any similar case. Unless the investigators of such cases have a detailed knowledge of the normal variations to be found in the conduction tissues of neonates and infants they are unlikely to determine accurately the causes of sudden death in infancy. Our own opinion at present is that only a very small proportion of such cases can justifiably be explained on the basis of structural abnormalities of the conduction pathways. The subject of conduction disturbances in the adult will be dealt with in Part B of this volume.

MALFORMATIONS OF THE CORONARY ARTERIES

As with all the systems discussed in this chapter, anomalies of the coronary arteries are often an integral part of the many congenital malformations already described and discussed where relevant. At this point we are concerned with primary abnormalities of the coronary arteries of congenital origin.[33] The time when these lesions were classified as 'major' and 'minor'[34] is long past, since it is now known that virtually all can produce clinical disease. An anatomical categorization whereby the anomalies conveniently can be considered in terms of variations in origin, number and branching of the coronary arteries is the best approach.[35] Abnormal communications between the arteries and adjacent structures can also be congenital. Previously,[35] we unified our categorization of all these lesions on the basis of their presumed morphogenesis. Studies since that time[36] have revealed to us the simplistic and fallacious nature of our speculations, showing only too clearly the errors that are always inherent in concepts based upon embryogenesis.

Coronary arteries may take an abnormal origin either from the pulmonary trunk or from the aorta. Anomalous origin from the pulmonary trunk is by far the more serious lesion. Rarely, both coronary arteries take their origin from the pulmonary trunk rather than the aorta but usually it is either the right or the left coronary artery which is anomalously connected. Aberrant origin of the right coronary artery is much the rarer and, usually, is of no clinical significance although cases have been reported with sudden and unexpected death in which the right coronary artery took origin from the pulmonary trunk rather than the aorta.[37] If there is uncertainty about the significance of anomalous origin of the right coronary artery, there is no such doubt concerning origin of the left artery from the pulmonary trunk. Known eponymously by the names of Bland, Garland and White,[38] the consequences of this lesion are well established. Usually it is the entire left coronary artery which takes anomalous origin, although in some cases only the anterior interventricular branch may be

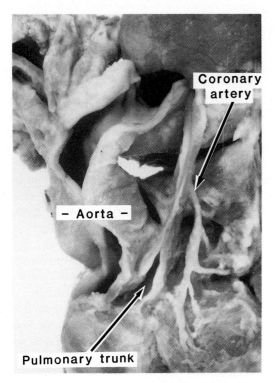

Fig. 23.14 This dissection shows anomalous origin of a solitary coronary artery from the pulmonary trunk in a case of tetralogy of Fallot.

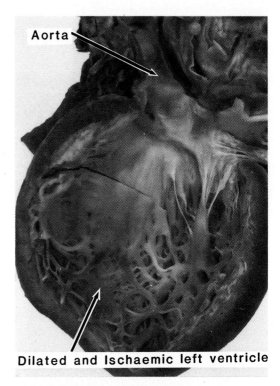

Fig. 23.15 This left ventricle shows the ischaemic consequences of anomalous origin of the left coronary artery from the pulmonary trunk (compare with Fig. 23.4).

involved.[39] The clinical consequences are more severe when the entire artery is anomalously connected. Usually it arises from a sinus of the pulmonary trunk adjacent to the aorta, although its position within that sinus can vary. More rarely, the artery may take origin from the pulmonary trunk itself (Fig. 23.14) or even from a pulmonary arterial branch. The problems produced by the anomalous connexion become manifest only after birth, when the drop in pulmonary arterial pressure together with the decreased content of oxygen within the pulmonary arterial blood, tend to produce myocardial ischaemia and infarction. If severe, this can lead to mitral insufficiency as a consequence of dysfunction of the papillary muscles. The results of these changes are usually evident in specimens (Fig. 23.15), and post-mortem angiograms usually show widespread formation of collateral channels (Fig. 23.16).

Anomalous origin of the coronary arteries from the aorta is much more frequent than from the pulmonary trunk, but the consequences are less frequently manifest. In the 'normal' arrangement, the right and left coronary arteries arise from the two aortic sinuses which 'face' the pulmonary trunk, and do so within the aortic sinus (see Ch. 1). Any deviation from this rule might be considered an anomalous origin of a coronary artery from the aorta. As an arbitrary criterion, however, it is usually considered that an artery must arise at least one centimetre above the sinutubular bar before being considered anomalous. Such high origin imposes an oblique course on the artery as it runs towards the atrioventricular grooves and the ventricular mass. This arrangement, although its effects are not yet proven, can give rise to narrowing of the arterial orifice and, hence, diminished myocardial perfusion. Several possibilities exist for anomalous origin of the coronary arteries within the aortic sinuses. It is rare for a coronary artery

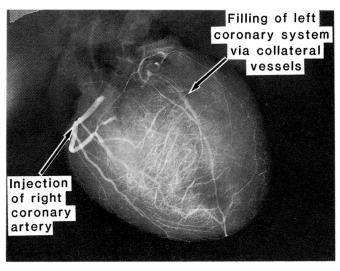

Fig. 23.16 This post-mortem angiogram shows the collateral circulation in a case of anomalous origin of the left coronary artery from the pulmonary trunk.

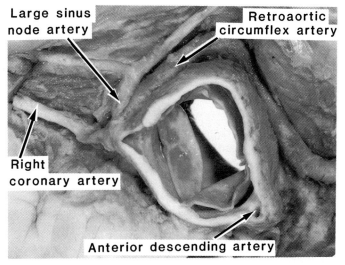

Fig. 23.17 This dissection shows anomalous retro-aortic origin of the circumflex coronary artery from the right coronary artery in an otherwise normal heart.

to arise from the non-facing aortic sinus, but the arrangement does exist. Well-documented examples of anomalous aortic origin within the facing sinuses[40-43] include origin of the circumflex artery from the right-hand facing sinus or the right coronary artery (Fig. 23.17), origin of the anterior interventricular artery from the right coronary artery and origin of both

coronary arteries from either the right-hand or the left-hand facing sinus. Of these, the ones probably of most functional significance are those in which the left coronary artery is sandwiched between the aorta and the pulmonary trunk, or in which it takes an extended intramural course as it leaves the aorta.

The number of coronary arterial orifices varies

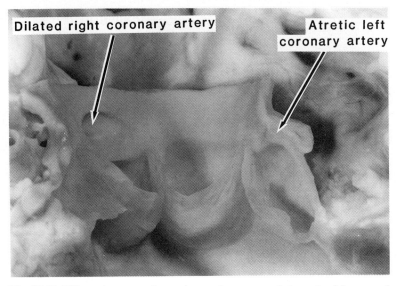

Dilated right coronary artery

Atretic left coronary artery

Fig. 23.18 This section across the aortic root shows congenital atresia of the stem of the left coronary artery. Note the enlarged orifice of the right coronary artery.

markedly within the normal population. Thus, in about 50% of all hearts there is a second small orifice within the right-hand facing aortic sinus which gives rise either to the infundibular branch of the right coronary artery or to the artery of the sinus node. In contrast, dual orifices for the branches of the left coronary artery are exceedingly rare.[44] Dual orifices, of whatever artery, are rarely, if ever, of functional significance. In contrast, a solitary origin of the coronary arteries is of much more significance, and this anomaly has branching from the solitary artery of two varieties. The artery may originate from the right-hand facing sinus, encircle the tricuspid and mitral valves following the anticipated pathways of the right and circumflex arteries and then terminate as the anterior interventricular artery. This is the rarer variety of single coronary artery. More commonly, the solitary artery, having originated from the right-hand facing sinus, divides immediately into right and left coronary arteries which then follow their anticipated course, the left coronary artery either passing in front of or behind the arterial trunks before branching into anterior interventricular and circumflex branches. In some circumstances, as may also happen when the anterior interventricular artery originates from the right coronary

artery, the anomalous vessels may pass between the aorta and the pulmonary trunk, rarely buried within the substance of the ventricular septum. The arrangement of a solitary coronary artery can also be produced when there is congenital atresia of the main stem of the left coronary artery (Fig. 23.18), what should be the branches of the left coronary artery then being supplied through collateral channels.[45] As with all the variations described above, the major significance of this anomaly is its association with sudden and unexpected death.

Fistulous communications from the coronary arteries to adjacent structures can occur with otherwise normally structured arteries or when the arteries themselves take an anomalous origin. Such communications are so frequent when there is ventricular outflow atresia with an intact ventricular septum that they can be considered as part of the malformation (see Chs 7 and 8). In normally structured hearts, the fistulous extensions connect most frequently to the right ventricle, followed, in decreasing order of frequency, by the right atrium, the pulmonary trunk, and the left atrium.[46] Rarely, the arteries may communicate with most unusual sites such as the peripheral branches of the pulmonary arteries.[47] If severe, the fistulous communications may produce a left-to-right shunt, eventually leading to myocardial decompensation and, if untreated, to death.[48]

REFERENCES

1. Factor SM. Endocardial fibroelastosis found on transventricular endomyocardial biopsy in children. Arch Pathol Lab Med 1979; 103: 214–219.

2. Levin S. Parvovirus: a possible etiologic agent in cardiomyopathy and endocardial fibroelastosis. Hum Pathol 1980; 11: 404–405.

3. Chen SC, Thompson NW, Rose V. Endocardial fibroelastosis: family studies with special reference to counselling. J Pediatr 1971; 79: 385–392.

4. Becker AE, Anderson RH. The endocardium. In: Pathology of congenital heart disease. London: Butterworths, 1981; 391–395.

5. Edwards JE. Primary endocardial sclerosis. In: Gould SE, ed. Pathology of the heart. 2nd ed. Springfield, Illinois: Charles C Thomas, 1960; 419–20.

6. Ursell PC, Neill CA, Anderson RH, Ho SY, Becker AE, Gerlis IM. Endocardial fibroelastosis and hypoplasia of the left ventricle in neonates without significant aortic stenosis. Br Heart J 1984; 51: 492–497.

7. Uhl HSM. A previously undescribed congenital malformation of the heart: almost total absence of the myocardium of the right ventricle. Bull Johns Hopkins Hosp 1952; 91: 197–205.

8. Vecht RJ, Carmichael DJS, Gopal R, Philip G. Uhl's anomaly. Br Heart J 1979; 41; 676–682.

9. Thiene G, Nava A, Corrado D, Rossi L, Pennelli N. Right ventricular cardiomyopathy and sudden death in young people. N Engl J Med 1988; 318: 129–133.

10. Cantrell JR, Haller JA, Ravitch MM. A syndrome of congenital defects involving the abdominal wall, sternum, diaphragm, pericardium and heart. Surg Gynecol Obstet 1958; 107: 602–614.

11. Chesler E, Goffe N, Schamroth L, Meyers A. Annular subvalvular left ventricular aneurysms in the South African Bantu. Circulation 1965; 32: 43–51.

12. Fenoglio JJ Jr. McAllister HA Jr, Ferrans VJ. Cardiac rhabdomyoma: a clinicopathologic and electron microscopic study. Am J Cardiol 1976; 38: 241–251.

13. Becker AE, Anderson RH. Cardiac tumours or tumour-like lesions. In: Pathology of congenital heart disease. London: Butterworths,1981; 419–430.

14. MacMahon EH. Infantile xanthomatous cardiomyopathy. Pediatrics 1971; 48: 312–315.

15. Bove KE, Schwartz DC. Focal lipid cardiomyopathy in an infant with paroxysmal tachycardia. Arch Pathol 1973; 95: 26–36.

16. Witzleben CL, Pinto M. Foamy myocardial transformation of infancy. Arch Pathol Lab Med 1978; 102: 306–311.

17. Ferrans VJ, McAllister HA Jr, Haese W. Infantile cardiomyopathy with histiocytoid change in cardiac muscle cells. Circulation 1976; 53: 708–710.

18. Amini M, Bosman C, Marino B. Histiocytoid cardiomyopathy in infancy: a new hypothesis. Chest 1980; 77: 556–558.

19. Blanc WA, Franciosi RA, Cadotte M. L'infarctus et la fibrose du myocarde en pathologie foetale et infantile. [Infarct and fibrosis of the myocardium in fetal and infantile pathology]. Med Hyg 1966; 24: 216–230.

20. Esterly JH, Oppenheimer EH. Some aspects of cardiac pathology in infancy and childhood. I. Neonatal myocardial necrosis. Bull Johns Hopkins Hosp 1966; 119: 111–191.

21. Berry CL. Myocardial ischemia in infancy and childhood. J Clin Pathol 1967; 20: 38–41.

22. Anderson RH, Macartney FJ, Shinebourne EA, Tynan M. Abnormal positions and relationships of the heart. Paediatric cardiology, vol. 2. Edinburgh: Churchill Livingstone, 1987; 1057–1072.

23. Nasser WK. Congenital defects of the pericardium. In: Fowler NO, ed. The pericardium in health and disease. Mount Kisco, New York: Futura, 1985; 51–78.

24. Anderson RH, Davies MJ, Becker AE. Atrioventricular ring specialized tissue in the normal heart. Eur J Cardiol 1974; 2: 219–230.

25. Ho SY, Mortimer G, Anderson RH, Pomerance A, Keeling JW. Conduction system defects in three perinatal patients with arrhythmia. Br Heart J 1985; 53: 158–163.

26. Anderson RH, Ho SY, Smith A, Wilkinson JL, Becker AE. Study of the cardiac conduction tissues in the paediatric age group. Diagn Histopathol 1981; 4: 3–15.

27. Ho SY, Esscher E, Anderson RH, Michaelsson M. Anatomy of congenital complete heart block and relation to maternal anti-Ro antibodies. Am J Cardiol 1986; 58: 291–294.

28. Scott JS, Maddison PJ, Taylor PV, Esscher E, Scott O, Skinner RD. Connective tissue disease, antibodies to ribonucleoprotein, and congenital heart block. N Engl J Med 1983; 4: 209–212.

29. Becker AE, Anderson RH, Durrer D, Wellens HJJ. The anatomical substrates of Wolff–Parkinson–White syndrome: a clinico-pathologic correlation in seven patients. Circulation 1978; 57: 870–879.

30. James TN. Sudden death in babies: new observations in the heart. Am J Cardiol 1968; 22: 479–506.

31. Ho SY, Anderson RH. Conduction system and SIDS. Ann NY Acad Sci 1988; 533: 176–190.

32. Anderson RH, Bouton J, Burrow CT, Smith A. Sudden death in infancy: a study of the cardiac specialized tissue. Br Med J 1974; 2: 135–139.

33. Angelini P. Normal and anomalous coronary arteries: definitions and classification. Am Heart J 1989; 117: 418–434.

34. Ogden JA. Congenital anomalies of the coronary arteries. Am J Cardiol 1970; 25: 474–479.

35. Becker AE, Anderson RH. Coronary artery anomalies. In: Pathology of congenital heart disease. London: Butterworths, 1981; 369–378.

36. Bogers AJJC, Gittenberger-de-Groot AC, Dubbeldam JA, Huysmans HA. The inadequacy of existing theories on development of the proximal coronary arteries and their

connexions with the arterial trunks. Int J Cardiol 1988; 20: 117–123.

37. Wald S, Stonecipher K, Baldwin BJ, Nutter DO. Anomalous origin of the right coronary artery from the pulmonary artery. Am J Cardiol 1971; 27: 677–681.

38. Bland EF, White PD, Garland J. Congenital anomalies of coronary arteries: report of unusual case associated with cardiac hypertrophy. Am Heart J 1933; 8: 787–801.

39. Schwartz RP, Robicsek F. An unusual anomaly of the coronary system: origin of the anterior (descending) interventricular artery from the pulmonary trunk. J Pediatr 1971; 78: 123–126.

40. Liberthson RR, Dinsmore RE, Bharati S et al. Aberrant coronary artery origin from the aorta. Diagnosis and clinical significance. Circulation 1974; 50: 774–779.

41. Zijlstra JP, Duren DR, Tan SL, Yacoub ML, Durrer D. Operatieve behandeling van de aberrante corsprong van de A. coronaria sinistra bij een 12-jarige jongen. [Operation treatment of the aberrant origin of the left coronary artery in a 12 years old boy]. Ned Tijdschr Geneeskd 1979; 123: 1681–1685.

42. Kragel AH, Roberts WC. Anomalous origin of either right or left main coronary artery from the aorta with subsequent coursing between aorta and pulmonary trunk: analysis of 32 necropsy cases. Am J Cardiol 1988; 62: 771– 777.

43. Roberts WC, Kragel AH. Anomalous origin of either the right or left main coronary artery from the aorta without coursing of the anomalistically arising artery between aorta and pulmonary trunk. Am J Cardiol 1988; 62: 1263–1267.

44. Zumbo O, Fain K, Jarmolych J, Daoud AS. Coronary atherosclerosis and myocardial infarction in hearts with anomalous coronary arteries. Lab Invest 1965: 14: 571 (abstract).

45. Debich DE, Williams KE, Anderson RH. Congenital atresia of the orifice of the left coronary artery and its main stem. Int J Cardiol 1989; 22: 398–404.

46. de Nef JJE, Varghese JP, Losekoot TG. Congenital coronary artery fistula. Analysis of 17 cases. Br Heart J 1971; 33: 857–862.

47. Macchi RJ, Fabregas RA, Chianelli HO, Bourdet JCB, Lhez O, Stagnaro R. Anomalous communication of the left coronary artery with a peripheral branch of the right pulmonary artery. Chest 1976; 69: 565–568.

48. Effler DB, Sheldon WC, Turner JJ, Groves LK. Coronary arteriovenous fistulas: diagnosis and surgical management. Report of 15 cases. Surgery 1967; 61: 41–50.

The Vascular System: Basic Principles

Morphology and pathophysiology of the vascular system

INTRODUCTION

It is remarkable that it was not until the seventeenth century that William Harvey[1] in his classic treatise described the circulation of the blood. Even so, there was a tendency subsequently to regard the arterial and venous systems as passive conduits with control of the circulation being vested largely in the action of the heart. During the present century the vascular system has been shown to be exceedingly complex and subject to a variety of physical and chemical interacting influences, none of which is yet fully understood. It is impossible, in the space available, to discuss in detail all known aspects of the subject and we must restrict our comments to those essentials relevant to the understanding of diseases of blood vessels and to the involvement of the vascular system in systemic disorders.

Blood is expelled from the heart in pulsatile fashion by ventricular contraction; the systolic pressure is the highest pressure coinciding with the end of contraction and the diastolic pressure is the lowest pressure occurring near the end of ventricular relaxation. The pressure within the arterial system is the product of the forces generated in the heart and the inherent resistance of the arteries, particularly in the smaller arteries and arterioles which are known as the pre-capillary resistance vessels. The large arteries, the aorta and its major branches, are distensible. Their distensibility enables them to accommodate the cardiac output after each contraction and, by their elastic recoil, to modulate the central pulsatile expulsion of blood to a smoother continuous flow in the peripheral smaller arteries. After passing

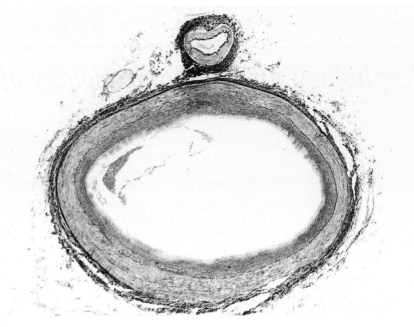

Fig. 24.1 Transverse section through a muscular artery with prominent medial smooth muscle separated from a concentrically thickened intima by a distinct internal elastic lamella. The intimal thickening is due to proliferation of myointimal cells. The adventitia is composed of a looser arrangement of collagen and elastic tissue and although there is focal condensation of the latter no true lamella is formed.
Elastica/Van Gieson × 17.5

through the capillary bed (the exchange vessels) blood enters the venules, the post-capillary resistance vessels, which play an important part in determining the pressure within the capillary bed, reciprocating the action of the pre-capillary arterioles. Thus, constriction of the pre-capillary arterioles decreases capillary pressure while constriction of the post-capillary venules has the opposite effect. Similarly, dilatation of the venules leads to decreased capillary pressure and dilatation of the arterioles has the opposite effect. Obviously, haemodynamic disturbances that affect the resistance arterioles and venules will interfere with fluid and solute exchange and filtration in the capillary bed and will upset the Starling equilibrium of hydrostatic and osmotic pressure gradients in relation to capillary permeability. A good example is the tissue oedema found in congestive cardiac failure.

The large veins are capacitance vessels, acting as reservoirs of de-oxygenated blood. Skeletal muscular activity acting on vein walls, aided by the venous valves preventing retrograde flow, returns blood to the heart. The quantity of blood reaching the heart is an important determinant of cardiac output, succinctly expressed by Swales[2] in the axiom that 'the heart can only put out the blood it is receiving'.

STRUCTURE OF BLOOD VESSELS

All blood vessels have an inner layer, the intima, lined by endothelium with subjacent connective tissue; a middle layer, the media, composed of smooth muscle, elastic tissue and collagen embedded in ground substance; and an outer layer, the adventitia, composed of elastic and fibrous tissue (Fig. 24.1). The composition and structure of the vessel wall vary considerably amongst the different categories of vessel so it is prudent to review briefly the properties and functions of individual components before describing the morphology of each category of

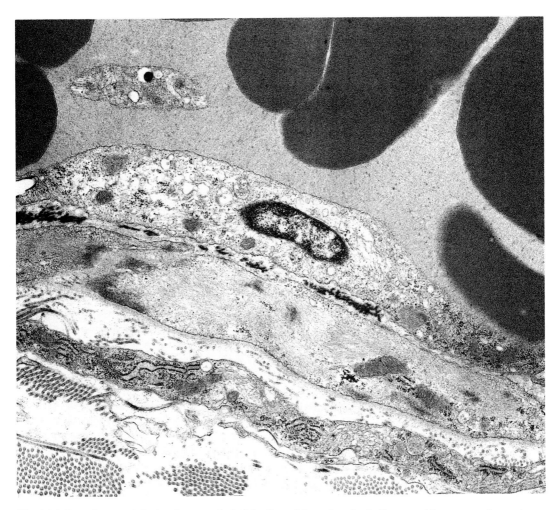

Fig. 24.2 Part of an arteriole showing an endothelial cell overlying a few elastin fibres, a subjacent smooth muscle cell and bundles of collagen fibres.
Electronmicrograph × 16 000

artery and vein. The important subject of the nerve supply to blood vessels will be dealt with later.

Endothelium

The endothelium[3] is a monolayer of elongated epithelium-like cells (Fig. 24.2) that forms the inner lining of the heart, arteries, capillaries, veins and lymphatics, the individual cells being oriented with the long axis in the line of blood flow. Adjacent cells are connected by tight and gap junctions, the number and proportion of each varying in different parts of the vascular system and in different segments of vessels. In the visceral capillary beds there are fenestrations between individual cells. The pattern of cell junctions is related to the permeability, metabolic and exchange requirements in the different parts of the vascular system; in some parts it is 'tight', as in large arteries, in others it is 'leaky' as in arterioles, capillaries and venules, permitting the protein-rich and cell-rich exudate in inflammation.

An important function of endothelium is the prevention of thrombosis, an almost invariable consequence of a significant breach in continuity of the otherwise smooth lining.[4] The subjacent

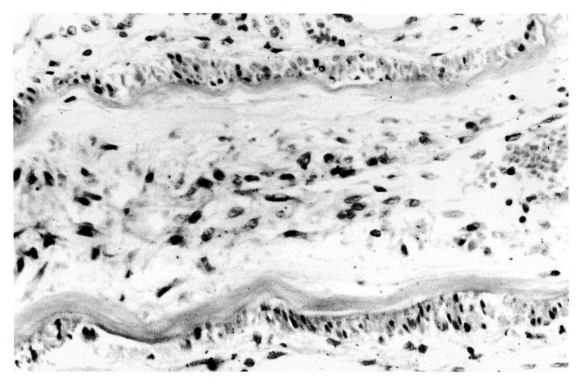

Fig. 24.3 Longitudinal section of a small intrarenal artery from a case of hypertension showing marked proliferation of myointimal (smooth muscle) cells which have migrated from the media.
Haematoxylin–eosin × 450

intimal tissues are highly thrombogenic, quickly initiating platelet adhesion and agglutination followed by fibrin deposition. The luminal aspect of the normal endothelium repels platelets and other blood cells, which tend to be concentrated in the axial blood stream with the plasma flowing over the surface electronegative glycocalyx of the endothelium. The anti-thrombotic property of endothelium is probably enhanced by a recently identified factor, the endothelium-derived relaxing factor (EDRF),[5] a locally produced vasodilator. The active principle is nitric oxide,[6] synthesized from L-arginine by the vascular endothelium, and in addition to its vasodilating properties, it inhibits platelet aggregation and adhesion. Endothelium also produces prostacyclin, a potent inhibitor of platelet aggregation, and fibrinolytic factors which would appear to vary in different arterial and venous systems depending on physiological and pathological circumstances.[7]

Smooth muscle

The ability of blood vessels to accommodate or influence changes in blood flow and intraluminal pressure by contraction or relaxation rests largely with the smooth muscle component of their wall, moderated by connective tissue elements and a complex of vasoactive substances and the autonomic nervous system.[8] At one time smooth muscle was thought to be restricted to the media of vessels but with the advent of electron microscopy and other technological advances such as immunocytochemistry it was established that the so-called 'transitional' or 'myointimal' cells (Fig. 24.3), a prominent component of the intima in normal adult blood vessels and also of atherosclerotic lesions, are smooth muscle cells.

The individual smooth muscle cell[3] is spindle-shaped and surrounded by a closely applied basement membrane; it contains thick myosin

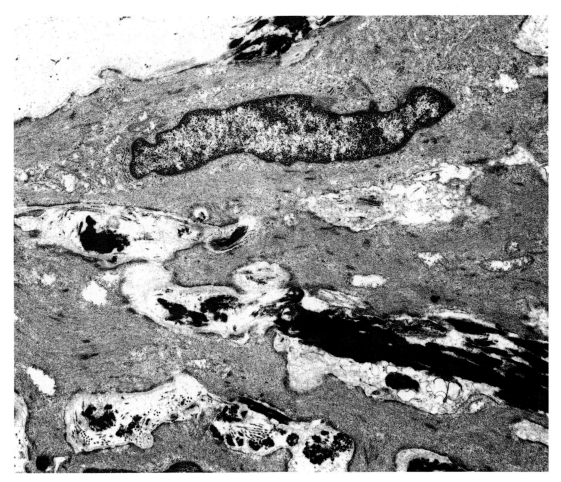

Fig. 24.4 The media of a muscular artery showing smooth muscle cells invested by elastin fibres and ground substance. Note the dense bodies associated with myofilaments in the smooth muscle and dense zones on the internal aspect of the cell membrane acting as anchoring points for the myofilaments. Electronmicrograph × 9 000

and thin actin filaments imparting contractile properties. The cytoplasm also contains non-contractile intermediate filaments of the vimentin and desmin type as part of the cytoskeleton. The dense bodies scattered throughout the sarcoplasm are analogous with the Z lines of skeletal muscle, acting as zones of attachment for contractile filaments, while the dense bands on the internal aspect of the plasma membrane are the anchoring sites for the contractile filaments (Fig. 24.4). This arrangement provides the mechanism whereby smooth muscle cells can considerably alter their shape in response to stimuli and produce the

contractile force in vessel walls. The coordinated action within the vessel wall is achieved through junctional complexes between adjacent cells, gap junctions (adherence or intermediate junctions), which correspond to, but differ structurally from, the desmosomes of epithelial cells. In addition, glycoproteins such as fibronectin act as transmitters of contractile forces from smooth muscle cells to the investing stroma of collagen and elastic tissue. Smooth muscle, in contrast to skeletal or cardiac muscle, will replicate and proliferate under appropriate stimuli as is seen for example in repair processes, in response to

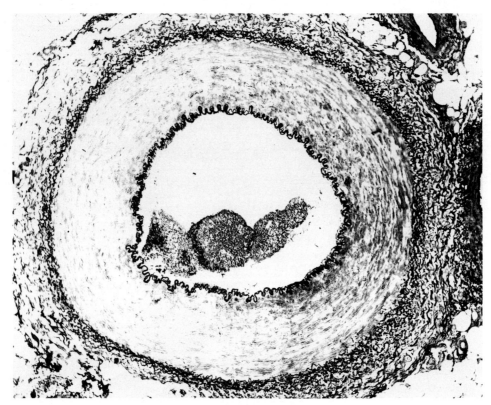

Fig. 24.5 Transverse section of a radial artery from a young man to show the well-defined internal elastic lamina (lamella) separating an inconspicuous intima from the bulky media. There is also condensation of elastic tissue between the media and surrounding adventitia.
Elastica/Van Gieson × 30
Reproduced by kind permission of Sir Theo Crawford from 'Arteries, veins and lymphatics'. In: Symmers W St C, ed. Systemic Pathology, 2nd ed. Edinburgh: Churchill Livingstone, 1976; 1: 120–169 [Fig. 3.1].

inflammation, in altered haemodynamic conditions such as hypertension, and in atherosclerotic lesions.

Connective tissues

Collagen and elastic tissue, the main fibrous proteins, are embedded in a complex ground substance of proteoglycans (acid mucopolysaccharides) and glycoproteins such as fibronectin, already referred to, and laminin, the basement membrane glycoprotein.[9] Of the eleven types of collagen described, types I and III of the so-called interstitial collagens are the major fibrous proteins of the walls of larger blood vessels; they are produced mainly by the fibroblasts of the adventitia but also by smooth muscle cells of the media.

These collagens provide the tensile strength of the vessel wall, putting a constraint on its distensibility. Types IV, V and VI collagens have also been isolated from vessel walls, the first two in particular association with the basement membranes of the endothelium and smooth muscle cells; type VI has been found in both intima and media. The 'reticulin' identified by older histological techniques that demonstrate argyrophilia is now thought to consist of fine type III collagen fibres coated with proteoglycans and glycoproteins.

Elastic tissue (the elastica) is another fibrous protein (elastin). It is a prominent component of vessel walls, particularly well shown by appropriate staining methods where it is concentrated to form the fenestrated lamella (internal elastic

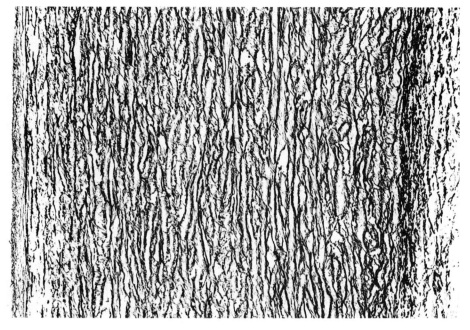

Fig. 24.6 Section through the wall of the aorta to show abundance of elastic tissue between medial smooth muscle cells, which are unstained.
Elastica × 90

membrane or lamina) (Fig. 24.5). This lamella is a porous tube, demarcating the intima from the media in large and medium-sized arteries. A less well defined lamella has been described in some arteries as the external elastic membrane: it indicates the junction between media and adventitia but its elastic fibres are more randomly distributed amongst the adventitial collagen. No such discrete lamellas are present in veins. In addition to the thicker lamellas in arteries, finer elastic fibres are distributed throughout the media, again in lamellar arrangement, the sheets of elastica enclosing helically oriented units of smooth muscle cells. Collagen and ground substance invest the lamellar units of elastica and smooth muscle. The elasticity inherent in all blood vessels is not determined by elastic tissue only, as the name of that tissue would seem to imply, but is a synergistic function of the contractile smooth muscle with its associated elastic tissue and matrix. Collagen, which is much less elastic, is the tensile element that serves to prevent overdistension of vessels.

STRUCTURE OF VARIOUS TYPES OF ARTERIES, ARTERIOLES AND CAPILLARIES

A distinction is made between elastic and muscular types of arteries. Elastic arteries, such as the aorta and its major branches, are characterized by an abundance of fibres of elastin in the media (Fig. 24.6). These fibres form concentrically layered and fenestrated membranes, the number of which varies with age and with the segments of elastic artery involved. For instance, the proximal part of the aorta contains more of these elastic lamellas than does the abdominal part of the aorta. Irrespective of the number of elastic lamellas, there is smooth muscle between each with the smooth muscle being connected to the elastin fibres by collagen. Thus, units are formed which consist of two elastic lamellas sandwiching layers of smooth muscle and collagenous tissue (Fig. 24.7). This architecture is the basis for the elastic properties of the major arteries whose principal role is transportation and the transformation of the discontinuous ejection of

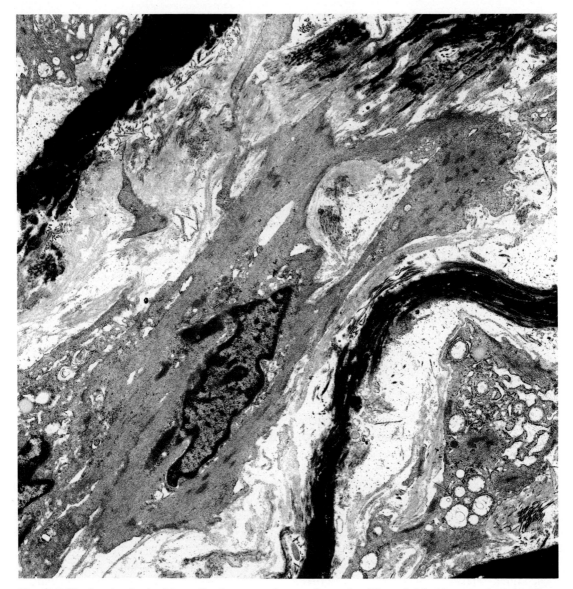

Fig. 24.7 The functional unit of the media of an artery: the smooth muscle cell is sandwiched between elastic lamellae associated with bundles of collagen fibres and ground substance.
Electronmicrograph × 9 000

blood from the heart to a continuous flow in the systemic circulation.

Muscular arteries, such as the coronary arteries and other arteries of similar calibre, have a different medial architecture. The main constituent is smooth muscle cells, which form concentric and coiled layers. Elements of collagenous connective tissue are present between the smooth muscle cells, as are elastic fibres, but not to the extent seen in elastic arteries. The muscular media is demarcated from the intima by a distinct internal elastic lamina. The intima thickens with age, due principally to the addition of smooth muscle cells which migrate from the media to form a so-called musculo-elastic layer. The thickness of the media varies in the arterial systems, being prominent, for example, in the coronary arteries and much thinner in the intracranial arteries. The external boundary of the media shows a condensation of collagen and elastin fibres, which occasionally gives the impression of an external elastic lamina; however, except in the muscular pulmonary arteries, no true external elastic lamina is formed.

At the level of the arterioles the media is much reduced in thickness and eventually is composed of a single layer of smooth muscle cells, spiralling around the lumen. The smooth muscle cells are separated from the endothelial cells by fragments of elastin (Fig. 24.2), reminiscent of the internal elastic lamina in larger-sized muscular arteries.

Capillaries constitute the smallest component of the vascular system and play an important role in the exchange of gases, fluids and nutrients. They consist of a single layer of endothelial cells which rests on a basal lamina produced by the cell itself. The different arrangement of the endothelial cells has led to a sub-classification of capillaries. A frequent type, known as capillary type I, shows a continuous layer of endothelial cells (Fig. 24.8). The cytoplasm of the cells forms a flat layer and adjacent cells have intimate contacts. At the site of each nucleus there is an apparent bulge into the lumen. This pattern contrasts with the so-called type II capillary, known also as 'fenestrated capillaries', which is characterized by gaps between the endothelial cells (Fig. 24.9). These gaps allow easy communication between the lumen and the subendothelial tissues despite the fact that an electron-dense diaphragm bridges the gap. The third type of capillary is the so-called sinusoidal capillary, its main characteristic being a wide luminal diameter.

Associated with many capillaries are cells closely applied to the outer aspect of the endothelium, known as adventitial cells or pericytes (Fig. 24.9). The pericyte is now considered to be a 'reserve' cell which may transform to a smooth muscle cell under appropriate stimulation, and it has a major role in angiogenesis. Pericytes have cytoplasmic filaments, as do endothelial cells, so the contribution made by each cell type in

contraction of capillaries is debated. Contraction of capillaries is an important physiological property as, in normal circumstances, only part of a capillary network is perfused by way of preferential routes. When there is a local demand for more blood, as in inflammation and other disorders, the collapsed capillaries will open up and fill with blood to produce hyperaemia.

STRUCTURE OF VEINS AND VENULES

Large veins possess a medial layer composed of bundles of smooth muscle cells embedded in connective tissues. The content of connective tissue exceeds that of the smooth muscle cells. In some of the large veins, like the caval veins, the adventitia is thick and also contains an abundance of smooth muscle cells, usually with a longitudinal orientation. By contrast, the intima is thin in these large veins. The muscular nature of the media is more evident in medium-sized veins but collagen and elastin fibres are prominent between the smooth muscle cells. The adventitia is composed mainly of collagen, again usually oriented in longitudinal fashion, and it appears to be the thickest layer of the wall. The intima is relatively inconspicuous.

In venules, the layer of smooth muscle cells is discontinuous, this discontinuity being particularly evident in the post-capillary venules (Fig. 24.10). There is a gradual transition of the architecture of capillaries towards venules containing a layer of smooth muscle cells. The collecting veins, of a diameter from 30–50 μm, are the first ones that show smooth muscle cells underneath the layer of endothelial cells. These smooth muscle cells gradually increase in number with concomitant increase in size of the venules and, eventually, form a continuous layer. Somewhat larger collecting veins, with a diameter of approximately 200 μm, have a true media with focal multilayering of smooth muscle cells. The efficient functioning of the venous system depends upon the competence of valves. These thin endothelium-lined structures are so constructed as to support the venous return to the heart against the action of gravity.

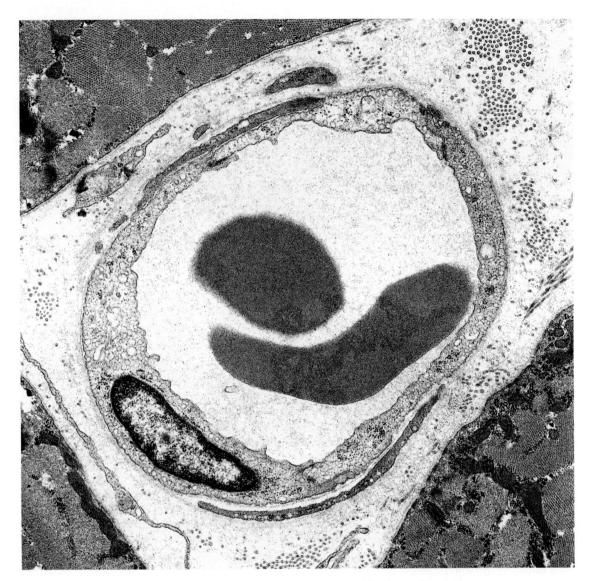

Fig. 24.8 A type I capillary with a continuous layer of endothelial cells closed by junctional complexes. Electronmicrograph × 19 000

NEURAL AND HORMONAL INFLUENCES ON BLOOD VESSELS

The earlier concept that the entire neural control of the vascular system was provided by the mutually antagonistic sympathetic and parasympathetic parts of the autonomic nervous system has been considerably elaborated in recent years to reveal a great complexity of interacting agents and mechanisms.[8] In the light of expanding knowledge, it has become simplistic to assume that the sympathetic system only causes vasoconstriction while the parasympathetic system only causes vasodilatation. There is good evidence that a single nerve may store and release more than one neurotransmitter. Furthermore, the receptors for vasoactive substances in nerve endings and on effector cells are proving to be variable in their agonistic and antagonistic effects.

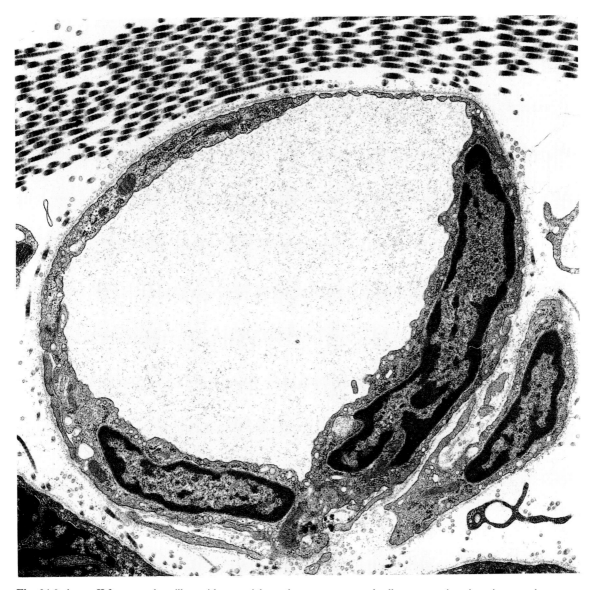

Fig. 24.9 A type II fenestrated capillary with potential gaps between attenuated cell processes. A pericyte is seen at bottom right.
Electronmicrograph × 19 000

The autonomic nerves to blood vessels terminate in bulbous 'varicosities' and form a branching complex in the outer media. This complex invests the circumferential layer of smooth muscle so that the whole coat, not just individual cells, reacts to neurotransmitters. The response is then transmitted by way of the gap junction or nexus apparatus that connects contiguous smooth muscle cells so that the entire media reacts appropriately to a particular stimulus. In general terms, the density of innervation of the vessels varies inversely with their calibre, being greatest in small arteries and arterioles, and thus corresponding to the contribution that the vessels make to peripheral resistance in the vascular system. This pattern is reflected on the venous side where the innervation, while less than that on the arterial side, is more concen-

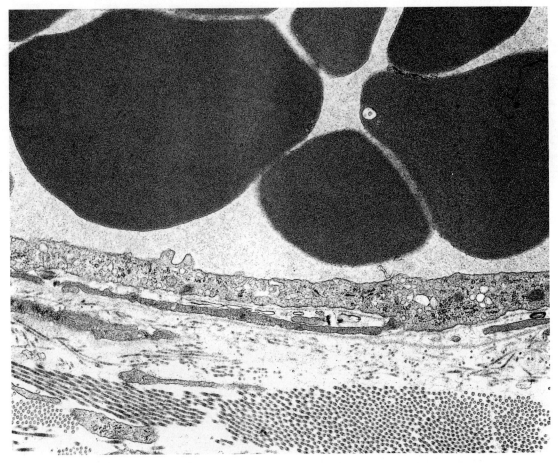

Fig. 24.10 A small venule with endothelial cell processes overlying attenuated processes of smooth muscle cells and collagen. No elastin fibres can be seen (compare with Fig. 24.2).
Electronmicrograph × 16 000

trated in venules and small veins than in the larger capacitance veins.

Sympathetic adrenergic fibres predominate in the nerve supply to blood vessels, inducing vasoconstriction by the release of stored noradrenaline which binds with adrenoreceptors on the effector smooth muscle cell membrane to promote contraction. In the receptor complex of the synapse between nerve and muscle the α_1-receptors are mainly responsible for the pressor effects; subsets of these receptors (α_2) have the property of inhibiting noradrenaline release to provide a negative feedback mechanism. There are also some α_2-receptors on the post-synaptic membrane. The β-receptors, in the presence of low levels of noradrenaline, stimulate increased release of the neurotransmitter thereby providing a positive feedback mechanism. The pattern of adrenergic receptors on the synapse between autonomic nerve varicosities and the effector smooth muscle cells (Fig. 24.11) varies in different vascular beds. Furthermore, the complex is influenced also by angiotensin, acetylcholine, prostaglandins and other vasoactive substances including the action of degrading enzymes. Pharmacological manipulation of this receptor system is the basis of the use of blocking agents in the treatment of hypertension and other cardio-vascular disorders.

Cholinergic (acetylcholine) vasodilatory effects on blood vessels, thought at one time to be restricted to the parasympathetic system, are now

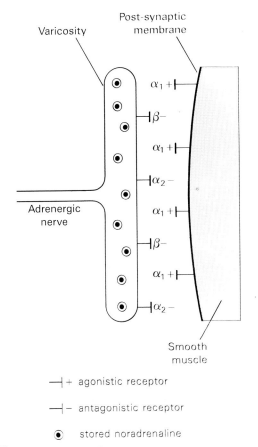

Fig. 24.11 Diagram of an example of the pattern of adrenergic receptors of the synapse between sympathetic nerves and smooth muscle. The pre-synaptic β-receptors in the presence of low levels of noradrenaline in the synaptic space stimulate noradrenaline release from the varicosity while the α_2-receptors inhibit release. The α_1-receptors on the post-synaptic membrane combine with noradrenaline to induce contraction of smooth muscle.

known to be generated also by some fibres of the sympathetic system in certain vascular beds. The main parasympathetic inhibiting influence on the cardiovascular system, however, is on the heart, via the vagus nerve, activation of which leads to bradycardia and a decrease in stroke volume, effects that are opposite to those of adrenergic stimulation.

CENTRAL NERVOUS SYSTEM CONTROL OF BLOOD PRESSURE

Control by the central nervous system of neural influences on the cardiovascular system, and hence of the regulation of arterial pressure, is vested in a complex of nuclei in the midbrain, medulla and cortex and in their associated neural pathways.[10] This integrated system is sensitive not only to circulating and locally produced catecholamines but also to other vasoactive substances such as angiotensin II, dopamine, vasopressin, serotonin (5-hydroxytryptamine) and an ever-increasing list of peptide neurotransmitters and modulators including the recently isolated neuropeptide Y (NPY),[11] a potent vasoconstrictor. The influence of the higher central nervous system control is exemplified by the variation in blood pressure during sleep and arousal and in stressful circumstances. Equally important for control and regulation by the central nervous system are the messages relayed to it by the baroreceptor system which comprises stretch receptors located in the heart and large arteries such as those in the carotid sinus. These receptors are activated by changes of blood pressure beyond a certain range; they indicate to the central nervous system that the pressure has risen or fallen outside that range and so evoke a rapid response to restore homeostasis. Thus (Fig. 24.12), a sharp rise in blood pressure activates stretch receptors in the carotid sinus to relay the message to the nucleus solitarius in the medulla (nucleus of the tractus solitarius, NTS). The NTS, through neural connexions, excites the vasomotor centre (VMC), a diffuse complex containing the vagal nuclei in the medulla. This leads to efferent parasympathetic stimulation of the conduction system of the heart resulting in slowing of the heart rate and a reduction in stroke volume. Simultaneously, through neural connexions between the NTS and vasomotor centre and the sympathetic centres in the spinal cord, there is inhibition of sympathetic efferent activity on the heart and blood vessels, leading to a reduction in blood pressure. Conversely, a significant drop in blood pressure detected by the baroreceptors excites the nucleus of the tractus solitarius and the vasomotor centre to inhibit vagal (parasympathetic) activity on the heart and to stimulate sympathetic activity on the heart and blood vessels to raise blood pressure. It is important to note that the baroreceptors, under the influence

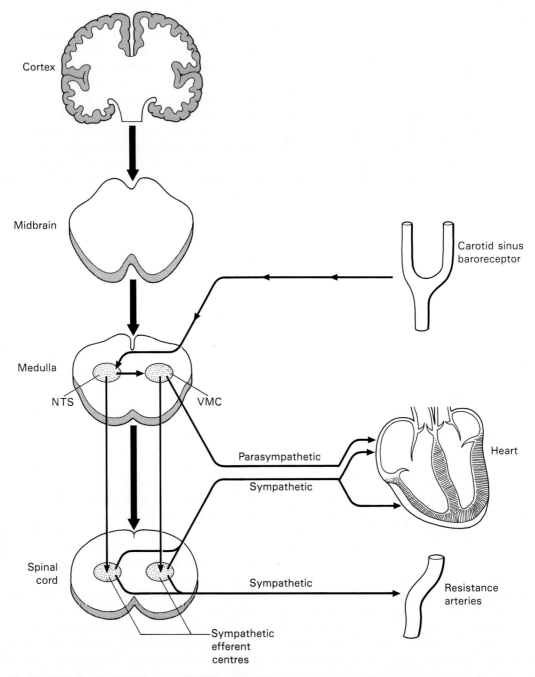

Fig. 24.12 In this simplified diagram of CNS control of blood pressure, many of the complex neural pathways in the cortex, midbrain and medulla are not shown. The effector pathways triggered by the baroreceptors are described in the text.

of a prolonged change in pressure, as in established hypertension, will reset to a higher range of response.

RENIN-ANGIOTENSIN SYSTEM

The enzyme renin is secreted by the juxtaglomerular apparatus of the kidney[12] into the circulation where it hydrolyses the α_2-globulin, angiotensinogen or renin substrate, to produce angiotensin I, a decapeptide. A converting enzyme (kininase II) then hydrolyses the decapeptide to the vasoconstrictor angiotensin II, an octapeptide. Although the converting enzyme is present in plasma, it is particularly concentrated in the lungs and it is found also in the kidneys and in vascular endothelium. The half-life of the active angiotensin II is very short, at most one or two minutes, because it is quickly metabolized by enzyme activity and uptake by effector tissues. In addition to the angiotensin II produced in the circulating blood, angiotensin I is probably converted in situ to the active octapeptide by the converting enzyme produced by the endothelium of the vessels. Indeed, it has been argued recently[13] that the start of the cascade is effectively in the target tissues by the delivery of renin and angiotensinogen to the tissues where angiotensin I and II are produced locally. Angiotensin II exerts its vasoconstrictor effect directly on the smooth muscle of the media, inducing contraction, but it also appears to facilitate the release of noradrenaline from nerve endings to enhance pressor effects in general.

Another important action of angiotensin II is the stimulation of secretion of aldosterone from the zona glomerulosa of the adrenal cortex. Aldosterone induces sodium and water resorption in the distal tubules of the kidney, thereby restoring the extracellular fluid volume in circumstances in which it is depleted. Angiotensin II in small amounts also promotes sodium and water retention by local action within the kidneys. Angiotensin II is also involved in the complex central nervous system blood pressure regulation system referred to above.

Juxtaglomerular apparatus

In normal humans the juxtaglomerular apparatus (JGA)[14] is inconspicuous and much of the information about its structure and function has been derived from experimental animals such as the rat. Where the afferent arteriole to the glomerulus abuts against a specialized segment of the distal tubule, the macula densa, the contiguous smooth

muscle cells are swollen and granulated. The granules are stores of renin and the specialized smooth muscle cells act as stretch receptors, that is, as baroreceptors which are sensitive to changes in perfusion pressure. When pressure falls in the afferent arteriole, renin is secreted into the circulation to produce a rapid pressor effect to restore the pressure.

The juxtaglomerular apparatus is sensitive also to changes in fluid volume and electrolyte levels. It is probable that the macula densa of the distal tubule acts as a chemoreceptor, reacting to the composition of the glomerular filtrate that it receives from the proximal nephron. Initially it was thought that the concentration of sodium ions in the filtrate (urine) was the determining factor, with renin secretion inversely proportional to the level of sodium above and below the norm, but it now seems that the level of the chloride ion is the main trigger. Whatever the exact mechanism ultimately proves to be, sodium and chloride depletion associated with a reduced extracellular fluid volume stimulates the juxtaglomerular apparatus to increase renin production.

Figure 24.13 gives a diagrammatic representation of the interrelationships between the blood pressure, renin activity, the autonomic nervous system, baroreceptors, tissue salt and water content and aldosterone.

ELECTROLYTE METABOLISM IN VASCULAR ACTIVITY

In the last analysis, allowing for the complex regulating mechanisms already mentioned, blood pressure in man is determined by the activity of the smooth muscle in arteries, particularly that in the pre-capillary resistance vessels. The smooth muscle cells functioning as a syncytium, because of the connecting gap junctions or nexuses between adjacent cells, effect a coordinating action in response to stimuli. Vascular smooth muscle is able to regulate blood flow, contracting when flow and pressure rise and relaxing when flow and pressure fall (autoregulation).

Contraction in smooth muscle would appear to be initiated by a rise in intracellular calcium content.[15] Calcium is stored, probably protein-

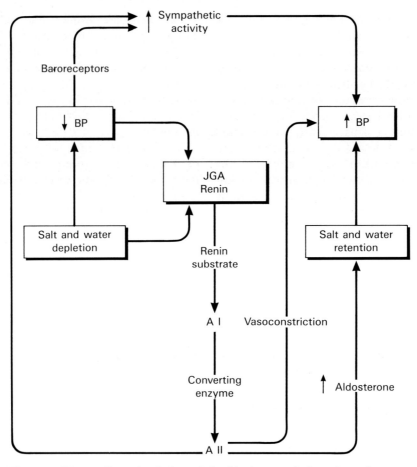

Fig. 24.13 Diagram illustrating the interrelationships between the juxtaglomerular apparatus (JGA), renin, angiotensin, salt and water content of tissues, aldosterone, sympathetic activity and the blood pressure (BP).

bound, in the endoplasmic reticulum of the cell and its transport across the cell membrane is intimately involved with sodium and potassium influx and efflux. There is a high potassium ion concentration and a relatively low sodium ion concentration in cells; the opposite pertains in extracellular fluid. The maintenance of this disparity, essential for normal cell function, requires the activity of the 'sodium pump' as there is a passive permeability of the cell membrane to cation movement. The pump, in essence, is an active transport system for sodium and potassium mediated by adenosine triphosphatase (ATPase): the details of this system are outside the scope of this text. Calcium transport in smooth muscle is

linked in some way to that of sodium and there is evidence that an increase in intracellular sodium concentration leads to release of free calcium ion from its binding sites in the cell. It will therefore be evident that electrolyte disturbance at the cellular level is yet another factor that has to be taken into account in many cardiovascular disorders, a subject that was discussed in Chapter 2.

This brief account of neural, hormonal and other influences on vascular reactivity has excluded many factors which may yet prove to be crucial to a full understanding of the complex regulating system and to the elucidation of vascular disorders. The parts played by amines such as serotonin, the hormone vasopressin (antidiuretic hormone, ADH) and numerous peptides have still to be determined.[16] There are, too, many agents which act on blood vessels locally in circumstances such as inflammation and thrombosis. These include endothelium-derived relaxing factor, the prostaglandins (in particular prostacyclin), the potent vasodilator bradykinin, and histamine but it is not known whether these and other agents have systemic effects that are important in homeostasis of the vascular system.

VASCULAR RESPONSE TO ALTERED HAEMODYNAMICS AND TO INFLAMMATION

The structure of blood vessels is determined to a large extent, from fetal life well into adult life, by the haemodynamic requirements of the vessel in question.[17] The distensible aorta, designed to accommodate the cardiac output after each ventricular contraction, has a high content of the scleroproteins collagen and elastin to provide the necessary strain-bearing tensile strength and elasticity. In contrast, the smaller resistance arteries and arterioles have a lower collagen and elastin content, smooth muscle being the dominant tissue. In general, the ratio of thickness of vessel wall to lumen diameter varies directly with the level of intraluminal pressure.

The vascular system, both arteries and veins, can compensate for temporary fluctuation in haemodynamic forces without structural modification but, if there is a prolonged alteration as in established hypertension, adaptive morphological changes take place which, in the longer term, are detrimental to function and may accen-

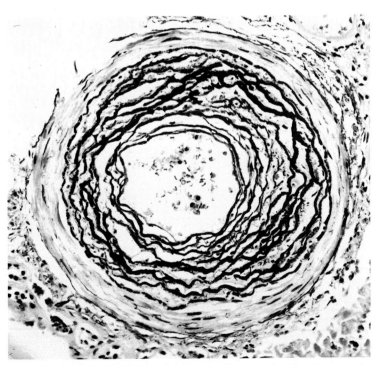

Fig. 24.14 Small intrarenal artery from a case of hypertension showing marked intimal fibroelastosis with narrowing of the lumen.
Elastica/Van Gieson × 150

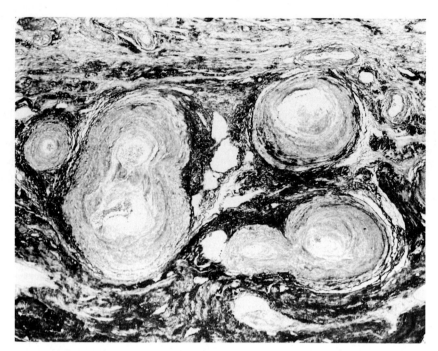

Fig. 24.15 Section from the uterus of an elderly multigravid woman. The involution of the arcuate arteries is indicated by multilayered intimal fibrous tissue with gross reduction in the lumen. There is abundant elastic-type tissue around the vessels.
Elastica/Van Gieson × 20

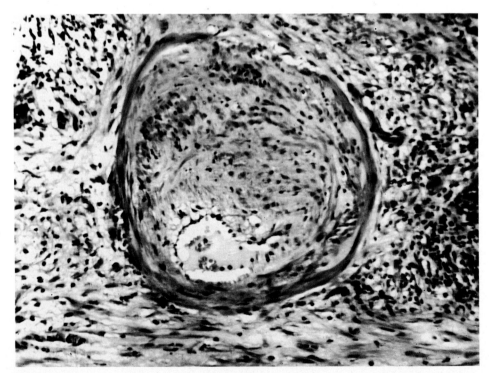

Fig. 24.16 Section of a small artery at the base of a chronic peptic ulcer of the stomach. The chronic inflammation has induced marked proliferative changes in the intima to produce the picture of endarteritis obliterans.
Haematoxylin–eosin × 180
Reproduced by kind permission of Sir Theo Crawford from 'Arteries, veins and lymphatics'. In: Symmers W St

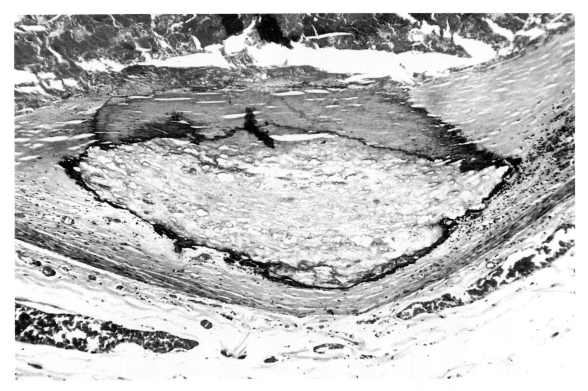

Fig. 24.17 Dystrophic calcification in an atherosclerotic plaque overlying the thinned media of a femoral artery. Partially decalcified tissue; haematoxylin–eosin × 40.
Reproduced by kind permission of Sir Theo Crawford from 'Arteries, veins and lymphatics'. In: Symmers W St C, ed. Systemic Pathology, 2nd ed. Edinburgh: Churchill Livingstone, 1976; 1: 120–169 [Fig. 3.13].

tuate the disease process that initiated the changes. Rising intraluminal pressure is a potent stimulus for collagen and elastin production in vessel walls, increasing the thickness but, in the earlier stages, preserving distensibility and, contrary to what might be expected, reducing the strain throughout the wall. Hypertrophy of smooth muscle cells also occurs, adding to the thickening and promoting increased synthesis of the scleroproteins.

The response to increased luminal pressure in the smaller arteries and arterioles, the muscular resistance vessels, is somewhat different in that hyperplasia in addition to hypertrophy of smooth muscle is a feature; this also leads to increased collagen and elastin synthesis by the medial and myointimal cells, ultimately producing the characteristic 'onion-skin' hyperplastic arteriosclerosis of small vessels

(Fig. 24.14). In these circumstances peripheral resistance, already raised, is increased because of the high ratio of wall thickness to luminal diameter and loss of compliance. The structural changes also amplify pressor responses. It is thought that these adaptive changes, a form of vicious circle, are responsible in the later stages of hypertension for the loss of the lability of the disorder and for the decreased perfusion of organs such as the kidney and heart.

Hypertension is by no means the only condition in which apparently hyperplastic arteries can be seen. In the involution of certain organs, such as the ovary and uterus after the menopause, the parenchymal arteries develop concentric laminar intimal thickening to reduce the calibre of the lumen (Fig. 24.15). Here there is a structural adaptation analogous to that in hypertension but the response is occasioned by reduced blood flow

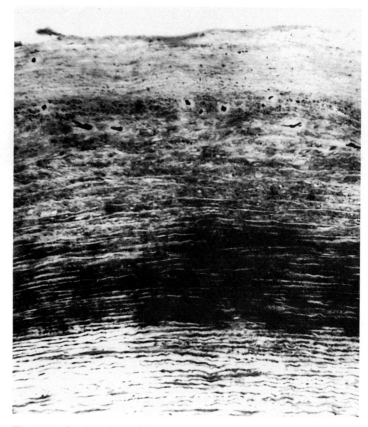

Fig. 24.18 Section of a brachial artery showing Mönckeberg's sclerosis. The media is heavily calcified while the intima shows only a few granules of calcified material.
Von Kossa × 75
Reproduced by kind permission of Sir Theo Crawford from 'Arteries, veins and lymphatics'. In: Symmers W St C, ed. Systemic Pathology, 2nd ed. Edinburgh: Churchill Livingstone, 1976; 1: 120–169 [Fig. 3.5].

to the involuting organ, presumably at a low or normal pressure. The mechanism by which these changes are brought about is unknown.

Blood vessels, being metabolically active tissue, respond to inflammation in or adjacent to the vessel wall in the same way as other tissues. Acute microbial infection and immunologically determined acute inflammatory processes are accompanied by variable degrees and types of necrosis, cellular exudation, oedema, fibrin deposition and all the other features of the acute inflammatory response; they will be dealt with in detail in the appropriate sections of Part B of this volume.

Similarly, chronic inflammation in and around vessels provokes a proliferative response, principally of fibrous tissue, and is accompanied by a cellular exudate, the composition of which depends upon the nature of the agent provoking the inflammation. A particular example of the response of blood vessels to chronic inflammation is seen in the base of active peptic ulceration of the stomach or duodenum (Fig. 24.16).

AGEING CHANGES IN BLOOD VESSELS

Clifford Allbutt[18] many years ago wrote, 'We recognise now, all of us, that in the lapse of man's years one long reckoning of his mortality is, and from all known ages has been, written on the walls

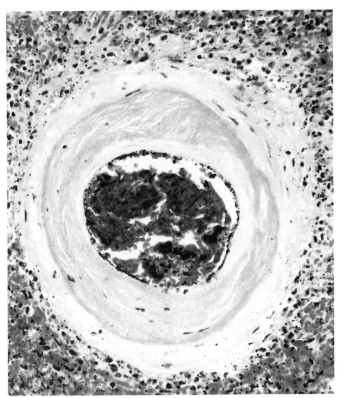

Fig. 24.19 Advanced hyaline change in a splenic arteriole.
Haematoxylin–eosin × 140
*Reproduced by kind permission of Sir Theo Crawford from 'Arteries, veins and
lymphatics'. In: Symmers W St C, ed. Systemic Pathology, 2nd ed.
Edinburgh: Churchill Livingstone, 1976; 1: 120–169 [Fig. 3.19].*

of his vessels'. He was referring, of course, to the progressive 'wear and tear' changes that occur, albeit with considerable individual variation, with age compounded by the lesions of arteriosclerosis and atherosclerosis. Indeed, some would aver[19] that such changes commence in infancy with a gradual increase in the thickness of the intima and some fraying of the internal elastic lamina, seen particularly well in the coronary arteries of otherwise normal young people.

The intimal thickening comprises an increase in elastic fibrils, collagen, glycosaminoglycan ground substance and myointimal cells (modified smooth muscle cells migrating through the fenestrations of the internal elastic lamina). Somewhat later, changes can be detected in the media with fragmentation of elastic fibres, accumulation of ground substance and increase in collagen fibres. In large arteries of the elastic type, these age-related changes lead to loss of elasticity, sclerosis of the wall, progressive distension and, in some vessels, tortuosity—in sum, the senile ectasia described by Aschoff[20] and now often referred to as arteriomegaly.[21] Usually, but to a variable degree, the ageing and degenerative changes are complicated and compounded by atherosclerotic lesions, the intimal damage creating further damage to the underlying media. Overt dystrophic calcification, a common feature of advanced atherosclerosis (Fig. 24.17), is not a frequent accompaniment of vascular medial degeneration but is seen in classic form in Mönckeberg's sclerosis of arteries such as the iliac, femoral and brachial (Fig. 24.18) and in the uterine arteries of elderly multigravid women.

The smaller muscular arteries down to the level of the arterioles also show progressive ageing changes. The intima tends to thicken concentrically with increased collagen and elastic fibrils produced by myointimal cells while the media undergoes hyalinosis with loss of smooth muscle and elastic tissue and their replacement by collagenous fibrous tissue. The hyaline ('glassy') change (Fig. 24.19) has long defied a satisfactory pathogenetic explanation but is now regarded as a form of plasmatic vasculosis,[22] that is, the insudation of complex protein material from the plasma into the vessel wall and its deposition there in ageing collagen. These age-related degenerative changes in small blood vessels frequently present problems of histological interpretation when they are seen in cases of recognized disease since certain disorders, such as hypertension and chronic inflammatory conditions, accentuate the features.

Age-related changes occur also in veins and are familiar to even the casual observer in the arms and legs of elderly people, particularly when there are varicosities of the leg veins. Sclerosis of the vessel wall and, most important, the development of incompetent venous valves underlie much of the pathology of veins, which will be dealt with in Part B of this volume.

REFERENCES

1. Harvey W. The works of William Harvey: translated by Willis R. Philadelphia: University of Pennsylvania Press, 1989.
2. Swales JD. Clinical hypertension. London: Chapman & Hall, 1979.
3. Hüttner I, Kocher O, Gabbiani G. Endothelial and smooth muscle cells. In: Camilleri J-P, Berry CL, Fiessinger J-N, Bariéty J, eds. Diseases of the arterial wall. London: Springer-Verlag, 1989: 3–41.
4. Legrand YJ, Drouet LO. The arterial wall and the haemostatic process. In: Camilleri J-P, Berry CL, Fiessinger J-N, Bariéty J, eds. Diseases of the arterial wall. London: Springer-Verlag, 1989: 127–141.
5. Leading Article. EDRF. Lancet 1987; 2: 137–138.
6. Collier J, Vallance P. Physiological importance of nitric oxide. Br Med J 1991; 302: 1289–1290.
7. Noordhoek Hegt V. Distribution and variation of fibrinolytic activity in the walls of human arteries and veins. Haemostasis 1976; 5: 355–372.
8. Dhital KK, Burnstock G. Adrenergic and non-adrenergic neural control of the arterial wall. In: Camilleri J-P, Berry CL, Fiessinger J-N, Bariéty J, eds. Diseases of the arterial wall. London: Springer-Verlag, 1989: 97–126.
9. Robert L, Birembaut P. Extracellular matrix of the arterial vessel wall. In: Camilleri J-P, Berry CL, Fiessinger J-N, Bariéty J, eds. Diseases of the arterial wall. London: Springer-Verlag, 1989: 43–54.
10. Brody MJ, Barron KW, Faber JE, Hartle DK, Lappe RW. Central nervous system control of blood pressure. In: Sleight P, Freis E, eds. Cardiology 1: Hypertension. London: Butterworths, 1982: 199–215.
11. Tatemoto K, Carlquist M, Mutt V. Neuropeptide Y—a novel brain peptide with structural similarities to peptide YY and pancreatic polypeptide. Nature 1982; 296: 659–660.
12. Barajas L, Salido E. Juxtaglomerular apparatus and the renin-angiotensin system. Lab Invest 1986; 54: 361–364.
13. Samani NJ. New developments in renin and hypertension. Tissue generation of angiotensin I & II changes the picture. Br Med J 1991; 302: 981–982.
14. Heptinstall RH. Pathology of the kidney, 4th ed, Vol I. Boston: Little, Brown, 1992: 68–71.
15. Blaustein MP. Sodium ions, calcium ions, blood pressure regulation, and hypertension; a reassessment and a hypothesis. Am J Physiol 1977; 232: c165–c173.
16. Alhenc-Gelas F, Corvol P. The vascular wall and hormonal control of vasomotor function. In: Camilleri J-P, Berry CL, Fiessinger J-N, Bariéty J, eds. Diseases of the arterial wall. London: Springer-Verlag, 1989: 97–126.
17. Berry CL. Organogenesis of the arterial wall. In: Camilleri J-P, Berry CL, Fiessinger J-N, Bariéty J, eds. Diseases of the arterial wall. London: Springer-Verlag, 1989: 55–70.
18. Allbutt TC. Diseases of the arteries including angina pectoris. London: Macmillan, 1915.
19. Levene CI. The early lesions of atheroma in the coronary arteries. J Pathol Bacteriol 1956; 72: 79–82.
20. Aschoff L. Lectures on pathology. New York: Hoeber, 1924.
21. Tilson D, Dang C. Generalized arteriomegaly: a possible predisposition to the formation of abdominal aortic aneurysms. Arch Surg 1981; 116: 1030–1032.
22. Lendrum AC. The hypertensive diabetic kidney as a model of the so-called collagen diseases. Can Med Assoc J 1963; 88: 442–452.

Hypertension

INTRODUCTION

Hypertension, literally 'overstretched', is the word now used universally to denote raised pressure within a vascular system, despite past attempts to introduce the etymologically more correct term hyperpiesia.[1] In this chapter we are concerned only with raised pressure in the systemic circulation, pulmonary hypertension being dealt with in Chapter 26 while portal hypertension, raised pressure in the portal venous system, is considered in the volume of this series dealing with the pathology of the liver (Volume 11).

The pathology of systemic hypertension has to be considered from two viewpoints. First, the aetiological and pathogenetic factors involved in the development of the condition, including the part, if any, played by the cardiovascular system itself in the genesis of abnormally high blood pressure. Second, the effects of the raised pressure on the cardiovascular system and on other systems and organs. It may be that we are dealing with a so-called vicious circle in which the effects of hypertension on the heart and blood vessels themselves aggravate the condition; there is certainly evidence for this in longstanding cases of hypertension.

The subject is complicated by problems of terminology, definition and classification. It is customary to label all cases of raised blood pressure as 'essential' when there is no demonstrable accepted cause or predisposing disorder. Essential, used by most writers in preference to primary, is nowadays a somewhat incongruous term, derived from the original meaning of being of the essence of a phenomenon or intrinsic to its nature. When first used in 1911 in this context by Frank[2] the word essential was the equivalent of idiopathic, namely of unknown cause. When essential hypertension is of mild or moderate degree and even of many years' duration it is frequently prefixed by benign to distinguish this state from the more sinister accelerated phase of hypertension which, if untreated, may lead to overt malignant hypertension.

A satisfactory definition of hypertension has not been reached for a number of reasons. Blood pressure is a dynamic variable in most individuals, depending on the mental and physical state of the individual at the time of measurement. The very act of recording blood pressure may cause an increase in levels, the alerting response, 'clinic' or 'white coat' hypertension familar to clinicians. In westernized societies blood pressure tends to rise with age so that readings which are regarded as normal at the age of 60 would be considered as abnormally high at the age of 30. There is, too, the problem of categorizing individuals with a high systolic reading but a normal diastolic level and, vice versa, those with high diastolic readings and only marginal rises in systolic pressure. It would be convenient if the normal upper limits were accepted as 120 mmHg systolic and 80 mmHg diastolic but these would be too restrictive for a physiological state that is inherently very labile and responsive to many exogenous and endogenous influences. The World Health Organization has produced definitions[3] which are useful in enabling comparability in epidemiological and population studies but they are of little help to clinicians dealing with individual patients. They are: (a) normal blood pressure—140/90 or below; (b) borderline blood pressure—between 140/90 and 160/95; and (c) hypertensive—160/95 and above.

Some 30 years ago two authorities, Pickering[4] and Platt,[5] engaged in a debate as to whether in a population the distribution of blood pressure levels is unimodal or bimodal. Pickering argued forcibly for a unimodal distribution and insisted that hypertension be classified quantitatively as a continuous variable about the norm like many human characteristics such as height and weight. Platt held the view equally strongly that the distribution of blood pressure levels is bimodal,

implying that hypertension is a distinct entity qualitatively different from the blood pressure in normal individuals. The debate continues to this day. Population studies identifying individuals and families genetically predisposed to hypertension[6] add weight to the bimodal view of the distribution of hypertension in populations. On the other hand, advances in the knowledge of the genetic make-up of man seem to point to genetic factors in almost every disease. Perhaps the two sides of the debate rest on differences that are more apparent than real or relevant.

The next immediate question is what level of hypertension is significant in causing pathological effects in the short and longer terms. As somewhere in the region of 15–20% of the populations of westernized developed countries are categorized as hypertensive, this question is crucial for the clinician as the answer will determine whether or not treatment should be instituted. The massive actuarial data produced by insurance companies[7] and other large group studies[8,9] show that the incidence of cardiovascular disorders such as coronary (ischaemic) heart disease and cerebrovascular accidents rises pari passu with incremental rises in blood pressure above the modest level of 140/90. Mortality statistics reveal a similar deterioration with rising levels of blood pressure. The implications, in terms of cost and the employment of medical manpower, of preventative drug treatment have provoked much debate on the long-term efficacy of such prophylaxis.[10]

EPIDEMIOLOGY

Epidemiological studies, of which there are many, have clearly established that there are significant differences in the mean levels of blood pressure amongst populations throughout the world. Populations leading a tribal life at a basic subsistence level, which has been their mode of life for centuries, have low blood pressure levels which rise little, if at all, with increasing age.[11,12] This contrasts strongly with the higher average readings of so-called civilized or westernized societies in whom there is a significant rise in blood pressure with advancing age.[13] The prevalence and incidence of cardiovascular disease reflect the difference in mean blood pressure levels between the two types of population, primitive societies having very low incidences of coronary heart disease and cerebrovascular accidents while in westernized societies cardiovascular diseases as a group are the major causes of morbidity and mortality. The demonstration that migration of people from primitive rural environments to more affluent urban surroundings leads to a progressive rise in blood pressure in the migrants indicates the part played by environmental factors in determining the level of blood pressure.[14] This is reinforced by comparing the levels of blood pressure recorded in tribal, rural Africans[12] with those reported in their descendants in succeeding generations in the West Indies[15] and in the United States of America.[13] In the USA, the black population has a higher mean level of blood pressure than the white population and both suffer much the same high incidence of cardiovascular diseases.[16]

While the stress of living in affluent westernized societies, a difficult factor to quantify, is considered important in influencing blood pressure, most attention has been directed to dietary factors and, in particular, to the salt content of the diet. There is ample evidence from epidemiological studies[17] that populations consuming low levels of salt in their diet have lower mean blood pressures than populations with a high salt content in the diet. The relation of salt ingestion to hypertension is discussed later.

Epidemiological studies would seem to show that adverse environmental factors are crucial aetiological agents in the genesis of hypertension. While they are obviously important, other factors must play a part as the majority in populations exposed to these adverse environmental factors, whatever they may prove to be, do not develop sustained significantly high levels of blood pressure. As already mentioned, family studies indicate also a genetic factor, further evidence for this coming from studies on identical twins who retain the same pattern of blood pressure even though they have lived in different environments for many years.[6] For the moment then, the evidence available would support the view that hypertension results from environmental factors operating upon individuals genetically predisposed to react more strongly to those factors. Such a view accords well with the variability in blood pressure levels between and within different geographical populations, including the variability among age groups.

AETIOLOGY AND PATHOGENESIS OF ESSENTIAL HYPERTENSION

Although it is customary in describing diseases to separate aetiology, the factors initiating disorders, from pathogenesis, the evolution of a disease from its initiation to its fully developed form, this approach is impossible with hypertension because of the complexity of interaction of the many factors and agents initiating, promoting and aggravating a rise in blood pressure. Systemic blood pressure can be expressed as the product of cardiac output and total peripheral vascular resistance and this section will deal with the various theories that have been proposed to explain the deviations from the norm that lead to the development of hypertension.

Increased peripheral vascular resistance

While there is evidence that cardiac output is increased in people in the early stages of essential hypertension and in normotensive first-degree relatives, it is generally agreed that in established hypertension the significant defect is increased peripheral vascular resistance.[18] Factors which initiate a rise in blood pressure are not necessarily the same as those that sustain a high blood pressure and from the practical clinical point of view, the latter may be regarded as more important. The small peripheral arteries and arterioles, the resistance vessels, respond to many biochemical and electrophysiological agents acting on the smooth muscle which is their dominant component and it has been postulated that in hypertensive individuals there is an enhanced pressor response to vasoconstricting agents and a diminished response to vasodilators.[19] Prolonged vasoconstriction allied to increased luminal pressure leads to hypertrophy and hyperplasia of vascular smooth muscle and an increase in collagen and elastic tissue in the walls of the resistance vessels. The increased bulk of smooth muscle may explain the increased response of the resistance vessels to vasoconstrictors such as noradrenaline and angiotensin II but an intrinsic defect in vascular smooth muscle in those with essential hypertension[20] has not been ruled out. The significant decrease from the normal in peripheral vascular compliance in young people with mild hypertension and in their normotensive first-degree relatives is supportive evidence for a primary defect in the resistance vessels in essential hypertension.[21]

Be that as it may, it is at this early stage that the vicious circle can be considered to have started with factors initiating the rise in blood pressure and resultant structural changes in small arteries leading to permanently increased peripheral resistance and a sustained high blood pressure.

Increased response to sympathetic nervous activity

The known hypertensive effects of catecholamines acting on the heart and peripheral vessels and the benefits of autonomic blocking agents in the treatment of hypertension are the basis of the theory that hyperreactivity of the target vessels to sympathetic stimulation is a cause of hypertension. In a proportion of patients with essential hypertension there are increased plasma concentrations of noradrenaline,[22] implying overactivity of the sympathetic nervous system. The increased plasma concentrations in such patients may be due not so much to excess production of catecholamines but to altered handling and clearance of these agents because of structural alterations in the resistance vessels.[23] There is also the possibility that in hypertensives with normal plasma levels of noradrenaline the peripheral vessels may over-react due to a defect in the vascular smooth muscle, inherent or acquired. As stated in the previous section, hypertensive people show a greater response than normotensive people to the same intravenous doses of angiotensin II and noradrenaline.

Salt and water retention

Epidemiological studies have shown quite conclusively that there is a good correlation between the mean blood pressure of populations and the consumption of salt: the higher the intake the higher is the mean pressure.[17] The correlation does not hold, however, for individuals within a given population[24] and this has led to the postulate that only individuals with a genetic predisposition to defective handling of salt and water will develop hypertension when exposed to diets with a high salt content, a return to Platt's assertion of the bimodal distribution of hypertension in populations. The basis of the salt theory is that there is a congenital defect in the kidney rendering it less efficient in secreting sodium, with resultant expansion of the extracellular fluid compartment and triggering of the renin-angiotensin-aldosterone and other regulatory systems to re-establish homeostasis but with 'compensatory' hypertension as the inevitable outcome. The theory has been refined by the suggestion that essential hypertension may be due to the effects of excess quantities of a circulating hormone, the natriuretic factor.[25] According to this hypothesis, the high levels of the natriuretic hormone depress the sodium pump at the cellular level, increasing the influx of calcium into vascular smooth muscle cells with resultant constriction of the resistance vessels and hypertension. While the theory is attractive in offering an explanation for the genetic, epidemiological and other features of hypertension, it still falls far short of proof in humans and is not universally accepted.

Autoregulation

In each vascular bed there is a regulatory mechanism which ensures that when the perfusion pressure rises or falls outside a certain range, the resistance vessels constrict or distend as appropriate to maintain a constant blood flow. One theory of hypertension incriminates the autoregulatory mechanism throughout the body, postulating that there is increased cardiac output due to an increased venous return to the heart, in turn induced by sodium retention associated with an expanded extracellular fluid volume.[26] The increase in cardiac output then triggers vasoconstriction in all the resistance arteries, leading to a rise in systemic blood pressure which, if prolonged, would induce structural changes in the peripheral arteries to keep the pressure raised even if other regulating mechanisms effected natriuresis by resetting the threshold for sodium excretion to correct the sodium imbalance and restore the extracellular fluid volume to normal.

Renin-angiotensin system

Because angiotensin II is a potent vasoconstrictor and causes hypertension in acute experiments, it is to be expected that overproduction of renin should be considered a key factor in the genesis of essential hypertension. The idea received a considerable boost over 50 years ago when Goldblatt and his colleagues[27] described the production of hypertension in the dog by various combinations of renal artery clipping and nephrectomy. However, subsequent research has shown[28] that while the renin-angiotensin system is involved in the early stages of the experimentally-produced hypertension other factors, including salt retention, operate to sustain the high blood pressure. Furthermore, in man, essential hypertension is associated with low plasma renin levels in a minority of cases and with higher than normal levels in a further minority.[29] In effect, there is no consistent pattern nor does sodium depletion consistently induce renin production in hypertensive subjects. The available evidence suggests that the renin-angiotensin system is involved in the mechanisms promoting and sustaining the hypertension but that this system is not the seat of the fundamental defect and that its involvement is a secondary phenomenon.

From this summarized review of the current theories of the genesis of essential hypertension it will readily be appreciated that there is considerable overlap amongst the theories, an inevitable consequence of the inter-relationships of the many complex mechanisms controlling blood pressure in man. It may be that there is not a single entity, essential hypertension, but that the condition that is so named is a collection of heterogeneous disorders with related, but discrete, defects that eventually lead to a clinical pattern with similar features and consequences in all cases, irrespective of the differences between the underlying defects.

ACCELERATED PHASE OR MALIGNANT HYPERTENSION

For reasons that are unknown, a small minority of people with established hypertension enter a rapidly progressive phase of the disorder, the accelerated phase, with diastolic pressures quickly climbing to 130 and above. Unless treatment is instituted, this phase will culminate in overt malignant hypertension characterized by the development of severe headaches, visual disturbance due to retinal damage, dyspnoea from left ventricular failure, and signs of deterioration in renal function.[30] The retinal changes — papilloedema, flame haemorrhages and exudates — are considered pathognomonic of malignant hypertension. In untreated cases, or cases refractory to treatment, death within two years of onset from renal failure, hypertensive encephalopathy or cerebral haemorrhage is almost inevitable. Fortunately, the development of effective antihypertensive drugs over the last three decades has considerably reduced the incidence of overt malignant hypertension and of its serious complications[31] so that the condition is now seen mainly in patients suffering from secondary, particularly renal, hypertension.

Because of treatment, it is now uncommon for malignant hypertension to be seen as a consequence of benign essential hypertension; when this does occur, it is usually in untreated people between the ages of 30 and 50 years. It affects men more than women (although fulminating pre-eclampsia during pregnancy is analogous) and it is commoner in the black than in the white races. It tends to occur in the 'high renin' groups of hypertensives. In cases supervening on secondary hypertension the main underlying diseases are rapidly progressive proliferative glomerulonephritis, polyarteritis, Wegener's disease, scleroderma with renal involvement, systemic lupus erythematosus and renal artery stenosis.

OTHER TYPES OF HYPERTENSION

The vast majority, in excess of 95%, of all individuals with raised blood pressure are categorized as having essential hypertension. In the others the hypertension is due to a detectable underlying disorder and is described as secondary.

Renal hypertension

Richard Bright,[32] in 1836, was the first to connect high blood pressure with chronic renal disease and it is interesting that his observations antedated by quite some time the distinction between renal and essential hypertension, the latter being unrecognized as an entity until Allbutt[33] described it some 60 years later. The demonstration by Goldblatt and his colleagues,[27] in 1934, that hypertension could be caused by clipping the renal arteries in dogs to produce renal ischaemia led to the differentiation of renal hypertension in man into two types, one due to chronic ischaemia and the other to chronic parenchymal disease of other causation (the original Bright's disease). The two types are commonly labelled renovascular and renoprival respectively.

Renal ischaemia

The two main causes of acquired stenosis of the renal arteries are fibromuscular dysplasia and atherosclerosis, the former occurring as a relative rarity, usually in women in the third and fourth decades of life, the latter more commonly in older men. Various subtypes of fibromuscular dysplasia have been described,[34] depending upon whether the intima, media or adventitia of the arteries bears the brunt of the excessive collagen depositions, but the net effect is the same — severe ischaemia of the kidneys and hypertension. Atherosclerosis of the more distal portions of the main renal arteries is uncommon but severe atherosclerosis of the aorta may involve the ostia and extend into the first few millimetres of the renal arteries, thereby producing stenosis and consequent renal ischaemia (Fig. 25.1). Atheromatous stenosis may be unilateral only or unequally bilateral, whereas fibromuscular stenosis is more usually bilateral.

The mechanism producing the hypertension is almost certainly stimulation of the renin-angiotensin system by the ischaemic kidney(s) leading to high plasma renin levels in most, but not all, patients with renovascular hypertension. Furthermore, surgical correction of the arterial defect leads, in most cases, to return of the blood pressure to normal levels and corresponding reversal of the plasma renin levels. In the minority who do not respond to surgical treatment it is probable that the hypertension is sustained by chronic damage inflicted on the kidney(s) or induced irreversible changes in the peripheral resistance vessels or a combination of both, whereby mechanisms already discussed, other than the renin-angiotensin system, are activated.

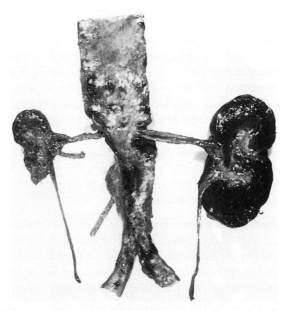

Fig. 25.1 Atherosclerosis of the aorta causing severe stenosis of the ostium of the left renal artery with resultant ischaemia and atrophy of the kidney leading to renovascular hypertension.

Hypertension in chronic renal disease

There is a long list of chronic renal disorders, unilateral and bilateral, that have been described as causes of secondary hypertension. The evidence for many of these associations is secure, for others debatable, and it has to be borne in mind during the assessment of such cases that individuals with essential hypertension, known or unknown, are not immune from contracting renal disease. There is, too, the consideration that those genetically susceptible to the development of essential hypertension may have that susceptibility enhanced and declared by the development of renal disease whereas those without the genetic defect may remain normotensive despite the renal disease. An analogous situation is encountered in the hypertensive disorders of pregnancy, to be discussed later.

Glomerulonephritis

Hypertension is a feature of most cases of glomerulonephritis, whatever the aetiology and pathogenesis of the latter. The observations made here apply to the glomerular diseases associated with streptococcal and other infectious agents, autoimmune disorders such as polyarteritis, systemic sclerosis (scleroderma), systemic lupus erythematosus and Henoch–Schönlein purpura, and other glomerulopathies of known and unknown aetiology.

While most patients with chronic glomerulonephritis develop hypertension at some stage, usually later in the disease, the mechanisms involved are complex and incompletely understood. The hypertension characteristic of acute post-streptococcal glomerulonephritis is probably generated by sodium and water retention associated with oliguria and oedema. Simultaneous activation of the renin-angiotensin system may also be a factor, the trigger being the acute ischaemia induced in the kidneys by the glomerular damage; however, plasma renin levels are not usually raised. The severity of hypertension in chronic glomerulonephritis correlates in general with the severity of the renal disorder, particularly in those with progressive renal failure associated with sodium and fluid retention.

Additionally, the renin-angiotensin system may be involved because the secondary damage to the afferent arterioles causes increased vascular resistance within the kidneys. In effect, the hypertension could be both renoprival (loss of kidney substance) and renovascular.

Malignant hypertension secondary to renal disease

Malignant hypertension occasionally may supervene in any form of renal hypertension but, as stated earlier, it is particularly associated with the fulminating form of acute proliferative glomerulonephritis, with rapidly progressive polyarteritis, the late renal manifestations of systemic sclerosis and systemic lupus erythematosus, and in hypertension secondary to renal artery stenosis.

Chronic pyelonephritis

There is uncertainty about the relation of chronic pyelonephritis to secondary hypertension and pathologists are particularly to blame for this situation. In the past, and still today, there is an unwarranted readiness to label non-specific scarring with round cell infiltrates in the kidney as 'chronic pyelonephritis', whether in renal biopsies or in autopsy specimens. This non-specific histological feature is amongst the commonest of incidental findings at autopsy. While the label may be terminologically justified it unfortunately carries the implication that the lesion is the result of bacterial infection at some time in the past and in the great majority of cases there is no supporting evidence for the supposition.[35] Undoubtedly there is an association between hypertension and the condition labelled, for want of a definitive diagnosis, chronic pyelonephritis, particularly where there is severe unilateral disease with a small scarred kidney (Fig. 25.2) and when, in some cases but by no means in all, the hypertension is corrected by removal of the diseased kidney. Interestingly, there is evidence from family studies that people with essential hypertension and their normotensive blood relatives are more prone to develop 'chronic pyelonephritis' than those with no genetic predis-

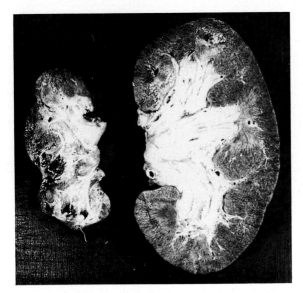

Fig. 25.2 Female aged 50 with chronic hypertension: at autopsy the left kidney was shrunken but with a patent renal artery—histology showed the features of chronic pyelonephritis.

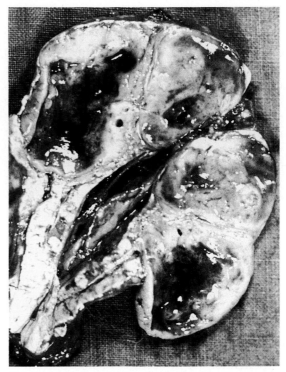

Fig. 25.3 Haemorrhagic necrosis of a phaeochromocytoma of the adrenal medulla. Incidental finding at autopsy from a patient dying of intracerebral haemorrhage.

position to essential hypertension.[35] This may be an example of the unmasking of hypertension, already referred to, by an acquired disorder.

Secondary (renal) hypertension has been reported in a variety of disorders of the urinary system, including renal tuberculosis, diabetic nephropathy, gouty nephropathy, irradiation damage to the kidneys, urinary tract obstruction, particularly when unilateral, and polycystic disease of the kidneys. The pathology of these conditions is dealt with in the volume of this series devoted to disorders of the urinary system (Volume 8).

Endocrine hypertension

Because of the role of the endocrine system in cardiovascular regulation it is to be expected that certain disorders of that system are accompanied by high blood pressure, induced by a variety of mechanisms.

Phaeochromocytoma

This catecholamine-producing tumour is perhaps the best-known example of an endocrine cause of hypertension.[36] The tumour arises from the chromaffin cells of the adrenergic system, the adrenal medulla (Fig. 25.3) accounting for 90% of cases with the paraganglionic cells of the sympathetic system and the para-aortic organ of Zuckerkandl as the minority sites. The autopsy incidence of phaeochromocytoma has been estimated to be 0.1%, a somewhat surprisingly high figure in view of the relatively rarity with which the tumour is diagnosed in the clinical investigation of patients with hypertension. It has to be said, however, that there is no more regrettable circumstance than when this tumour, eminently curable and undiagnosed in life, is found at autopsy when death has been due to, say, an intracerebral haemorrhage. The hypertension associated with phaeochromocytoma is the direct result of the secretion of large amounts of vasopressor amines, noradrenaline being the major component. In 50% of cases the hypertension is paroxysmal; this probably accounts for

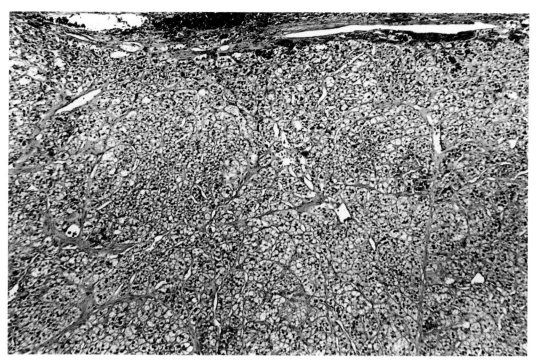

Fig. 25.4 Section of an adenoma of the zona glomerulosa of the adrenal cortex from a case of Conn's syndrome. Haematoxylin–eosin × 90

some of those tumours revealed only at autopsy since in cases in which the hypertension is persistent, although fluctuating, the tumour can be diagnosed by appropriate clinical investigations such as urinary estimation of catecholamine metabolites, normetanephrine and vanillylmandelic acid (VMA), and radiological imaging techniques. About 10% of cases are familial and in a small proportion there is an association with medullary carcinoma of the thyroid, parathyroid adenomas and neurofibromatosis. About 20% of cases have multiple tumours and in 5% of all cases metastases have been reported. The presence of metastatic deposits is the only means of distinguishing the malignant phaeochromocytoma from the benign as the pathological features of the two are otherwise the same.

Primary aldosteronism (Conn's syndrome)

This uncommon condition is due to an adenoma (Fig. 25.4) or bilateral hyperplasia of the zona glomerulosa of the adrenal glands.[37] The resultant excess secretion of aldosterone causes increased resorption of sodium by, and loss of potassium from, the renal tubules together with expansion of the extracellular fluid volume. The hypokalaemia accounts for the pronounced muscle weakness characteristic of the condition. Because expansion of the extracellular fluid volume reflexly leads to suppression of renin production, the hypertension cannot be attributed to angiotensin II hyperactivity. Persistence of the elevated extracellular fluid volume, in association with sodium retention, and a direct pressor effect by mineralocorticoids on the resistance vessels have been suggested in explanation of this form of secondary hypertension but, as yet, the exact mechanism is undetermined.

While surgical removal of the offending adenoma or of adrenal cortical tissue in cases of hyperplasia may correct the electrolyte imbalance, cure of the hypertension may not be achieved, particularly in those with adrenal cortical hyperplasia.

Cushing's syndrome

Hypertension is present in most cases of this disorder, which is due to excess adrenocortical secretions from an adrenal tumour or from cortical hyperplasia (Fig. 25.5) or to adrenocortical overactivity resulting from corticotrophin secretion by a pituitary adenoma.[37] The features of the syndrome include adiposity of the upper half of the body, diabetes mellitus, osteoporosis, dusky complexion and, in women, amenorrhoea, hypertrichosis and cutaneous striae, all induced by oversecretion of glucocorticoid and, in some cases, of mineralocorticoid hormones. Similar features, including hypertension, may complicate glucocorticoid therapy ('steroid therapy') in certain chronic diseases, such as Still's disease (juvenile rheumatoid arthritis). As in aldosteronism, the cause of the hypertension is undetermined. It is not due to excess renin production, as the plasma renin is usually in the normal range, nor to sodium retention as there is no evidence of suppression of the renin-angiotensin system as would occur with sodium overload. The suspicion is that a direct pressor effect of either mineralocorticoid or glucocorticoid hormones, or both, is involved.

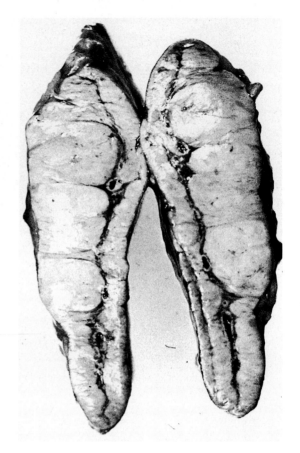

Fig. 25.5 Marked hyperplasia, focally nodular, of the adrenal cortex in a case of Cushing's syndrome.

Congenital adrenal hyperplasia

In this rare congenital disorder there are deficiencies in the enzymes involved in the synthesis of cortisol which lead to compensatory hyperplasia of the adrenal cortices resulting in overproduction of mineralocorticoid hormones.[37] Two forms have been described. The first is 11β-hydroxylase deficiency which is characterized by infantile virilism (pseudo-hermaphroditism) due to excess secretion of adrenal androgens. The second is 17α-hydroxylase deficiency which is not associated with virilism but, in girls, with failure of secondary sexual development at puberty. In both forms the occurrence of hypertension is attributed to the overproduction of mineralocorticoids.

Hypertension is reported in a smaller proportion of cases of other endocrine disorders, including acromegaly, hyperparathyroidism and myxoedema. The mechanisms of production of hypertension in these cases, and indeed the relevance of the endocrine disturbance, are debatable.

Oral contraceptives

Synthetic oestrogens and progestagens in various combinations used for contraceptive purposes are the factors that most frequently predispose to hypertension in young women. The qualification 'predisposing' has to be used as, in many cases, there is a family history of hypertension and the suspicion must arise that in these women the genetic predisposition to hypertension has been enhanced by the steroidal preparations. Furthermore, the majority of these women are diagnosed incidentally as hypertensive when attending general practitioner or hospital clinics for other reasons and an unknown number may have been in the borderline zone of hypertension before starting contraceptive medication. Nevertheless, withdrawal of the steroids leads to the return of normal blood pressure in most cases. The oestrogen component of the pill is thought to be the promoter of hypertension by causing increased production of renin substrate by the liver and by enhancing sodium resorption in the kidneys and so leading to expansion of the extra-cellular fluid volume.[38] The progestagen component may also be involved. The whole subject of hypertension in association with the contraceptive pill is ambiguous and under-researched.

Other associations with hypertension

Central nervous system lesions

In view of the complex and anatomically widespread regulatory influence of the central nervous system on the cardiovascular system it is not surprising that lesions in the central nervous system may be associated with a rise in blood pressure.

It is well known that mental stress, in normotensives as well as in hypertensives, can cause significant elevation of the blood pressure; even the procedure of blood pressure measurement can have this effect, which is why random blood pressure readings cannot be regarded as the true level in any individual. Rapid rise in intracranial pressure from whatever cause—intracranial haemorrhage, intracranial tumour, or severe trauma to the brain—is associated with a rise in blood pressure, the Cushing response, which is thought to be a reflex response of the sympathetic system causing vasoconstriction. Lesions of the brainstem and of the upper part of the spinal cord may produce the same response.

Hypertension in pregnancy

The various hypertensive disorders of pregnancy are of major concern to obstetricians as they are associated with an increase in fetal and neonatal morbidity and mortality. In the United Kingdom, the complications of hypertension, as a group, are the single largest cause of maternal mortality,[39] fortunately now an uncommon event.

The subject is confused by lack of agreement on criteria for diagnosis and on definitions, particularly in relation to the pre-eclampsia/eclampsia syndrome.[40,41] Two distinct groups can be identified. The first comprises women known to have hypertension, whether essential or secondary, before pregnancy; the second comprises women known to be normotensive before pregnancy and early in its course who, after the 20th week of gestation, develop hypertension with proteinuria as overt pre-eclampsia. Between these two groups there are a number of women who develop hypertension without proteinuria, referred to variously by different authorities as pregnancy-induced hypertension or gestational hypertension. There is, too, the problem of categorizing women with hypertension established before pregnancy, with or without proteinuria, whose condition worsens during pregnancy; they are usually regarded as having pre-eclampsia superimposed upon essential hypertension or upon secondary, usually renal, hypertension. The differentiation between the last two categories depends upon whether the patients had proteinuria in the early weeks of pregnancy (renal hypertension plus pre-eclampsia) or developed proteinuria after the 20th week of gestation (essential hypertension plus pre-eclampsia). As with other forms of hypertension, there is good evidence from family studies that women with a genetic predisposition to essential hypertension may have the condition unmasked by pregnancy, particularly those women who develop hypertension without proteinuria during pregnancy.

The pre-eclampsia/eclampsia syndrome has been named 'the disease of theories' and its aetiology continues to baffle investigators. It is a disorder usually occurring in first pregnancies; those women who suffer recurrent pre-eclampsia in subsequent pregnancies are suspected of having latent renal disease or a predisposition to essential hypertension. Long-term follow-up studies confirm that many such women develop chronic hypertension in later life. Manifestly, pre-eclampsia is associated in some way with an abnormal reaction by the pregnant mother to the trophoblast of her fetus. The condition occurs only in pregnancy and resolves quickly and completely after removal of the fetus and placenta

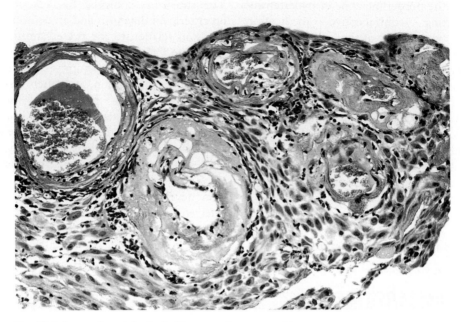

Fig. 25.6 Acute atherosis in the decidua vera of a woman with severe pre-eclampsia in the third trimester of pregnancy. The spiral arteries show fibrinoid necrosis and the damaged walls contain vacuolated lipophages. There is a mild infiltrate of round cells related to the vasculopathy. Haematoxylin–eosin × 200

although eclamptic fits may occur in the puerperium even, on occasions, when the pre-eclampsia during pregnancy and labour has been relatively mild. Many abnormalities of renal function, of response to vasoactive agents, of the coagulation system, of the immunological system and of other parameters have been described but full understanding of the nature of the disorder is not yet in sight.

Whatever the aetiology and pathogenesis may prove to be, the only significant morphological lesions are found in the spiral and uteroplacental arteries of the pregnant uterus.[42] In established pre-eclampsia these arteries develop a characteristic necrotizing vasculopathy called acute atherosis (Fig. 25.6), the name deriving from the foam cells present in the fibrinoid arterial wall. The lesion is analogous in some respects to the arterial fibrinoid necrosis of malignant hypertension but acute atherosis develops in many cases of pre-eclampsia at blood pressure levels well below those of malignant hypertension. Two other features deserve comment. First, in women with

essential or renal hypertension complicating pregnancy, the spiral arteries of the uterus, which are converted to uteroplacental arteries in pregnancy, may show a surprising degree of hyperplastic arteriosclerosis (Fig. 25.7), far in excess of that in arteries of similar calibre in other organs. This may be due to the altered haemodynamic requirements of the pregnant uterus, where a tenfold increase in blood supply is ultimately needed and is effected in the presence of a higher than normal blood pressure. Second, a renal glomerular lesion has been described as characteristic of pre-eclampsia and labelled as 'glomerular endotheliosis' or 'intracapillary cell swelling'. It can be seen satisfactorily only by electronmicroscopy of renal biopsies performed during pregnancy or immediately post partum.

Coarctation of the aorta

The various forms and associated lesions of this congenital disorder are described in Chapter 13 of

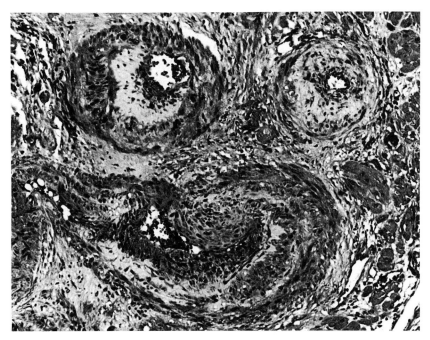

Fig. 25.7 Myometrial segments of spiral arteries in late pregnancy of a woman of 30 years with essential hypertension who subsequently developed pre-eclampsia. The arteries show a surprising degree of hyperplastic arteriosclerosis, presumably due to the effect of the hypertension on arteries adapting to the requirements of the pregnant uterus.
Haematoxylin–eosin × 250

this volume. Suspicion of the existence of coarctation may be aroused by the finding of a raised blood pressure in a child, particularly when high readings are obtained in the arms with normal or low readings in the legs. In a minority of cases the child may present with quite severe and progressive hypertension. All young adults who are found to have hypertension should be investigated by appropriate methods to exclude, or confirm, the presence of coarctation, a relatively rare condition that is amenable to surgical correction. Premature death from cardiovascular complications is inevitable if the obstruction of the aorta is not corrected before there has been irreversible damage to the circulatory system.

The genesis of hypertension in cases of coarctation is not as straightforward as it might seem. It is reasonable to assume that, initially at least, raised pressure in arteries proximal to the coarctation is the result of increased cardiac effort to overcome the obstruction. The fact, however, that in a sizeable minority of cases, including infants, the blood pressure does not return to normal after surgical correction of the coarctation indicates that other mechanisms are involved.[43] Some have suggested that the coarctation has an effect analogous with the Goldblatt renal artery clip rendering the kidneys ischaemic so that in the early stages the hypertension is renin induced. There may also be reflex efferent activity of the sympathetic system as part of autoregulatory mechanisms. The sympathetic effect may be seen dramatically immediately following corrective surgery. In some cases, due it is thought to rapid triggering of the sympathetic response by baroreceptor readjustment to the sudden fall in pressure in the arteries previously subject to hypertension, plasma catecholamine levels rise sharply leading to a temporary elevation of blood pressure to the extent that acute necrotizing changes may be induced in vessels previously functioning in a low pressure system distal to the coarctation.

MISCELLANEOUS ASSOCIATIONS WITH HYPERTENSION

Alcohol

It is perhaps not surprising in populations with high prevalences of both hypertension and alcoholism that an association between the two has been detected.[44] It would appear that in those predisposed to hypertension and in those with established hypertension, consumption of excess alcohol promotes or aggravates the hypertension. Those hypertensives who drink heavily can lower their blood pressures significantly by abstaining from alcohol. The exact mechanism by which alcohol influences blood pressure is unknown[45] but it is probably complex and involves cerebral centres and the autonomic nervous system.

Drugs

There are many drugs which have been reported to cause or aggravate hypertension.[38] These include corticosteroids, mineralocorticoids and anabolic steroids reproducing features of naturally occurring disorders of the endocrine system that are dealt with above. Non-steroidal anti-inflammatory drugs may induce hypertension by promoting salt and water retention. Hypertension associated with oral contraceptives has been discussed earlier in this section.

EXPERIMENTAL HYPERTENSION

Over the last 50 years a large number and variety of experimental procedures have been developed and refined to investigate the pathogenesis of hypertension.[46] The animals used, in most instances, have been the dog, rat or rabbit. While experimentally produced hypertension has been useful in elucidating mechanisms of production of high blood pressure in the animal concerned, the relevance of the findings to the commonest form of hypertension in man, essential hypertension, must be questioned. There is, too, the problem of differences between species in their response to procedures and agents producing hypertension; infusion of renin raises the blood pressure in

rats but it does not do so in dogs. Caution must therefore be exercised in extrapolating causal findings in the experimental animal to man.

Renal ischaemia

In 1934 Goldblatt and his colleagues[27] produced hypertension in the dog by constricting one renal artery, and subsequently both, with adjustable silver clips. The consequent rise in blood pressure in the dog is only mild to moderate and short-lived, and the blood pressure quickly returns to normal after removal of the clips. In contrast, in the rat, severe and sustained hypertension is produced by this procedure, analogous to the situation in man when renal artery stenosis is the cause of hypertension. In the rat, removal of the intact unclipped kidney worsens the hypertension and ensures its persistence. Variations in this type of experiment[46] include production of hemi-infarction in the unclipped kidney and the addition of salt to the drinking water or diet. The hypertension induced by experiments in the rat where only one kidney is clipped would appear to be due initially to excess production of renin by the ischaemic kidney accompanied by retention of sodium and water and hypokalaemia. If the high blood pressure continues for long enough arteriosclerotic changes develop in the small blood vessels of the intact kidney: these may produce ischaemia in that kidney, so enhancing and sustaining the hypertension. At this stage plasma renin levels and electrolyte levels have reverted to normal.

Experimentally, kidneys may be rendered ischaemic by enclosing them in plastic wrapping, which stimulates perirenal inflammation, or by X-irradiation. In both circumstances the causal mechanism and the natural history of the induced hypertension are thought to be the same as those induced by renal artery constriction.

Salt and deoxycorticosterone acetate (DOCA)

The association of hypertension with a high salt intake in certain human populations has already been referred to and this situation is mirrored in some strains of rats but not in dogs and rabbits fed on high salt diets. The hypertensive effect of a high salt diet in the rat is augmented by the administration of the mineralocorticoid deoxycorticosterone acetate,[47] mimicking in many respects the hypertension associated with adrenal cortical disorders in man such as primary aldosteronism and congenital adrenal hyperplasia. The hypertensive effect of the administration of excess salt and of deoxycorticosterone acetate to rabbits and dogs is much less than that in rats.

Infusions of pressor agents

Renin, angiotensin II and catecholamines, particularly noradrenaline, are known to raise blood pressure in man and it could be anticipated that infusion of these substances into animals would have similar effects.[46] This proves to be so but, once again, there are differences among species in the level of response. For example, renin infusion is a potent hypertensive agent in rats and less so in rabbits, while in dogs it does not raise the blood pressure.

In recent years selective breeding has produced strains of rats that develop spontaneous hypertension.[29] These genetically hypertensive animals have been used extensively as models for the study of mechanisms in the genesis of hypertension.

EFFECTS OF HYPERTENSION

As stated earlier, actuarial and other statistics show beyond any doubt that the segment of a population with hypertension, of whatever type or cause, has a greater than average incidence of morbidity and of premature mortality. Because the effects of hypertension are systematized, there is scarcely an organ in the body that may not be

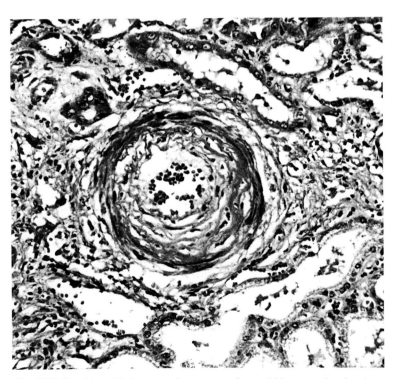

Fig. 25.8 Renal interlobular artery from a case of essential hypertension showing hyperplastic arteriosclerosis with increased collagen and elastic tissue in the wall and early hyaline change.
Haematoxylin–eosin × 250

damaged in the long or short term by the raised blood pressure itself and also by the damage induced, or enhanced, in small and large blood vessels. It is, therefore, appropriate to discuss the pathology of large and small blood vessels in relation to hypertension before dealing with the effects on systems and organs.

Atherosclerosis

In Chapter 24 allusion was made to the effect of ageing and of hypertension on the aorta, leading to degenerative changes in the media, sclerosis and ectasia. Of equal, and probably more, importance is the influence hypertension has on the natural history of atherosclerosis, the intimal disease that now underlies the commonest cause of death in affluent countries.

Several studies have shown that the extent and severity of atherosclerotic lesions in the aorta and in the coronary and cerebral arteries are greater in people with hypertension than in those with a normal blood pressure. Perhaps the most illustra-tive study of this kind was the International Atherosclerosis Project[48] in which aortas and coronary and cerebral arteries from autopsies were assessed for atherosclerosis. The partici-pating centres were located in North, Central and South America, the Caribbean, Europe, Africa and Asia. Consistently in all geographical locations, it was shown that hypertension increased the extent and severity of atheroscle-rosis irrespective of age, sex and race.[49] This deleterious effect of hypertension is further illus-trated by the fact that significant atheroma is seen in the pulmonary arteries only in the presence of pulmonary hypertension.

Arteriosclerosis

The sequence of events in small blood vessels, particularly the resistance arteries, in hypertensive people has already been touched upon in this chapter and in Chapter 24. It is advantageous to consolidate these observations here. The persis-tent vasoconstriction inherent in the hypertensive

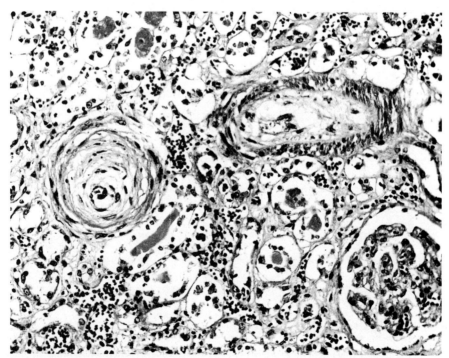

Fig. 25.9 Accelerated phase of essential hypertension with 'onion-skin' hyperplastic change (endarteritis fibrosa) of a renal interlobular artery. Haematoxylin–eosin × 200

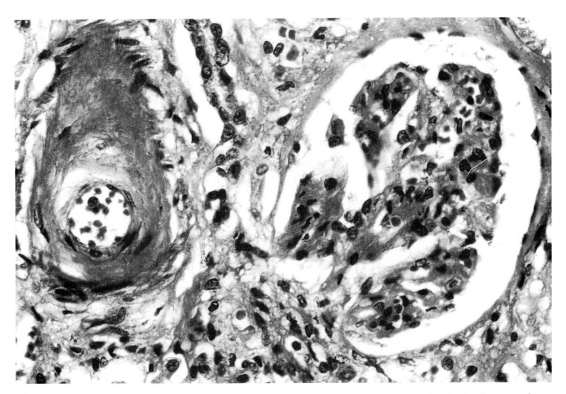

Fig. 25.10 Essential hypertension: tangential section of a glomerular afferent arteriole showing the development of hyaline change, the presence of amorphous material in the vessel wall. Haematoxylin–eosin × 450

state, allied to the consequent increased intraluminal pressure because of the high ratio of wall thickness to lumen diameter, induces hypertrophy of smooth muscle cells and their hyperplasia (replication) also. The hypertrophied medial and myointimal cells, together with adventitial fibroblasts, produce more collagen and elastica, adding to the thickness of the vessel wall (Fig. 25.8) and thereby reducing elasticity and vascular compliance. Many regard this as the stage of establishment of the vicious circle which is only partially reversible by appropriate treatment of the hypertension. Continuation of the process leads to the characteristic 'onion-skin' appearance of small blood vessels exposed to longstanding hypertension (Fig. 25.9). The smaller arterioles develop a greater degree of hyaline change (Fig. 25.10) than is seen as a result of age only.

When malignant hypertension supervenes on benign hypertension the arteriosclerosis progresses rapidly and extensively in small arteries but the most characteristic feature is the development of fibrinoid necrosis in arterioles. While this necrotizing arteriopathy is traditionally described and illustrated in the kidneys (Fig. 25.11) it occurs also in vessels in many other sites including the peri-adrenal and pancreatic arterioles, in the intestinal arterioles (causing the uraemic colitis of malignant hypertension) and in small vessels in the brain in patients with hypertensive encephalopathy. The pathogenesis of the lesion correlates well with the rapidity and the level of the rise in blood pressure: it develops in younger people whose diastolic pressure rises quickly to a high level whereas it tends not to develop in older people whose equally high diastolic pressure has evolved over a period of many years. The pathogenesis of the lesion is probably the result of the rapid increase in intraluminal pressure in arterioles that have

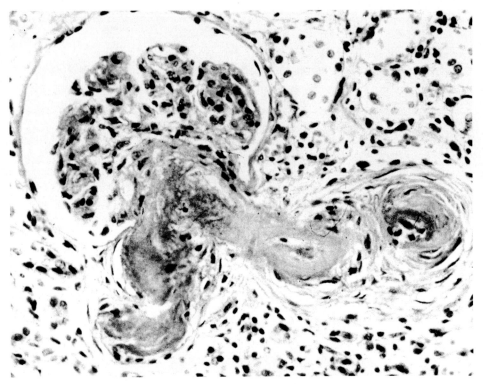

Fig. 25.11 Malignant hypertension: fibrinoid necrosis in the glomerular afferent arteriole extending into the efferent arteriole.
Picro–Mallory trichrome stain × 300

responded with vasoconstriction but have not had time to buttress themselves against the severe pressure by hypertrophy, hyperplasia and increased collagen content. The autoregulatory mechanism breaks down and endothelium and subjacent tissues are irreparably damaged, allowing insudation of plasma into the wall with deposition of fibrin, lipoproteins, immunoproteins and other plasma constituents, all of which can be demonstrated by appropriate histological and immunohistochemical techniques. The lesion is an example of acute plasmatic vasculosis.[50]

Cardiac hypertrophy

The general principles and mechanisms of cardiac hypertrophy have been discussed in Chapter 3. Because hypertension is so common, some 15–20% of the population of affluent countries

being affected, it is by far the commonest cause of left ventricular hypertrophy (Fig. 25.12); in the later stages of severe cases it is the commonest cause of generalized cardiomegaly. While this fact is universally accepted, the assessment of cardiac hypertrophy is by no means agreed upon. The common practice at autopsy of simply weighing the cleaned heart and measuring the thickness of the left ventricle at the base of the exposed left lateral papillary muscle has been severely criticized by many. This time-honoured procedure usually does not take account of whether the heart at autopsy is in a state of contraction or distension or whether or not there is generalized oedema of the body which influences the fluid content of the myocardium and therefore its weight and thickness. Also, it is seldom related to the age, height, weight and other bodily characteristics of the individual.[51] The values of heart weight and left ventricular thickness are then compared with

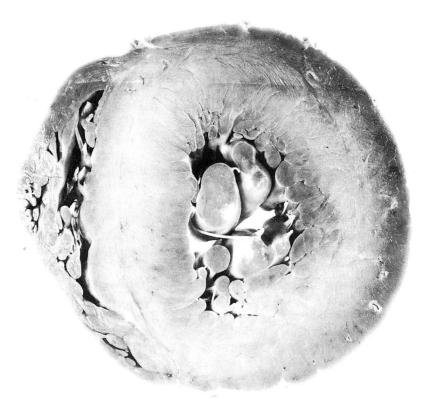

Fig. 25.12 Left ventricular hypertrophy in a case of longstanding severe essential hypertension.

arbitrarily set norms for male and female. Thus, on many occasions a dubious deduction is made that there is cardiac hypertrophy due to hypertension. More detailed and precise techniques such as dissecting and weighing the four chambers of the heart separately[52] are too tedious for the average pathologist: in practical terms one can only advise caution in the interpretation at autopsy of the degree of cardiac hypertrophy in relation to hypertension.

In hypertensive subjects cardiac hypertrophy can be tolerated for many years without apparent disability but, if it is progressive, a stage is reached when the myocardium of the left ventricle, particularly in the presence of co-existing coronary artery disease (see below), cannot meet the demands put upon it by the hypertensive state due to the sub-optimal coronary blood supply. Left ventricular failure ensues with dilatation of the ventricle, the first symptom in the patient usually being breathlessness because of pulmonary oedema. As the failure worsens, the right side of the heart comes under increasing strain and eventually, unless treatment is instituted, congestive cardiac failure supervenes with raised venous pressure and pulmonary and peripheral oedema. It should be noted that the enlarged congested 'nutmeg' liver, characteristically found at autopsy, owes its macroscopic appearances as much to deficient arterial perfusion as to the raised pressure in the hepatic venous system.

Coronary (ischaemic) heart disease

The detailed pathology of diseases of the coronary arteries is dealt with in Part B of this volume. The commonest single cause of death in Europe, North America and many countries in other continents is now coronary heart disease; this is also the commonest cause of death in those with hypertension in the same regions. This is not just a statistical coincidence: it is now well established that hypertension is a potent risk factor in relation to coronary heart disease, in that people with hypertension have a much higher incidence of coronary heart disease than their normotensive counterparts. It is important to note that the availability of effective treatment for hypertension has not effected a reduction of the incidence of coronary heart disease amongst hypertensives; this is in contrast to the reduction of incidence of cerebrovascular disorders complicating hypertension. As already stated, hypertension accentuates the extent and severity of atherosclerosis, presumably through mechanical factors, but this does not entirely explain why hypertensives should be more prone to develop coronary thrombosis, the acknowledged precipitator of most cases of myocardial infarction and sudden death in coronary heart disease. It may be that the haemodynamics of hypertension acting on a diseased intima cause a higher incidence of plaque fissuring and rupture, the immediate antecedent of coronary thrombosis;[53] this remains unproven. Hypertension also increases the morbidity and mortality in patients with a myocardial infarct; the incidence of cardiac failure, of rupture of the heart or of papillary muscles, and, in the longer term, the incidence of cardiac aneurysms are higher in those with hypertension than in normotensives.[54]

Aneurysms

For a detailed account of aneurysms of all types, the reader should refer to Part B of this volume.

The degenerative changes that regularly occur in the aorta and other large arteries with age are accentuated by hypertension and it is not surprising that the incidence of aneurysms, and of their complications, is much higher in people with hypertension than in those whose blood pressure is normal.[54] This applies to both saccular and fusiform aneurysms and to dissecting aneurysms of the aorta. However, the severity of intimal disease does not always correlate well with the presence or absence of an aneurysm. There is evidence that in a proportion of cases the

aneurysm may be a consequence of a chronic inflammatory process,[55] possibly autoimmune in nature, initiated by products of degenerating atherosclerotic plaques.[56] Whatever the basic cause of these aneurysms, hypertension augments their formation and promotes thrombosis in the sac and rupture of the wall. The association of hypertension with dissecting aneurysms of the aorta is even stronger: if cases of Marfan's disease and allied disorders are excluded, together with the rare occurrence of dissecting aneurysm in young pregnant women, almost all instances of this variety of aneurysm are in people who have hypertension.[54] Coarctation of the aorta may be complicated by dissection of the aortic segment under high pressure proximal to the stenosis.

It may be added here that the complications of atherosclerosis of the aorta and its major branches, such as thrombosis of the aortic bifurcation (Leriche syndrome), renal artery stenosis and claudication of the legs due to ilio-femoral arterial obstruction, have a higher incidence in hypertensives than in normotensives.[54]

Cerebrovascular disorders

Before the advent of effective drugs for the treatment of hypertension one of the major consequences was the occurrence of a 'cerebrovascular accident'.[57] Like the word stroke, cerebrovascular accident is a generic and non-definitive term which encompasses intracerebral haemorrhage, cerebral infarction, focal or lacunar softenings of the brain and subarachnoid haemorrhage when the precise diagnosis cannot immediately be established. In contrast to coronary heart disease, the incidence of these cerebrovascular complications of hypertension, particularly intracerebral haemorrhage, has been considerably reduced in consequence of therapeutic advances during the last three decades. However, because age is a potent factor in the genesis of cerebral softening, the problem of strokes is still of major importance among the ageing population of affluent countries. When trauma, vascular malformations, bleeding into tumours and the like are excluded, intracerebral haemorrhage is nearly always a result of high blood pressure. It is thought to be due to rupture of microaneurysms in the

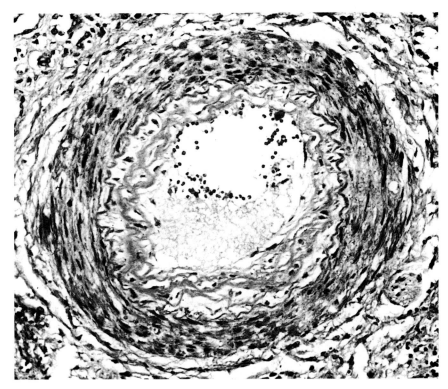

Fig. 25.13 A renal arcuate artery from a case of essential hypertension showing hyperplastic medial smooth muscle and reduplication of the elastica in the thickened intima. This accounts for the prominence of these vessels in benign nephrosclerosis.
Haematoxylin–eosin × 200

small parenchymal vessels (Charcot–Bouchard aneurysms), which are much more frequent in hypertensive than in normotensive people.[58]

The higher incidence in hypertensives of cerebral atherothrombotic infarction can be attributed to the increased extent and severity of atherosclerosis in the carotid and vertebral arteries and the circle of Willis. Subarachnoid haemorrhage, from rupture of a 'berry' aneurysm on one of the arteries at the base of the brain, occurs more often in people who are hypertensive than in those whose blood pressure is normal. Although these aneurysms are generally regarded as starting from a congenital defect in the arterial wall, the median age at which rupture occurs is about 50 years, indicating that age itself is a factor in their development. Certainly, hypertension contributes to their occurrence and to their rupture.

Hypertensive encephalopathy

When hypertension is severe, and particularly in malignant hypertension, the cerebral autoregulatory mechanism breaks down with dilatation of the small thin-walled intracerebral arteries and arterioles. Cerebral oedema results and, in the severest cases, focal softening and petechial haemorrhages. The affected patient becomes confused and dysphasic and may have fits and other neurological signs and, if treatment is not instituted, may suffer extensive cerebral infarction or massive intracerebral haemorrhage.

Retinal changes in hypertension

The retinal arteries, like arteries elsewhere in the body, constrict in response to rising blood pressure as part of the autoregulatory mechanism.[59] The fact that they can be visualized

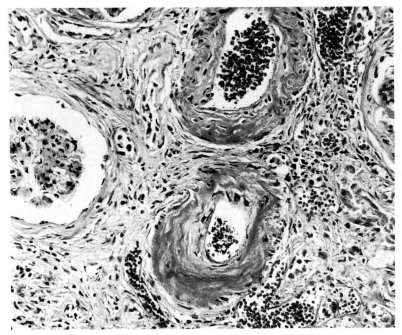

Fig. 25.14 Longstanding severe essential hypertension with thickened, partially hyalinized interlobular arteries, interstitial fibrosis, and glomerular damage with thickening of Bowman's capsule and atrophy of capillary tufts.
Haematoxylin–eosin × 150

through an ophthalmoscope provides the clinician with a means of monitoring vascular changes in hypertension in relation to the natural history of the disorder. In the early stages, the developing arteriosclerosis in the retinal arteries causes 'nipping' of the veins at the intimate crossing points of veins and arteries. On ophthalmoscopy the thickened arteries have a characteristic appearance, due to increased light reflex; this feature is called 'silver wiring' of the arteries. During the accelerated phase of hypertension vascular damage leads to retinal flame-shaped haemorrhages and exudates; in established malignant hypertension papilloedema is the pathognomonic feature.

Renal complications

Chronic renal failure in benign essential hypertension is uncommon unless the patient's circulatory system is compromised by other diseases. For example, a hypertensive individual who develops severe coronary heart disease with much myocardial damage and consequent impaired cardiac function will have inadequate perfusion of the kidneys. Existing renal damage due to longstanding hypertension will be aggravated to the extent that renal failure ensues. In contrast, renal failure is characteristic of malignant hypertension and is also the usual terminal event in hypertension secondary to chronic nephritis of all types.

In those with longstanding benign essential hypertension the kidneys may be of normal or slightly reduced size. Usually, when the renal capsules are stripped at autopsy, a fine surface granularity is revealed which, in appearance and feel, has been likened to morocco leather. Hemisection of the kidneys shows the granularity to be due to fine, relatively superficial, cortical scarring, the cortices themselves being thinned to a greater or lesser degree (benign nephrosclerosis). The cut arcuate arteries at the corticomedullary junction are prominent because of their thickened walls (Fig. 25.13). The reduction in

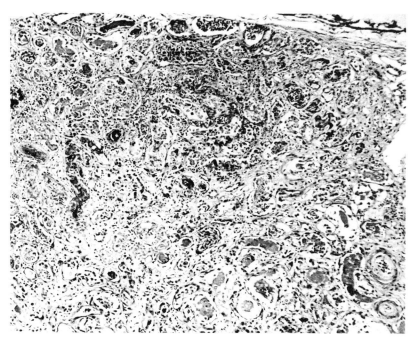

Fig. 25.15 Malignant hypertension: the histological counterpart of the 'flea-bites' seen on the surface of the kidneys. There is focal haemorrhagic necrosis of cortical glomeruli and tubules and proteinaceous material in tubular lumens. Haematoxylin–eosin × 100

total mass of renal parenchyma may be accompanied by an increase in peripelvic fat, particularly in obese subjects.

The histological features vary with the age of the individual and with the duration and severity of the hypertension. They range from the near normal for the age of the individual through various degrees of damage to arteries and ischaemic changes in glomeruli and tubules. It is not easy in assessing histological changes to determine how much is due to hypertension and how much to the ageing process, the latter being subject to considerable individual variation. The temptation to attribute the major share to the effects of hypertension must be resisted but in severe cases there can be little doubt that, for example, the arcuate arteries and their major branches show a degree of intimal and medial collagenous thickening well in excess of that due to ageing alone. Similarly in hypertensives, the severity and extent of hyaline change in the afferent arterioles exceeds that normally seen in normotensive individuals of the same age. In

relation to the most severely affected arterioles (Fig. 25.14) the glomeruli show a gradation of changes from thickening of the basement membrane of capillary loops and of Bowman's capsule, collapse and shrinkage of capillary tufts up to complete sclerosis of individual glomeruli. The tubules of damaged nephrons may also atrophy, showing thickened basement membranes with flattening; not infrequently, the lumens contain eosinophilic homogeneous proteinaceous material. It is not unusual to see mild infiltrates of round cells in these focal areas of damage and the picture should not be misdiagnosed as chronic pyelonephritis. This pitfall was discussed earlier.

The kidneys in cases of malignant hypertension look quite different. If malignant hypertension has developed from the benign condition, at autopsy the kidneys may be normal in size or, due to the parenchymal oedema associated with rapidly developed renal failure, they may be enlarged. In both circumstances, however, the surfaces are mottled in colour with punctate haemorrhages

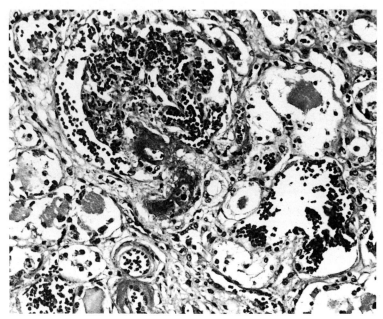

Fig. 25.16 Malignant hypertension: fibrinoid necrosis of an afferent arteriole extending into the hilum of the glomerulus with haemorrhage into the capsular space. There is damage also to surrounding tubules.
Haematoxylin–eosin × 200

producing the characteristic 'flea-bitten' appearance. In cases superimposed on renal disease, now the majority, the kidneys are usually symmetrically reduced in size due to the underlying chronic renal condition; they also show 'flea-bitten' surfaces. The mottled red-yellow discoloration of the surfaces of the cortices reflects alternating areas of haemorrhagic necrosis in glomeruli and surrounding tissue (Fig. 25.15) with areas of sublethal damage characterized by fatty change in tubular epithelium.

Histologically there is a marked hyperplastic change, 'onion-skinning' or endarteritis fibrosa, in small arteries but the most striking and virtually pathognomonic feature is fibrinoid necrosis of afferent arterioles, the necrosis often extending into the glomerulus itself (Fig. 25.16). The acute vascular lesions cause focal areas of haemorrhagic necrosis, the 'flea-bites' seen macroscopically. Reactionary acute inflammatory exudates may be seen in the surrounding necrotic areas.

The appearances, both macroscopic and microscopic, of the kidneys in cases of hypertension secondary to renal disease will depend upon the nature of the renal disorder. In chronic nephritis of some years' duration, both kidneys are often markedly and equally reduced in size and cortical scarring, because of more extensive parenchymal loss and damage, tends to be coarser than that of benign nephrosclerosis. The histological features will reflect the underlying renal disease but one problem common to all varieties is the interpretation of lesions in blood vessels. It is impossible in most instances to determine with any degree of precision the separate contributions made by the renal disease and by the secondary hypertension to the sclerosis and hyaline change seen in small arteries in such cases.

REFERENCES

1. Allbutt TC. Diseases of the arteries including angina pectoris. London: Macmillan, 1915.
2. Frank E. Cited by Pickering G. High blood pressure, 2nd ed. London: Churchill, 1968.
3. World Health Organization. Arterial hypertension. WHO Tech Rep Ser 628, 1978.
4. Pickering G. High blood pressure, 2nd ed. London: Churchill, 1968.
5. Platt R. The influence of heredity. In: Stamler J, Stamler R, Pullmann TN, eds. The epidemiology of hypertension. New York: Grune & Stratton, 1967: 9–17.
6. Platt R. Heredity in hypertension. Q J Med 1947; NS 16: 1111–1121.
7. Society of Actuaries. Build and blood pressure study. Chicago: Society of Actuaries, 1959.
8. Castelli WP. Hypertension: a perspective from the Framingham experience. In: Sleight P, Freis ED, eds. Cardiology 1: Hypertension. London: Butterworths, 1982: 1–13.
9. Hypertension Detection and Follow-up Program Co-operative Group. Five-year findings of the hypertension and follow-up program. 1. Reduction in mortality of persons with high blood pressure, including mild hypertension. J A M A 1979; 242: 2562–2571.
10. Alderman MH. The indications for treatment with antihypertensive drugs. In: Sleight P, Freis ED, eds. Cardiology 1: Hypertension. London: Butterworths, 1982: 229–247.
11. Lowenstein FW. Blood pressure in relation to age and sex in the tropics and subtropics. A review of the literature and an investigation in two Indian tribes in Brazil. Lancet 1961; 1: 389–392.
12. Shaper AG. Blood pressure studies in East Africa. In: Stamler J, Stamler R, Pullmann TN, eds. The epidemiology of hypertension. New York: Grune & Stratton, 1967: 139–149.
13. Acheson RM. Blood pressure in a national sample of US adults. Percentile distribution by age, sex and race. Int J Epidemiol 1973; 2: 293–301.
14. Poulter NR, Khaw KT, Hopwood BEC et al. The Kenyan Luo migration study: observations on the initiation of a rise in blood pressure. Br Med J 1990; 300: 967–972.
15. Miall WE, Kass EH, Ling J, Stuart KL. Factors influencing arterial pressure in the general population in Jamaica. Br Med J 1962; 2: 497–506.
16. Hypertension and Follow-up Program Co-operative Group. Five-year findings of the hypertension detection and follow-up program. II. Mortality by race, sex and age. J A M A 1979; 242: 2572–2577.
17. Parfrey PS. Salt in essential hypertension. In: Sleight P, Freis ED, eds. Cardiology 1: Hypertension. London: Butterworths, 1982: 322–339.
18. Folkow B. Physiological aspects of primary hypertension. Physiol Rev 1982; 62: 347–504.
19. Dickinson CJ. Neurogenic hypertension revisited. Clin Sci 1981; 60: 471–477.
20. Robinson BF, Dobbs RJ, Bayley S. Response of forearm resistance vessels to verapamil and sodium nitroprusside in normotensive and hypertensive men: evidence for a functional abnormality of vascular smooth muscle in primary hypertension. Clin Sci 1982; 63: 33–42.
21. Weber MA, Smith DHG, Neutel JM, Graettinger WF. Arterial properties of early hypertension. J Hum Hypertens 1991; 5: 417–423.
22. Goldstein DS. Plasma catecholamines and essential hypertension: an analytical review. Hypertension 1983; 5: 86–89.
23. Philipp TH, Distler A, Cordes U. Sympathetic nervous system and blood pressure control in essential hypertension. Lancet 1978; 2: 959–963.
24. Leading Article. Salt and blood pressure: the next chapter. Lancet 1989; 1: 1301–1303.
25. De Wardener HE, MacGregor GA. The natriuretic hormone and essential hypertension. Lancet 1982; 1: 1450–1453.
26. Guyton AC. Arterial pressure and hypertension. Philadelphia: Saunders, 1980.
27. Goldblatt H, Lynch J, Hanzal RF, Summerville WW. Studies on experimental hypertension. 1. The production of persistent elevation of systolic blood pressure by means of renal ischemia. J Exp Med 1934; 59: 347–379.
28. Swales JD. Clinical hypertension. London: Chapman & Hall, 1979: 92–96.
29. Bianchi G, Ferrari P, Cusi D. Renal models and their relation to human essential hypertension. In: Sleight P, Freis ED, eds. Cardiology 1: Hypertension. London: Butterworths, 1982: 37–55.
30. Kincaid-Smith P, McMichael J, Murphy EA. The clinical course and pathology of hypertension with papilloedema (malignant hypertension). Q J Med 1958; 27: 117–153.
31. Lee TH, Alderman MH. Malignant hypertension: declining mortality rate in New York City, 1958–1974. NY State J Med 1978; 78: 1389–1391.
32. Bright R. Cited in Swales JD, ed. Classic papers in hypertension, blood pressure and renin. London: Scientific Press, 1987: 27–47.
33. Allbutt C. Cited in Swales JD, ed. Classic papers in hypertension, blood pressure and renin. London: Scientific Press, 1987: 104–123.
34. Harrison EG, McCormack LJ. Pathologic classification of renal arterial disease in renovascular hypertension. Mayo Clin Proc 1971; 46: 161–167.
35. Leading Article. Hypertension in pyelonephritis. Lancet 1968; 2: 615–616.
36. Manger WM, Gifford RW. Pheochromocytoma. In: Sleight P, Freis ED, eds. Cardiology 1: Hypertension. London: Butterworths, 1982: 153–172.
37. Kater CE, Biglieri EG. Adrenocortical disease and hypertension. In: Sleight P, Fries E, eds. Cardiology 1: Hypertension. London: Butterworths, 1982: 135–152.
38. Crane MG. Iatrogenic hypertension. In: Genest J, Kuchel O, Hamet P, Cantin M, eds. Hypertension: physiopathology and treatment, 2nd ed. New York: McGraw-Hill, 1983: 976–988.
39. Report on confidential enquiries into maternal deaths in England and Wales, 1982–4. London: HMSO, 1989.
40. Chesley LC. Hypertensive disorders of pregnancy. New York: Appleton-Century-Crofts, 1978.
41. MacGillivray I. Pre-eclampsia: the hypertensive disease of pregnancy. London: Saunders, 1983.
42. Robertson WB, Brosens I, Dixon G. Uteroplacental vascular pathology. Eur J Obstet Gynecol Reprod Biol 1975; 5: 47–65.
43. Heptinstall RH. Pathology of the kidney, 4th ed. Boston: Little, Brown, 1992; 2: 1029–1095.

44. Smith WCS, Crombie IK, Tavendale RT, Gulland SK, Tunstall-Pedoe HD. Urinary electrolyte excretion, alcohol consumption, and blood pressure in the Scottish heart health study. Br Med J 1988; 297: 329–330.

45. Potter JF, Beevers DG. Pressor effect of alcohol in hypertension. Lancet 1984; 1: 119–122.

46. Bianchi G, Ferrari P. Animal models for hypertension. In: Genest J, Kuchel O, Hamet P, Cantin M, eds. Hypertension: pathophysiology and treatment, 2nd ed. New York: McGraw-Hill, 1983: 534–555.

47. Selye H, Hall CE, Rowley EM. Malignant hypertension produced by treatment with desoxycorticosterone acetate and sodium chloride. Can Med Assoc J 1943; 49: 88–92.

48. McGill HC. The geographic pathology of atherosclerosis. Baltimore: Williams & Wilkins, 1968.

49. Robertson WB, Strong JP. Atherosclerosis in persons with hypertension and diabetes mellitus. Lab Invest 1968; 18: 538–551.

50. Lendrum AC. The hypertensive diabetic kidney as a model of the so-called collagen diseases. Can Med Assoc J 1963; 88: 442–452.

51. Davies MJ. Atlas of cardiovascular pathology. Oxford University Press: Harvey Miller, 1986: 176–177.

52. Fulton RM, Hutchinson EC, Jones MA. Ventricular weight in cardiac hypertrophy. Br Heart J 1952; 14: 413–420.

53. Davies MJ, Thomas AC. Plaque fissuring: the cause of acute myocardial infarction, sudden ischaemic death and crescendo angina. Br Heart J 1985; 53: 363–373.

54. Roberts WC. Cardiovascular consequences of systemic hypertension: a morphologic survey. In: Sleight P, Freis ED, eds. Cardiology 1: Hypertension. London: Butterworths, 1982: 78–91.

55. Walker DI, Bloor K, Williams G, Gillie I. Inflammatory aneurysms of the abdominal aorta. Br J Surg 1972; 59: 609–614.

56. Mitchinson MJ. Chronic periaortitis and periarteritis. Histopathology 1984; 8: 589–600.

57. Graham DI. Vascular disease and hypoxic brain damage. In: Weller RO, ed. Nervous system, muscle and eyes. Systemic Pathology, 3rd ed. Edinburgh: Churchill Livingstone, 1990; 4: 89–124.

58. Cole FM, Yates PO. The occurrence and significance of intracerebral microaneurysms. J Pathol Bacteriol 1967; 93: 393–411.

59. Chaine GJ, Kohner EM. Hypertensive retinopathy. In: Sleight P, Freis ED, eds. Cardiology 1: Hypertension. London: Butterworths, 1982: 92–116.

Pathology of the pulmonary vasculature

INTRODUCTION

Diseases of the heart, whether congenital or acquired, may lead to changes in the pulmonary vascular circuit, changes which themselves may have further consequences for the heart. Moreover, diseases of the lung, whether parenchymal or vascular, may adversely affect the heart and, eventually, may lead to overt cardiac disorders. Consequently, full understanding of the pathology of the heart cannot be isolated from an understanding of the pathology of the pulmonary vascular bed.

Sections of this chapter, therefore, will be devoted to pulmonary vascular changes associated with congenital heart disease; pulmonary vascular changes that may occur in the setting of acquired heart disease; and lung diseases producing or associated with pulmonary vascular changes that affect the heart. Finally, a section will be devoted to the grading of pulmonary vascular pathology in the evaluation of lung biopsies in relation to heart disease.

CONGENITAL HEART DISEASE

For ease of description, we will discuss under three headings the changes in the pulmonary circulation that may occur in patients with congenital heart disease. First, we will consider those that occur in the setting of a left-to-right shunt, characterized by an increase in flow within the pulmonary vascular circuit. Bronchial compression due to pulmonary arterial dilatation

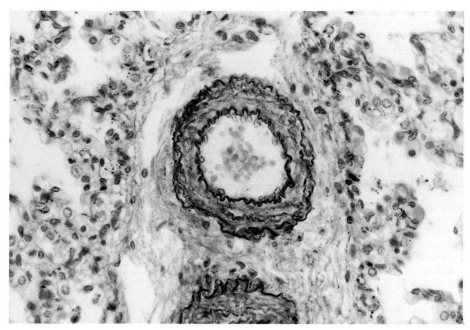

Fig. 26.1 Muscular pulmonary artery with marked medial hypertrophy.
Elastic tissue stain × 350.
Reproduced with permission from Becker A E, Anderson R H. Pathology of congenital heart
disease. *London: Butterworths, 1981; Fig. 35.1a.*

will be considered also in this context. Second, we will consider the changes that occur when there is obstruction of the pulmonary outflow tract leading to a decrease in flow. Third, we will discuss the changes that occur in cases of cardiac malformations with increased pressure within the left side of the heart promoting raised pulmonary venous pressure.

Pulmonary vascular changes with left-to-right shunts

Left-to-right shunts (intracardiac as well as those that occur with patency of the arterial duct, a common arterial trunk or an aortopulmonary window) may lead to pulmonary vascular changes which, collectively, have been termed 'plexogenic pulmonary arteriopathy'.[1] The term describes a sequence of changes with the plexiform lesion occurring as an end-result (see below). These alterations are not limited to congenital heart disease with a left-to-right shunt, but occur also in patients with so-called primary pulmonary hyper-

tension (see later in this Chapter).[2] The primary defect and precise mechanisms remain unknown, but almost certainly relate to abnormalities of vascular growth and remodelling.

Early changes

The early changes of a left-to-right shunt have been described classically as hypertrophy of the media of the muscular pulmonary arteries (Fig. 26.1). Subtle alterations may also occur in the pulmonary arterial tree and may easily escape notice unless searched for carefully: the conditions to be looked for include collapse of alveolar vessels, muscularization of arterioles (Fig. 26.2) and a decrease in the ratio of alveoli to arteries. It has been noted that, during the early changes of pulmonary hypertension, muscularization of arterioles may occur without medial hypertrophy of larger arteries.[3] In these instances, the raised pressure was considered a phenomenon of increased flow, rather than having a structural basis. The changes, therefore, were considered

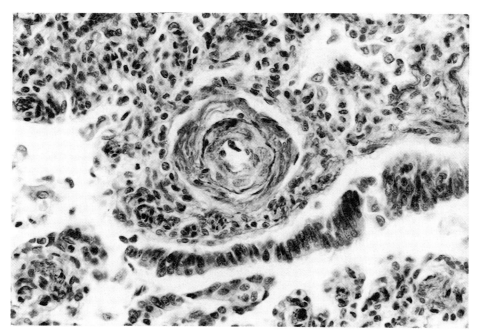

Fig. 26.2 Muscularization of an arteriole less than 60 µm in external diameter.
Elastic tissue stain × 350.
Reproduced with permission from Becker A E, Anderson R H. Pathology of congenital heart disease.
London: Butterworths, 1981; Fig. 35.1b.

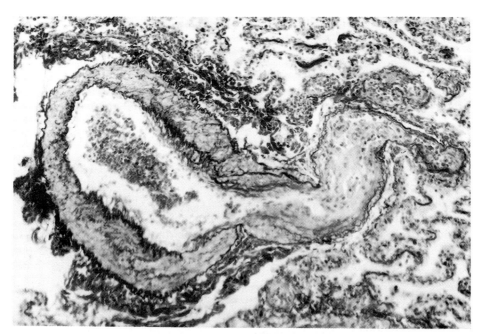

Fig. 26.3   Cellular intimal proliferation in a branch from a muscular pulmonary artery.
Elastic tissue stain × 230.

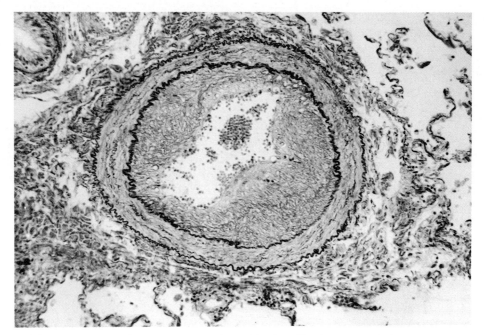

Fig. 26.4 Muscular pulmonary artery with cellular intimal proliferation, concentric in nature, showing an early stage of intimal fibrosis.
Elastic tissue stain × 140.
Reproduced with permission from Becker A E, Anderson R H. Pathology of congenital heart disease.
London: Butterworths, 1981; Fig. 35.4a.

potentially to be reversible. In cases in which the number of peripheral arteries was reduced, the raised arterial pressure was always considered to reflect an irreversible type of functional impairment.

It has now been demonstrated that, in terms of operability, the early changes may not necessarily be located within the intra-acinar arteries, but rather at a more proximal level.[4,5] Intimal thickening of the side branches at a pre-acinar level may cause serious impairment of flow at the acinar level although not accompanied by structural changes in the intra-acinar arteries. When a biopsy is inadequate, therefore, the pathologist may be misled into believing that there are no structural arterial changes. On the other hand, the interpretation of medial hypertrophy as a solitary 'simple' vascular change of no direct importance may also be potentially dangerous, since such hypertrophy may provoke postoperative hypertensive crises.

The evaluation of lung biopsies in the early stages of raised pulmonary pressure in patients with left-to-right shunts is undoubtedly a difficult task, as the relation of lesions to altered function is still uncertain. The pathologist should be aware of these problems and, hence, be extremely cautious in coming to firm conclusions.

Cellular intimal proliferation

This change is characterized by proliferation of smooth muscle (myointimal) cells within the intimal lining: the proliferating cells are derived from the media (Fig. 26.3).[6] The intimal cellularity may vary from site to site, both in degree and in extent. Careful examination, correlating the findings with the clinical presentation, is mandatory for proper evaluation of the functional significance of this condition. Potentially, a cellular intimal change is reversible and, hence, should not militate against the possibility of surgical repair. Indeed, there is evidence that a cellular lesion, which may contain some collagenous deposits, may regress to a stage at which it can still be recognized using the light microscope, although making minimal or no contribution to pulmonary resistance.

Intimal fibrosis

Intimal fibrosis most likely represents a more advanced form of cellular intimal proliferation (Fig. 26.4). In some instances, the intimal thickening is mainly composed of elastin fibres (Fig. 26.5). The lesions usually are concentric, often showing various stages of maturation (Fig. 26.6). Occasionally, 'onion-skinning' may be seen (Fig. 26.7), most likely as an expression of rapid evolution. Similar changes may be observed in cases of primary pulmonary hypertension (see later in this Chapter).[2]

Intimal fibrosis may vary considerably in degree and extent. Again, the overall picture, including clinical presentation, should be taken into account when making a functional evaluation. The consensus is that these changes should be considered non-reversible. There are firm indications, however, that, following corrective surgery, the intimal process may not progress further.

It is important to re-emphasize that concentric intimal fibrosis should be differentiated from other causes of intimal fibrosis, such as an organized thrombus or thrombo-embolus. In the latter circumstances, the intimal thickening tends to be cushion-like rather than concentric and laminar.[7] On the other hand, cushion-like intimal thickenings may occur as part of the sequence of plexogenic pulmonary arteriopathy, occurring at branching points (Fig. 26.8). The latter circumstance, however, is not always immediately evident from cross sections and the pathologist should thus always be cautious in interpreting cushion-like intimal fibrous lesions.

Plexiform lesions

The term 'plexogenic pulmonary arteriopathy' indicates the presence of plexiform changes, aptly named from its histological appearance.

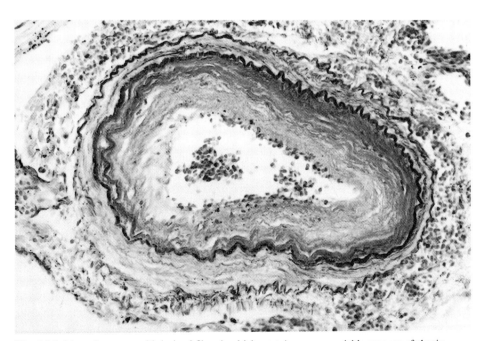

Fig. 26.5 Muscular artery with intimal fibrosis which contains an appreciable amount of elastin fibres.
Elastic tissue stain × 230.
Reproduced with permission from Becker A E, Anderson R H. Pathology of congenital heart disease.
London: Butterworths, 1981; Fig. 35.4b.

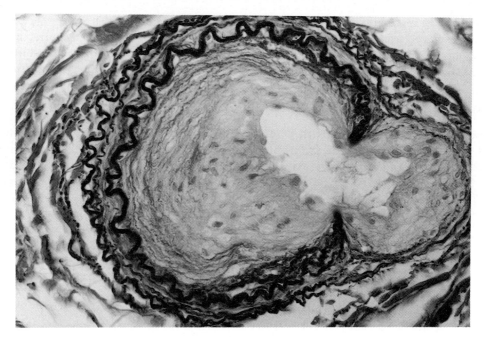

Fig. 26.6 Muscular pulmonary artery with intimal changes which at the luminal side are cellular in nature, whereas the sites closer to the media are characterized by a distinct laminar arrangement of collagen and elastin fibres.
Elastic tissue stain × 350.
Reproduced with permission from Becker A E, Anderson R H. Pathology of congenital heart disease. London: Butterworths, 1981; Fig. 35.5.

This type of change comprises a widely dilated and thin-walled segment of a muscular artery, almost always just beyond a point of branching (Fig. 26.9) and with proliferation of cells inside the lumen. These myointimal cells form cords and strands within the original lumen, often with fibrinoid material glueing them together and leaving slit-like spaces as the only luminal channels. Beyond the plexus, the artery continues as a widely dilated and extremely thin-walled and tortuous vessel. When seen in isolation, such vessels may easily be interpreted as dilatation lesions (see below).

The plexiform lesion is often associated with a distinct cellular inflammatory reaction and most likely represents a vascular response to fibrinoid necrosis of the wall of the vessel. This conclusion is supported by the observation that transitional forms may occasionally be seen (Fig. 26.10). The plexiform lesion should not be confused with a recanalized and organized thrombotic lesion. There is consensus that the plexiform lesion itself is beyond the stage of regression and correlates, therefore, with a grave prognosis.

Dilatation lesion

This change is characterized by the presence of dilated and thin-walled tortuous vessels (Fig. 26.11); the vessels lack an intraluminal plexus. Once such vessels are observed, serial sectioning is often required to rule out the plexiform lesion as the basis of the dilatation. On the other hand, there is not much difference between dilatation and plexiform lesions as far as prognosis is concerned. Both indicate a far-advanced state of plexogenic arteriopathy.

Bronchial compression

Many patients with congenital cardiac malforma-

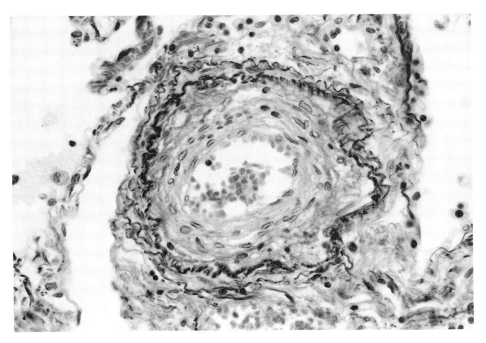

Fig. 26.7 Muscular pulmonary artery with concentric layering in the intima, known as 'onion-skinning'.
Elastic tissue stain × 350.
Reproduced with permission from Becker A E, Anderson R H. Pathology of congenital heart disease.
London: Butterworths, 1981; Fig. 35.6a.

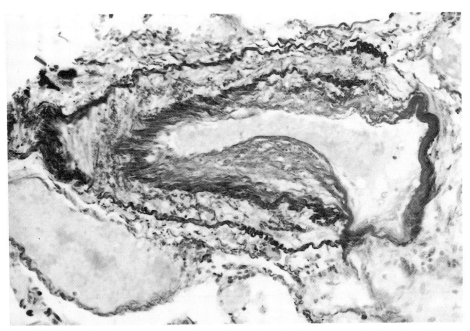

Fig. 26.8 Muscular pulmonary artery with a cushion-like intimal fibrosis, localized at a branching point, which in this patient occurred as part of plexogenic pulmonary arteriopathy.
Elastic tissue stain × 230.

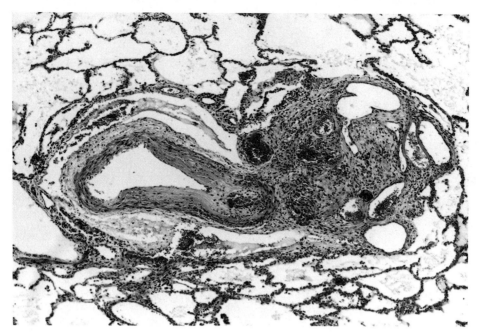

Fig. 26.9 Plexiform lesion in a muscular artery just beyond the site of branching.
Haematoxylin–eosin × 55.
Reproduced with permission from Becker A E, Anderson R H. Pathology of congenital heart disease.
London: Butterworths, 1981; Fig. 35.8a.

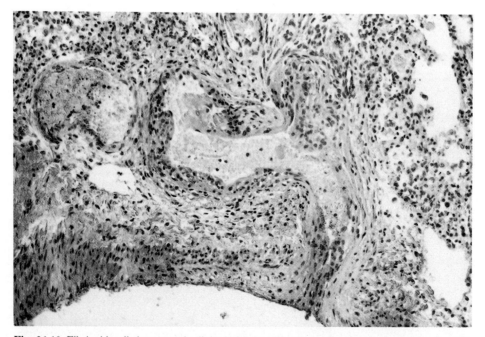

Fig. 26.10 Fibrinoid wall changes and cellular intimal proliferation in an arterial segment just beyond
a branching point, suggestive of an 'early' plexiform lesion.
Haematoxylin–eosin × 140.
Reproduced with permission from Becker A E, Anderson R H. Pathology of congenital heart disease.
London: Butterworths, 1981; Fig. 35.9.

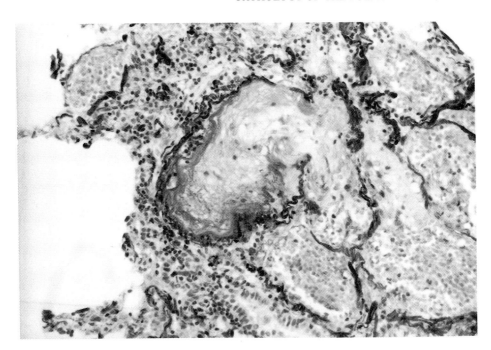

Fig. 26.11 Dilatation lesion, characterized by thin-walled dilated tortuous vessels which lack an intraluminal plexus.
Elastic tissue stain × 230.
Reproduced with permission from Becker A E, Anderson R H. Pathology of congenital heart disease.
London: Butterworths, 1981; Fig. 35.10.

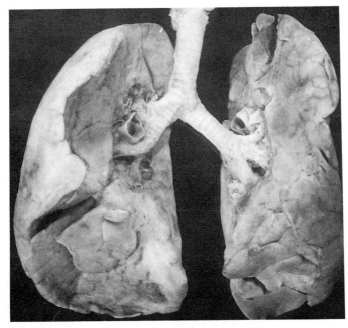

Fig. 26.12 The normal relationship of the main bronchi and main pulmonary arteries to exemplify potential sites of bronchial compression in case of dilatation of pulmonary arteries.
Reproduced with permission from Becker A E, Anderson R H. Pathology of
congenital heart disease. *London: Butterworths, 1981; Fig. 34.1a.*

tions suffer from shortness of breath, either at rest or during exercise. Most commonly, the respiratory difficulties are caused by decreased pulmonary flow or pulmonary venous congestion due to the underlying cardiac defect. Occasionally, however, the shortness of breath is caused by compression of bronchi by pulmonary arteries, the result being either atelectasis or hyperinflation of the corresponding lung segment.[8] It has been shown that the topographical anatomy of the pulmonary arteries relative to the tracheobronchial tree dictates that certain areas of the airways are always prone to compression subsequent to dilatation of the pulmonary arteries (Fig. 26.12). When the lungs are normal, the relationship is such that the right pulmonary artery gives off its branch to the right upper lobe with the bronchus above the artery.

The pulmonary artery then continues and crosses over the intermediate bronchial segment to descend posterior to the bronchus supplying the right middle lobe. The intermediate segment and the bronchus to the right middle lobe may then become compressed by dilatation of the right pulmonary artery (Fig. 26.13, left). On the left side the pulmonary artery crosses over the left bronchus, using the site of origin of the bronchus to the left upper lobe as a 'hinge', so that a dilated left pulmonary artery may compromise the main left bronchus and, in particular, its branch to the left upper lobe (Fig. 26.13, right).

Bronchial compression can be produced by any cardiac condition resulting in a left-to-right shunt of sufficient degree to produce dilatation of the pulmonary arteries and an increase in pulmonary

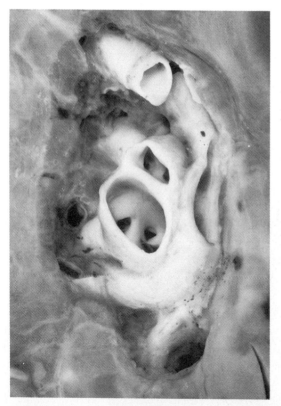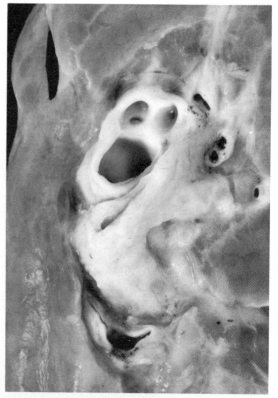

Fig. 26.13 Bronchial compression produced by dilated pulmonary arteries in a patient with a significant left-to-right shunt. The panel on the left shows the dilated pulmonary artery compressing the intermediate bronchus. The panel on the right shows compression of the left upper lobe bronchus.
Reproduced with permission from Becker A E, Anderson R H. Pathology of congenital heart disease. *London: Butterworths, 1981; Fig. 34.2b and c.*

arterial pressure. The commonest examples are ventricular septal defects, atrioventricular septal defects and patency of the arterial duct. An atrial septal defect may also lead to bronchial compression, although usually at a much later age. Other conditions associated with widely dilated pulmonary arteries, but not necessarily accompanied by raised arterial pressure, may also, on occasion, lead to bronchial compression. Examples are those patients with Fallot's tetralogy in whom bronchial compression may occur because of so-called 'absence' of the leaflets of the pulmonary valve (see Ch. 12).

Decreased pulmonary flow

In patients with decreased pulmonary flow, the pulmonary vascular bed will usually show more or less generalized atrophy of the vessel walls. The elastic arteries have a tortuous course and have thin walls with wavy elastin lamellae (Fig. 26.14). The muscular pulmonary arteries are extremely thin-walled (Fig. 26.15), the media sometimes

being no longer apparent. The basic condition presages secondary complications. Because of decreased flow, and the almost invariably increased haematocrit, intravascular thrombosis will occur. Organization of such thrombi may eventually lead to the bands and webs that are characteristically found in these conditions. Such bands and webs can be detected while dissecting the large hilar arteries but can be observed also in microscopic sections of smaller arteries (Fig. 26.16). Only rarely will these structural changes become so severe that they impede pulmonary flow to the extent of producing pulmonary hypertension.[9,10] Previous shunt procedures in these patients (such as Potts, Blalock–Taussig or Waterston shunts) may alter the pre-existent structural characteristics and may produce plexogenic pulmonary arteriopathy as the dominant feature.

Pulmonary venous congestion

Cardiac conditions that lead to venous congestion

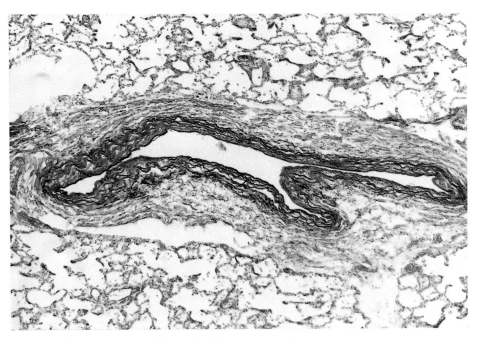

Fig. 26.14 Elastic type artery with atrophy of the media.
Elastic tissue stain × 55.
Reproduced with permission from Becker A E, Anderson R H. Pathology of congenital heart disease. London: Butterworths, 1981; Fig. 35.12b.

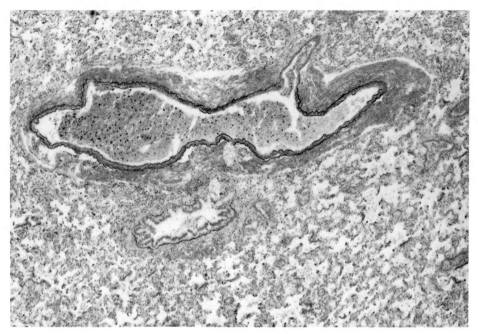

Fig. 26.15 Muscular artery but with distinct atrophy in the media.
Elastic tissue stain × 55.
Reproduced with permission from Becker A E, Anderson R H. Pathology of congenital heart disease.
London: Butterworths, 1981; Fig. 35.12c.

of the lungs are manifold. The histology of the lung in these circumstances is characterized by congestion and dilatation of the veins, often with oedema of interlobular septa together with dilated lymphatics. In longstanding cases the most striking structural alteration in veins is characterized by reduplication and reorientation of elastin fibres, together with medial hypertrophy. The result is a vein which has a distinct muscular media together with internal and external elastic laminae, to the extent that it resembles a muscular pulmonary artery, albeit less regular in appearance. The term 'arterialization' is used to describe this structural feature (Fig. 26.17). When arterialization is observed, it is almost certain that raised pulmonary venous pressure has existed for a long time. This is supported by the observation that the muscular pulmonary arteries in these cases usually exhibit medial hypertrophy. Moreover, the pulmonary lymphatics may be markedly dilated. Interestingly, in patients with an increased pulmonary arterial resistance caused by elevated left-sided pressure, the number of peripheral small arteries seems increased, rather than decreased as is described in patients with raised pulmonary pressure due to intracardiac left-to-right shunts.[11]

ACQUIRED HEART DISEASE

The most important lesions of the pulmonary vasculature in this context are consequences of disorders of the left side of the heart. Any condition that leads to an increase in left atrial pressure will result in pulmonary venous congestion and initiate a series of changes in the pulmonary vasculature. First, arteriolar vasoconstriction will occur, most likely in response to the increase in resistance on the venous side, in an attempt to protect the pulmonary capillary system from overdistension and irreversible damage. In longlasting conditions, the structure of the congested pulmonary veins will change because of

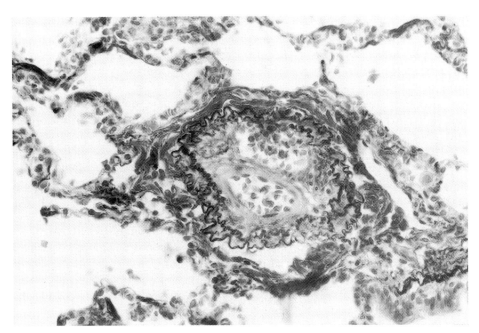

Fig. 26.16 Small-sized muscular pulmonary artery with an intraluminal band caused by organized and recanalized thrombus.
Elastic tissue stain × 350.

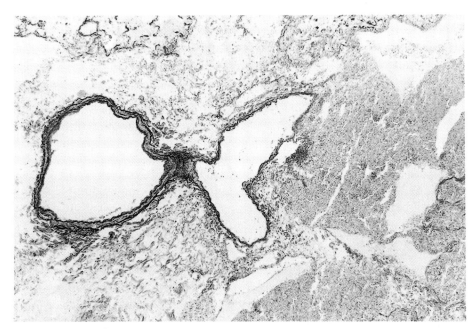

Fig. 26.17 'Arterialization' of a pulmonary vein in an intralobular septum.
Elastic tissue stain × 50.

medial hypertrophy and the development of intimal fibrosis. The changes are essentially similar to those observed in certain types of congenital heart disease. The pathologist, however, should be aware that, in the elderly, ageing changes characterized by some intimal fibrosis occur in pulmonary veins: these should not be taken as a sign of increased pulmonary venous pressure.

Persistent arteriolar vasoconstriction will gradually lead to hypertrophy of smooth muscle together with some accompanying intimal fibrosis. The latter is usually of a concentric type, but does not show the lamellar 'onion-skinning' as seen in congenital heart disease with a left-to-right shunt (see above). Nevertheless, progressive increase in pulmonary vascular resistance will occur and this will affect the right heart. Right ventricular hypertrophy will ensue and, eventually, right heart failure may follow. Under these conditions, thrombosis may occur in the right atrium, almost certainly associated with atrial fibrillation. Such thrombi may lead to pulmonary emboli and the pulmonary vascular pathology may become further complicated by embolic obstruction of the arterial circulation (see below). Despite such changes, the pulmonary vascular pathology usually is not a serious contraindication to an operative procedure designed to alleviate the obstructive effects of the lesion of the left side of the heart which led initially to the pulmonary venous congestion. Only occasionally will pulmonary vascular resistance be increased to such an extent that it affects the postoperative course.

In addition to these pulmonary venous changes, and the secondary arteriolar alterations, chronic increases in pulmonary venous pressure may induce fibrosis of the alveolar septa. This probably relates to the increase in fluid within the interstitial spaces, not necessarily clinically evident as pulmonary oedema.

Cardiac conditions that may underlie these pulmonary vascular consequences are varied, but the types most commonly involved are left heart failure, either of an ischaemic or a non-ischaemic nature, and abnormality of the mitral valve.

LUNG DISEASE

Various diseases of the lungs are associated with pulmonary vascular changes. Almost all forms of fibrotic lung disease, whether focal or diffuse, and the later stages of chronic obstructive airways disease, such as chronic bronchitis and emphysema, are associated with structural changes of the pulmonary vasculature. Inflammatory processes within the lung also affect the pulmonary vascular tree, either because of vasculitis or due to fibrosis of pulmonary parenchyma. Likewise, pulmonary thrombo-embolism, although not strictly a lung disorder, and other pulmonary vascular diseases, such as pulmonary veno-occlusive disease and idiopathic (primary) pulmonary hypertension, are accompanied by structural changes in the pulmonary vascular bed.

In general terms all pulmonary vascular changes mentioned above lead to an increase in pulmonary vascular resistance and, on that basis, have an effect on the heart. The major cardiac response is right ventricular hypertrophy which, eventually, may result in right heart failure.

Hypoxic pulmonary vascular disease

Lung diseases in which structural alterations occur at the alveolar-capillary level, leading to an impaired gas exchange, may cause arteriolar hypoxia and, eventually, pulmonary vascular pathology. The changes occur in the arterioles and the very small muscular pulmonary arteries. Hyperplasia of medial smooth muscle cells causes muscularization of the arterioles, while the larger-sized muscular arteries are virtually normal. In addition, longitudinally oriented smooth muscle cells may develop within the intima (Fig. 26.18).[12] The diffuse and widespread nature of these changes accounts for the development of pulmonary hypertension. A consequence of longstanding pulmonary hypertension is the development of atheroma in the pulmonary trunk and major pulmonary arteries, the only circumstance in which significant atheroma develops in the lesser circulation.

Other disease processes accompanied by arteriolar hypoxia may also lead to pulmonary vascular disease. These include muscle disorders with impaired respiratory movements, kyphoscoliosis and the Pickwickian syndrome. Similar

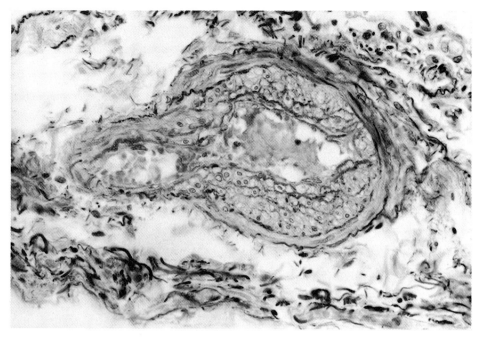

Fig. 26.18 Muscular pulmonary artery with longitudinally oriented smooth muscle cells in the intima. Elastic tissue stain × 350.

pulmonary vascular changes, moreover, may occur in those who live at high altitudes (such as inhabitants of the Andes).

Fibrotic lung disease

Any form of fibrotic lung disease, whether focal or interstitial, may cause pulmonary vascular changes. The latter consist of medial hypertrophy and intimal fibrosis of the muscular pulmonary arteries. In focal parenchymal disease, only arteries in the immediate neighbourhood are affected. Hence, clinically significant pulmonary hypertension under these circumstances is rare. Once severe diffuse interstitial lung disease is present, pulmonary hypertension is overt and right heart failure may eventually further complicate the clinical picture.

Pulmonary vasculitis

Vasculitis of the lung can be classified into three main categories: vasculitis with a known cause and confined to the lungs, vasculitis of unknown

cause with the lungs as the primary target organ, and systemic vasculitis that may involve the lungs.[13] Each category comprises several, often heterogeneous, conditions (see Table 26.1).

Among the conditions categorized as 'vasculitis of known cause and confined to the lungs', two are particularly notable. In severe necrotizing bronchopneumonia, direct extension of the inflammatory process to the pulmonary vasculature is a common finding. Second, septic thrombo-embolism may cause pulmonary vasculitis at the sites of lodgement of the emboli, often followed by infection of the affected lung parenchyma — this latter situation, in particular, induces a most serious clinical condition.

Pulmonary involvement in systemic vasculitis is uncommon but, when present, usually is considered an unfavourable prognostic indicator.

With respect to the conditions categorized as 'pulmonary angiitis and granulomatosis', overlap seems to occur with polyarteritis nodosa. It has been suggested that the necrotizing arteritis of Wegener's granulomatosis is essentially the same as the necrotizing arteritis characteristic of

Table 26.1 Classification of pulmonary angiitis and granulomatosis (according to JT Lie[13])

A. Vasculitis of known cause and confined to the lungs
    1. Infective vasculitis (bacterial, fungal, parasitic)
    2. Reactive vasculitis caused by embolic material (cotton, gauze, talc)
    3. Vasculitis of pulmonary hypertensive vascular disease

B. Vasculitis of unknown cause with lung as primary target organ (pulmonary angiitis and granulomatosis)
    1. Wegener's granulomatosis (classic and limited forms)
    2. Allergic granulomatosis and angiitis (Churg–Strauss syndrome)
    3. Necrotizing sarcoid granulomatosis
    4. Bronchocentric granulomatosis

C. Systemic vasculitis that may involve the lungs
    1. Polyarteritis nodosa
    2. Rheumatoid arteritis
    3. Systemic lupus erythematosus
    4. Scleroderma (systemic sclerosis)
    5. Dermatopolymyositis
    6. Mixed connective tissue disease
    7. Hypersensitivity vasculitis
    8. Behçet syndrome/Hughes–Stovin syndrome
    9. Takayasu arteritis
    10. Disseminated and isolated giant cell arteritis

---

polyarteritis nodosa. The only distinctive difference between the two conditions is the presence of granulomatous inflammation of the respiratory tract in Wegener's granulomatosis.[14] Presently, there is no consensus on the issue whether or not the term 'polyarteritis nodosa' can be used when there is non-granulomatous respiratory vasculitis of unknown cause. It is significant, particularly from a clinical viewpoint, that both conditions share the occurrence of anti-neutrophil cytoplasmic auto-antibodies which could indicate a similar pathogenetic pathway.

Pulmonary embolism

Some patients present with pulmonary hypertension on the basis of an increased pulmonary vascular resistance secondary to pulmonary embolism. Usually the source of these emboli is the deep veins of the leg. It is well recognized that individuals with severe obesity are particularly prone to this condition. Once pulmonary emboli occur, the clinical picture will largely depend on the size of the thrombo-embolus and the site of the occluded pulmonary artery.

Furthermore, the number of arteries involved becomes of vital significance. When small thrombo-emboli, usually from the veins of the calf, are distributed within the lung, the consequences are in most cases minimal, do not cause symptoms and are not detected clinically. The activation of the fibrinolytic system will clear the pulmonary vasculature of such microthrombi. If, however, the thrombo-embolus is more substantial in size, arising from the femoral or iliac veins, it may occlude a pulmonary artery at a level where it produces pulmonary infarction, particularly when the patient already has cardiac failure. There will usually be clinical evidence of this event. Should a large thrombus be dislodged from the veins of the leg, the chances are that it will obstruct one or both of the main pulmonary arteries, or even become coiled at the site of the bifurcation of the pulmonary trunk. These are serious manifestations and the patient will usually develop severe and rapid pulmonary hypertension, often leading quickly to progressive right heart failure and death.

In this context, it must be remembered that so-called silent pulmonary embolization also occurs. In patients with this condition, the first signs are those of pulmonary hypertension, when the cause may remain clinically unclear.

Pulmonary veno-occlusive disease

This is a rare condition of unknown cause that affects both children and adults. The pathology is characterized by an obliteration of pulmonary veins and venules by fibrous tissue having a loose texture and containing few cells. The muscular pulmonary arteries sometimes exhibit mild medial hypertrophy and occasionally may show a similar intimal change.[15] In some instances the pulmonary vascular changes appear in conjunction with respiratory infections.

Pulmonary veno-occlusive disease leads to pulmonary hypertension and is one of the three main conditions, together with 'silent' pulmonary emboli (see above) and idiopathic (primary) pulmonary hypertension (see below), that must be considered when patients present with pulmonary hypertension of no immediately obvious cause.

Idiopathic (primary) pulmonary hypertension

In some patients, pulmonary arterial hypertension is truly idiopathic. The disease predominantly affects young adults; the average age is between 20 and 30 years. In infants and children the sex ratio is equal, but in adults the disease has a strong predilection for women. The condition leads to severe respiratory distress and, eventually, right heart failure.

The changes within the pulmonary vasculature are those of plexogenic pulmonary arteriopathy (see earlier in this Chapter). Medial hypertrophy of muscular pulmonary arteries, concentric intimal fibrosis with a loose laminar structure ('onion-skinning') and plexiform lesions are the common pathological changes in the advanced stages of this disease.[16] Basically, these changes do not differ from those that occur in patients with congenital heart disease and a left-to-right shunt. It is likely that the process starts with constriction of pulmonary arterioles, which only at later stages becomes aggravated by structural alterations.

GRADING OF PULMONARY VASCULAR DISEASE

As long ago as 1958, Heath and Edwards[17] published a system of grading pulmonary vascular disease into six categories (Table 26.2). The Heath–Edwards system is still used as a method of estimating the potential reversibility or irreversibility of pulmonary vascular disease.[18,19] Others have repeatedly pointed out the fallacies inherent in this classification.[4,7,20–23]

A simple grading system has the advantage that comparisons can be made reliably between the

Table 26.2 The Heath and Edwards system of grading pulmonary vascular disease

Grade I	— medial hypertrophy of the pulmonary arteries
Grade II	— cellular intimal proliferation together with medial hypertrophy
Grade III	— occlusive intimal fibrosis
Grade IV	— plexiform lesions
Grade V	— dilatation lesions
Grade VI	— necrotizing arteritis

findings from different centres. Indeed, there is an almost worldwide consensus in terms of interpretation of advanced stages (Heath–Edwards grades III–VI) in relation to prognosis. The problems which arise reflect the oversimplification of reality by the system. It does not take into account the chronological sequence of structural changes and it is not sufficiently precise to meet the demands of the present era, particularly in the interpretation of pulmonary vascular changes in the very young. These drawbacks are particularly important when it comes to the interpretation of open lung biopsies. For example, even if only a solitary 'grade III' lesion is observed in a biopsy, the patient, for that reason alone, would be categorized as having a poor prognosis. This would be so despite the fact that all the other vessels observed in the sections studied may be less severely affected, or even normal. The Heath–Edwards system of grading, moreover, does not take into account the different types of intimal fibrosis. These may have completely different pathogeneses and, hence, vary in their significance. For instance, eccentric intimal fibrosis almost always is an expression of organized thrombosis (due to, for example, decreased pulmonary blood flow or an increase in blood viscosity consequent upon a critically elevated haematocrit). Concentric fibrosis, in contrast, relates almost without exception to structural changes induced by abnormal flows or pressures. Although both lesions may determine identical grades, it is crucial for pathologists to distinguish between these forms of intimal fibrosis.

The most important drawback of the Heath–Edwards system, however, is that, in disgnostic work and research studies, interest is now increasingly directed towards pulmonary vascular pathology in the very young. In other words, attention is now focussed on the changes within grades I and II of the traditional system. With the advance of cardiac surgery in neonates, the reliability of the interpretation of lung biopsies is under debate, largely because the traditional qualitative grading of lesions has proved inadequate in this category of patients. This is best illustrated by the fact that reversibility, as judged microscopically on the basis of low grade changes, does not necessarily relate to operability.[24,25]

Indeed, the pattern of growth and remodelling of pulmonary arteries may already be abnormal at birth in patients with congenital left-to-right shunts, such as 'simple' ventricular septal defects and ventricular septal defects complicating complete transposition.[24-26]

Because of these changes, a further grading of pulmonary vascular disease, described alphabetically (grades A–C), has been introduced.[22] Grade A is characterized by an abnormal extension of muscle into the small peripheral arteries that, normally, are non-muscular, such as those that accompany alveolar ducts. This process is due to a differentiation of pericytes and intermediate cells into smooth muscle cells. Grade B shows 'muscularization' as in grade A but in addition there is medial hypertrophy of arteries that normally have a muscular wall. Grade C is typified by a reduction in the concentration of arteries, in other words by an increased ratio of alveoli to arteries in a given section. It appears to involve the arteries in the alveolar walls first and to be associated with muscularization of intra-acinar arteries as described above.[27] These obliterative changes in alveolar arteries occur prior to the appearance of significant obliterative intimal changes in more proximal vessels. This reduction in the number of intra-acinar arteries has been shown to be associated with pulmonary hypertension of different causes.

The studies referred to above have shown that proper interpretation of open lung biopsies in cases of pulmonary hypertension produced by congenital left-to-right shunts can be achieved only when the biopsy includes tissue from deep within the lung and contains both pre-acinar and intra-acinar structures. Obviously, the early obliterative changes that lead to a shift in the ratio of alveoli to arteries can be observed only when intra-acinar structures are present. This will almost always be the case. Nevertheless, the pathologist must assess each and every artery in relation to its accompanying airway. It makes a significant difference, with respect to normal development and remodelling of the pulmonary vascular tree, whether the segment is at the level of the terminal bronchiole, the respiratory bronchioles or the alveolar ducts. When the number of arteries present at the alveolar level is reduced, and intimal hyperplasia is observed, early postoperative pulmonary hypertension is likely to occur. The diminished ratio of alveoli to arteries, moreover, may be one of the reasons why some patients, following successful repair of a congenital defect, suffer persistent, and even progressive, pulmonary hypertension.

Another important reason for taking a biopsy specimen that includes deep tissue of the lung is that the medial thickness of intra-acinar arteries may not correlate with the pulmonary arterial pressure and resistance.[4,28] This peculiar finding reflects the fact that obstruction of side branches may occur at the pre-acinar level, thus causing a diminished flow into the acinus while preventing structural changes usually associated with increased pulmonary vascular resistance. These pre-acinar lesions may give a false impression of the pulmonary vascular pathology present.

When investigating patients, therefore, the evaluation of the pulmonary vasculature must be included along with other parameters, such as assessment of the degree of cyanosis, the level of the haematocrit and the time-span of development of the rise in pulmonary arterial pressure.

REFERENCES

1. World Health Organization. Primary pulmonary hypertension. Report of Committee. Geneva, 1975.
2. Wagenvoort CA, Wagenvoort N. Pathology of pulmonary hypertension. New York: John Wiley, 1977.
3. Rabinovitch M, Haworth SG, Vance Z, Vawter G, Castaneda AR, Nadas AS, Reid LM. Early pulmonary vascular changes in congenital heart disease studied in biopsy tissue. Hum Pathol 1980; 11(suppl): 499–509.
4. Haworth SG. Pulmonary vascular disease in different types of congenital heart disease. Implications of interpretation of lung biopsy findings in early childhood. Br Heart J 1984; 52: 557–571.
5. Haworth SG, Sauer U, Bühlmeyer K, Reid L. Development of the pulmonary circulation in ventricular septal defect: a quantitative structural study. Am J Cardiol 1977; 40: 781–788.
6. Balk AG, Dingemans KP, Wagenvoort CA. The

ultrastructure of the various forms of pulmonary arterial intimal fibrosis. Virchows Arch [A] 1979; 382: 139–150.

7. Wagenvoort CA. Hypertensive pulmonary vascular disease complicating congenital heart disease: a review. Cardiovasc Clin 1973; 5: 43–60.

8. Stanger P, Lucas RV, Edwards JE. Anatomic factors causing respiratory distress in acyanotic congenital cardiac disease: special reference to bronchial obstruction. Pediatrics 1969; 43: 760–769.

9. Wagenvoort CA, Heath D, Edwards JE. The pathology of the pulmonary vasculature. Springfield, Illinois: Charles C Thomas, 1964.

10. Kinsley RH, McGoon DC, Danielson GK, Wallace RB, Mair DD. Pulmonary arterial hypertension after repair of tetralogy of Fallot. J Thorac Cardiovasc Surg 1974; 67: 110–120.

11. Haworth SG, Reid L. Quantitative structural study of pulmonary circulation in the newborn with pulmonary atresia. Thorax 1977; 32: 129–133.

12. Wagenvoort CA, Wagenvoort N. Hypoxic pulmonary vascular lesions in man at high altitudes and in patients with chronic respiratory disease. Pathol Microbiol 1973; 39: 276–282.

13. Lie JT. Classification of pulmonary angiitis and granulomatosis. Histopathologic perspectives. Sem Resp Med 1989; 10: 111–121.

14. Fahey J, Leonard E, Schurg J, Godman M. Wegener's granulomatosis. Am J Med 1954; 17: 168–179.

15. Wagenvoort CA, Wagenvoort N, Takahashi T. Pulmonary veno-occlusive disease. Involvement of pulmonary arteries and review of the literature. Hum Pathol 1985; 16: 1033–1041.

16. Wagenvoort CA, Wagenvoort N. Primary pulmonary hypertension. A pathologic study of the lung vessels in 156 clinically diagnosed cases. Circulation 1970; 42: 1163–1184.

17. Heath D, Edwards JE. The pathology of hypertensive pulmonary vascular disease: a description of six grades of structural changes in the pulmonary arteries with special reference to congenital cardiac septal defects. Circulation 1958; 18: 533–547.

18. Heath D, Helmholtz HF, Burchell HB, DuShane JW, Kirklin JW, Edwards JE. Relation between structural changes in the small pulmonary arteries and the immediate reversibility of pulmonary hypertension following closure of ventricular and atrial septal defects. Circulation 1958; 18: 1167–1174.

19. Frescura C, Thiene G, Franceschini E, Talenti E, Mazzucco A. Pulmonary vascular disease in infants with complete atrioventricular septal defect. Int J Cardiol 1987; 15: 91–100.

20. Wagenvoort CA, Wagenvoort N. Pathology of the Eisenmenger syndrome and primary pulmonary hypertension. Adv Cardiol 1974; 11: 123–130.

21. Yamaki S, Tezuka F. Quantitative analysis of pulmonary vascular disease in complete transposition of the great arteries. Circulation 1976; 54: 805–809.

22. Rabinovitch M, Haworth SG, Castaneda AR, Nadas AS, Reid LM. Lung biopsy in congenital heart disease: A morphometric approach to pulmonary vascular disease. Circulation 1978; 58: 1107–1122.

23. Haworth SG. Understanding pulmonary vascular disease in young children. Int J Cardiol 1987; 15: 101–103.

24. Haworth SG, Radley-Smith R, Yacoub M. Lung biopsy findings in transposition of the great arteries with ventricular septal defect: potentially reversible pulmonary vascular disease is not always synonymous with operability. J Am Coll Cardiol 1987; 9: 327–333.

25. Haworth SG. Pulmonary vascular disease in ventricular septal defect: structural and functional correlations in lung biopsies from 85 patients, with outcome of intracardiac repair. J Pathol 1987; 152: 157–168.

26. Hislop A, Haworth SG, Shinebourne EA, Reid L. Quantitative structural analysis of pulmonary vessels in isolated ventricular septal defect in infancy. Br Heart J 1975; 37: 1014–1021.

27. Haworth SG, Hall SM. Occlusion of intra-acinar pulmonary arteries in pulmonary hypertensive congenital heart disease. Int J Cardiol 1986; 13: 207–217.

28. Haworth SG. Pulmonary vascular bed in children with complete atrioventricular septal defect: relation between structural and hemodynamic abnormalities. Am J Cardiol 1986; 57: 833–839.

Index